It's Your Life!

It's *Your* Life!

A Gynecologist Challenges You to Take Control

JAMES A. SCHALLER, M.D.

BLUE DOLPHIN PUBLISHING

Published by Blue Dolphin Publishing, Inc.
P.O. Box 8, Nevada City, CA 95959
Orders: 1-800-643-0765

ISBN: 1-57733-004-8, soft cover, $16.95
ISBN: 1-57733-018-8, cloth, $24.95

Library of Congress Cataloging-in-Publication Data

Schaller, James A.
    It's your life : a gynecologist challenges you to take control /
James A. Schaller
        p.   cm.
    Includes bibligraphical references and index.
    ISBN 1-57733-004-8
    ISBN 1-57733-018-8
    1. Middle aged women—Health and hygiene.   2. Middle aged
women—mental health.   3. Menopause—Popular works
4. Women, Conduct of life.   I. Title.
    RA778.S278   1997
    613'.04244—dc21   96-40108
                                                              CIP

Cover design: Lito Castro

Printed in the United States of America by
Blue Dolphin Press

10   9   8   7   6   5   4   3   2

Dedication

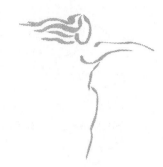

To my father, Francis Xavier (Frank) Schaller
who, as much as anyone I've ever known, reverenced women.
His loss left a personal void that required a long time to fill.

To Father Don Rinfret, S.J., whose concern for others was never
diminished by age or gender. Marianne and I delighted in his friendship
in life and treasure the memory, not only of many happy moments,
but also of the many challenging ones during his gallant, but final,
unsuccessful battle with cancer.

Contents

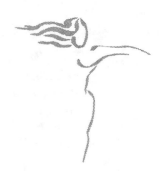

Preface

"Unless you love someone nothing else makes any sense."
—E.E. Cummings

The seeds for a book that challenges women to assume responsibility for every aspect of their own lives were planted many years ago:

My interest, love, and respect for women, and my fascination with them, began at home, sparked by my mother, a dynamo. My nine sisters provided me, from infancy, with a wealth of daily female contacts. Add thirty-seven years of marriage to my beloved Marianne, and the blessing of three All-American daughters, and this deep regard for women becomes almost inevitable. It was Marianne, after a year or two of marriage, who encouraged me to specialize in Obstetrics and Gynecology, because "I was good at it." (I never did discover exactly what she meant.)

In adolescence, I witnessed my mother's "change of life." Her appearance and personality were affected, to the extent that she became someone I didn't know. Physically, she went from 99 pounds to 170 pounds. Her beautiful dark curls became straight white strings. I can still vividly see my mother, pale and soaked with perspiration, even in the dead of winter, going to the kitchen cupboard for yet one more dose of **Lydia Pinkham's Compound**, the most-popular remedy then for the "change."[1] Those events have certainly influenced my attitudes toward the prevention and treatment of any hormonal deficiencies, especially at mid-life.

Luckily, the seventy pounds my mother gained in the five years after her periods stopped, provided her an alternative source of hormones, so that she rebounded physically and emotionally, and began a whirlwind career of new interests and activities that continued for forty years.

Unfortunately, my mother was just like ninety-eight percent of the women over sixty in America today, in that she stopped her gynecologic exams and pap tests. Despite her monthly visits to the doctor for her high blood pressure, she never mentioned a worsening gynecologic problem, and no one asked any questions or suggested an exam. The result of all this neglect was emergency surgery at age eighty-nine, during which she required fifteen pints of blood!

The challenge and privilege of being a women's doctor, and the tremendous opportunities this presents in providing preventive care, continues to motivate my life and give me great personal satisfaction. Yet a greater challenge comes from the knowledge that there are millions of women every day, who, like my mother, suffer unnecessarily, simply because much of what is known to the health care providers has not been made available to them. This book is my attempt to answer that larger challenge.

When I began this book, my intention was to amplify my patient-education booklets. However, it quickly became apparent that merely elaborating on the ways that women can maintain their health over a lifetime was not enough. However detailed and complete I made it, a book limited to health concerns alone can provide little help to the large number of women who possess good health but who are nevertheless discontent, angry, bored, resentful, or otherwise very unhappy with their lives and their relationships. Thus, my book includes information for these women, which might help them to understand and to heal their problems with parents, spouses, children, or co-workers, and, most important, help them to understand themselves.

In the search for causes of women's discontent, I found the greatest anger expressed for the "gender role" assigned to infant girls at birth. The unrelenting demands that women conform to the constraints of "femininity" follow them throughout their lives and assault their humanity.[2] One very poignant example of the effects of this rule for women was dramatically provided to me through the words of a poet. One New Year's Eve when my manuscript was still in its earliest draft, my wife and I were sharing dinner with close friends. Our host and hostess did not vary from their habit of engaging guests in a literary discussion, in this instance concerning a poem, "Warning" by Jenny Joseph. (See page 234.) In this poem, a woman envisions a return to her preadolescent wholeness and authenticity, when "she is old." She longs for the day when she might have the freedom to do "unfeminine" things.

Through the eyes of the poet, I saw more clearly than ever before the desirability of letting women themselves reveal what they want from their relationships, and to share what they believe can make their lives richer and more satisfying. Thus began a personal literary odyssey, to discover the techniques and the wisdom that women have used successfully to accomplish what they wanted most in their lives. Thus, one goal of my book is to spotlight what women themselves include in their agenda for happiness.

Also, having spent a lifetime in close contract with women in virtually every conceivable normal relationship, I have considered myself qualified to select or reject, edit or accept totally, and agree or argue with what women have written. I have purposely striven to make my book comprehensive—to discuss **all** the most important **active** choices now available to women (defined as those choices that require women to **do** something), especially in the areas of choosing ways to stay healthy and learning how to create loving relationships, but also with regard to getting the information to decide and embark upon their own career choices, and, along with other women and fair-minded men, selecting their own way to contribute to one or another of the feminists' goals.

This book also represents my attempt to say "thank you" to all the women in my life. I extend heartfelt gratitude and warmest affection to all those who have brought me joy or challenge, who have listened to me, who have taught me, who have given me their babies to hold, or who have brought their mothers, daughters, or friends for my care.

"Thank-you's" are extended to all those who have read at least one version of this book, a list that includes (in no particular order) Shirley Mulligan, Ayn Krebs, Joe Jakabcin, Eleanor and Bob Weirman, Helen and Harry Geib, Maryellen Dorsey, Jeanne O'Connor, and, of course, my wife and daughters—Marianne, Maureen, Michele, and Jean.

I respectfully "tip my hat" and give gratitude and affection to the fine and dedicated people at Blue Dolphin Publishing. Paul Clemens, the publisher, has invariably provided words of affirmation when they have been most needed. Both Paul and his lovely wife Nancy have devoted many years to making available fine books and journals intended to genuinely help people, young and old. My sincere appreciation is extended to my editor, Corinn Codye, who (besides being an accomplished teacher in the ancient arts of T'ai Chi and Qigong) has authored many scientific books for children. Paul, Nancy, and Corinn have graciously allowed me the freedom to summarize and interpret "what I think modern women are saying."

Acknowledgments and thanks are also due to all the other members of the Blue Dolphin "team": Linda Maxwell in text design and layout, John Mello in production, Lito Castro in cover design, Chris Comins and Lisa Horrell in distribution, marketing, and promotion, Beverly Craig in accounting, and Tom Pakham in shipping.

In additon to the guidance of Paul and Nancy Clemens and Corinn Codye, the format and final content of this book owe much to Mrs. Patricia Olley. Pat not only holds a Bachelor's degree in English and a Master's degree in American Studies and teaches English on the college level, but she is also a very active Christian-Feminist.

A special thank you is extended to my son, James Louis Schaller, an adult and adolescent psychiatrist, theologian, and published author. A special thank you as well to my brother, Francis Xavier, Jr., and to his lovely wife Marianne. All three have spent many hours reviewing a succession of manuscripts, making corrections, and offering many helpful suggestions. In 1952, Francis, who had just been discharged from three years obligatory army service overseas, gave me his last two hundred and fifty dollars to buy a microscope for college. Such kindness and generosity has always been typical of him, but that particular kindness remains a tender memory for me.

Pablo Casals said, ". . . the capacity to care is the thing that gives life its deepest significance." This thought I certainly share. Thus, my hope is that you will find care in the words that follow, and that what I have "learned," and now share, will be helpful to you in your own quest for happiness.

—J.A.S

Before Proceeding . . .

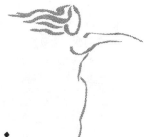

Women in the United States are over two-and-a-half times as likely as men to be diagnosed with **depression.** According to the American Psychiatric Association's 1990 Task Force on Women and Depression, this difference is due to the "specific problems" of being female in contemporary society.

This book aims to take these "specific problems" head on by dealing explicitly and at length with the interpersonal relationships that are more central than in men to a women's sense of self-esteem. Therefore, I strongly advise that the existence of a depression should be dealt with first by seeking professional counseling before proceeding with this book.[3]

In addition, in those areas of the book dealing with specific physical problems, I make no guarantees that the information is correct. The statement that "anyone can make mistakes" is especially true in medical diagnosis and treatment. **This disclaimer applies to every medical recommendation in this book.** In the face of any illness, personal professional consultation is very prudent, since generalities cannot replace individual attention.

Understanding the Message . . .

"If what you are doing gives you no joy, no pleasure,
no sense of purpose, no sense of fulfillment— it is **not** worth doing."
—Christiane Northrup, *Women's Bodies, Women's Wisdom*

The **selflessness** of women who subordinate their desires and needs to those of their husbands, mothers, children, friends, or co-workers, never giving themselves a break, wreaks havoc not only on their emotions but also on their health. Many of these same women act as though they don't deserve love, care, and compassion from anyone. **This book is especially written for them—to challenge them to be selfish in the highest sense of the word: by** 1) devoting significant time and effort every day to becoming **aware** of their own feelings and emotions; 2) totally **accepting** all that they discover through their exercise of awareness; and **3) honoring, loving, and respecting themselves** despite any faults and deficiencies.

Everyone's judgment on the "world" is a reflection of themselves and their own unique awareness of what they have experienced. Each person's sense of their own worth must **not** be dependent upon someone or something else outside them. Need becomes dependence only when we relinquish our responsibility to get our need satisfied.

By accepting but not **dwelling on** the negatives found by one's self-awareness, and then focusing on the positive feelings, emotions, and talents (I'm not talking here simply about the **power** of positive _thinking_, but rather the **power** of meditation and all the other techniques described throughout the book), one can **initiate improvements in both the mind and the body.** Thus begins the personal growth that brings with it inner freedom, creativity, vibrancy, and joy.

When the judgment a woman passes on herself is favorable, her thinking, motivation, feelings, behavior, and health will be considerably improved. Self-respect produces self-confidence to make one's own decisions, reducing dependence on or being controlled by others. **The ability to be assertive, rather than controlled, is the first step toward human well-being** and being open to life's possibilities, especially intimacy. It is well to remember that a woman's willingness to take care of her needs because she judges herself worthy of that care sends an important and positive message to the person who would love her—"I **am** worthy of your attention and your love." (Because the mind and body are inseparable and nourish each other, **the same positive message is sent to her body that "her body is well."**)

On the other hand, when a woman neglects to discover and nurture herself, it reflects her judgment that she does not deserve such attention.

There are few who will deny the logic and reasonableness in proclaiming that the woman who expects love and joy in her life must devote time every day to herself. To explain how best to use that time to maximum advantage is one of the main goals of this book. The more feelings she can appreciate in herself, the more alive she will become. Therefore, techniques for awareness and acceptance, then sharing and communicating (in the quest for greater joy and relatedness), will be found throughout the text. One such aid to making your life richer and more joyous is to keep a **daily journal** of the people, thoughts, or activities that help you feel wonderful. At the same time, writing down your daily feelings, thoughts, and emotions, as though you were talking to a friend, allows you to think your problems through and arrive at a plan to **do** something about them.

(**CAUTION:** If you are in a long-standing relationship and now wisely decide to provide time every day to address your own needs, try not to send the message to your mate that **he** is responsible for anything that you have been missing in the past. **You** were responsible then (though perhaps you were foolish) and you are going to be responsible—and perhaps wiser—now and in the future. **Never project yourself as a victim to the one who you would love and have love you.**)

Section 1
Staying Healthy

THE FIRST CHALLENGE:
*Selecting the Simplest and Least Expensive,
but Most Useful Health Strategies*

Introducing Section One . . . .

While the text separates most (but not all) of the care of the body (Section One) from care of one's inner self and one's relationships (Section Two), and from one's major career and moral choices (Section Three), there is no division whatsoever within the human person. Ample references are provided that prove that your thoughts and perceptions about your life totally affect your emotions and feelings, and that your fears, pain, anger, sadness, anxiety, or joy can direct or control your thoughts. When you smile, not only does the world smile with you, but you feel better and think more happy thoughts.

It has, in fact, been scientifically proven that confidence in a "higher value," beyond and distinct from the individual person, can greatly benefit both mind and body, not only in healing the body but in bringing to the person serenity and joy. (Sixty years of studies have repeatedly confirmed that if you believe in a "Healer," you are more likely to be healed.)

Most important, mental and emotional events do affect one's physical health. Dissatisfaction with one's job or marriage or children, or one's lot in life, are typically converted into physical problems. Women are more inclined than men in such instances to seek a medical cure. Unfortunately, doctors are just as poor as everyone else at reading minds, and it is rare for one to discover and address the woman's real problem. The result is the patient's eventual resort to an **alternative** method of treatment, some of which can be benefi-

3

cial for such problems, but others of which are not only a waste of money, but dangerous as well. Quoting Dr. Bernard Lown, one of the world's most famous cardiologists for the last forty years, "Beware of medical charlatans; your life could be at stake."[1]

While physical health is the subject matter for this first section of the book, please don't expect an encyclopedic listing of specific diseases, since **my purpose is to provide information to** _maintain_ **health.** Beginning with the general medical topics of skin care, respiratory hygiene, and bowel-friendly practices, then proceeding to the more specific gynecological concerns—breast or abdominal pain, menstrual difficulties, PMS, bladder malfunctions, and permanent estrogen loss at mid-life—the emphasis is on prevention of disease.

Some medical points will be repeated, often several times. Such repetition is primarily the result of the interconnectedness of good health practices. On the other hand, whenever a particular topic seems to be incompletely explained, the reader is invited to consult the subject index to see if it is mentioned again in some other Section of the book.

In Chapter Seven, an appropriate exercise program is presented that includes **relaxation** exercises designed to help you slow down enough that you might better gain awareness of "your heart," that is, the true feelings and emotions that are driving your body. The aerobic and anaerobic exercises described are intended to help you achieve your desired exercise goals efficiently, pleasantly, and most important, safely.

Chapter Eight follows with a program designed to help you develop a sensible and healthy attitude toward eating. Bingeing or starvation are equally capable of leading to the acquisition of body fat that is above the level of your genetic endowment. The topic of food and body image must be divorced from any concepts of rewards and punishments, good and bad, or shame and blame. The ultimate goal is seen as knowing when you are eating to satisfy the needs of your body and when you are eating to satisfy emotional needs. **Diets should be given their rightful place in your life and therefore put in the wastebasket**.

Chapter Nine concludes the basic suggestions for promoting health. In that chapter you will find information on five of the most common gynecological concerns of adolescence. The fifth case presented, in which a mother requests the birth control pill for her sexually-active teenager, prompts a brief discussion of a few of "the pill's" observed effects on the sexual activities of American adolescents.

Being Part of the Most Rapidly Growing Majority

Women now possess a markedly increased survival beyond the age when their lives should be driven by the need to be "feminine" (throughout the text, the negative and constricting connotations of that term will be made quite clear), and the now nearly **fifty** million American women over fifty certainly possess the potential **to be America's most powerful social and political force**.

The actual numbers of mature women at any age might surprise you. In fact, the number of women over 100 years of age is accelerating most rapidly. As recently as 1980, there were only 1000 women in America over 100 years of age. In the year 2000, there will be 100,000, with that number tripling within another decade. Some estimates place the figures at several million by 2050.

In fact, predicting the life expectancy of a twenty-five-year-old is not easy, because the medical advances are coming so rapidly, but a fifty-year-old woman who is a nonsmoker, a moderate drinker or a nondrinker, who is not obese, who does not have a chronic disease, and who follows simple health practices available now, should expect to live until ninety-two ! A woman at fifty-five, with the same caveats, will survive to age ninety-seven! And, for a twenty to forty-year-old, it should be ten or more years longer, at least.

Another certainty is that **good health practices** between the age of **twenty to sixty** will markedly **improve your quality of life between sixty and one hundred**. Even for those of you over sixty, be assured that it is never too late to start. Most women will have more birthdays than they expect, or, in many cases, desire. My only answer to the statement frequently expressed, "But I don't want to live that long!" is an honest "But you probably will!" These facts apply whether that "you" is twenty, forty, or eighty years of age.

George Burns probably summarized the point best: "If I had known I was going to live so long, I'd have taken better care of myself." Indeed, life is not over until you take your last breath. If you truly desire a good quality of life for each decade, you should start planning now. Chapters One through Nine will provide plenty of challenging suggestions.

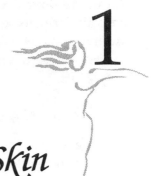

Being Kind to Your Skin

Listening to the Experts

Would you believe, problems with the skin are the number one gyn concern? The USA has more dermatologists than the rest of the world combined, and apparently for good reasons. One of our most eminent skin specialists has criticized the American obsession with skin "cleanliness" and expressed his mystification about our passion for "deep cleaning" and what that really accomplishes, if anything. The head of the company that produces **Neutrogena** once remarked that his products were better than most, "not for what they did to the skin, but for what they didn't do." A very famous hairdresser made a similar point in saying that the best shampoos are the "weakest" shampoos.

What are these very knowledgeable people really trying to tell us? Surely, there is a common message here!

Your First Line of Defense Against a Very Hostile World

Your skin and hair are your most important defense against our common environmental enemies—bacteria, viruses, fungi, and the myriad man-made chemicals like bleach, stain removers, pesticides, and the like. Despite the amazing natural protective function of the skin, we now need the pharmaceutical industry and the dermatologists more often than ever to help us heal all our skin problems. The sad truth is that a significant portion of our skin ailments are self-induced by our zeal for "clean" skin, which borders on the fanatic! Not all dermatological problems are self-inflicted; probably most are not. But certainly dermatologists would not need to be consulted quite so often if we made some simple changes in our cleansing habits.

More Is Not Always Better

In gynecologic practice, the occurrence of **discharge**, **itch**, **rash**, or **burning** is often related to the amount of effort spent cleaning. That means the cleaner you try to be or the more effort expended, the more problems you might create for yourself. For example, a cleansing douche, especially when performed as a routine practice, is more often harmful than helpful. Since the normal vagina is a "clean" and "self-cleaning" organ (as an effect of the female hormone estrogen, which causes the lining cells of the vagina to be constantly shed and replaced), no "washing" is necessary. Because the normal vagina promotes the growth of beneficial bacteria that keep the vagina very acid and thus free of harmful organisms, douching or antibiotics which remove the "protective" bacteria can do great harm. (Eating five ounces daily of yogurt *with active cultures* is said to prevent recurrent yeast infections and "bacterial vaginosis," the most common vaginal infection. There are only five grams of lactose in a whole cup of yogurt, so those women of nationalities with a high incidence of milk intolerance can still use this method.[1])

Hot water in bathing often removes too much of the skin's natural oils. As a consequence of losing our oil barrier, yeast or fungi, among other organisms, can begin to grow between the skin cells, where the oil has been removed, and produce an infection.

There are a number of other things that women can do to help themselves avoid problems with vaginal itch and discharge. While physicians generally try not to prescribe antibiotics for minor illnesses, and for various good reasons, some patients insist on them (for example, every time they get a sore throat or a chest cough), and the physician is influenced by diplomatic or legal reasons to acquiesce to their demands. Many women can attest to the nearly inevitable "yeast infection" and "itch" that results when the antibiotics prescribed destroy the vagina's beneficial bacteria. Gloria Steinem raised the question some years ago, in her own inimitable way, "Why don't the stupid doctors tell you that you are going to get a vaginal yeast infection when they prescribe antibiotics?" In fact, many of us do, and our warning is often not heard.

Deodorant soaps or **detergents** can produce many of the same unwanted results. Solving the riddle of recurrent yeast infections in my practice is often accomplished by simply changing the kind of washing bar that is used in the shower or bath. It is still amusing to me that after decades of medical training, the "high tech" solution in these cases is just changing soap!

Getting Rid of the Villains in the Laundry

The latest chemicals to cause **yeast-like infections** that are, in fact, not yeast infections at all, are **the laundry detergents that contain stain removers and bleach**. Unfortunately, this means most of them. When one popular brand that I had recommended for years was recently "improved" to include these two ingredients, the incidence of rash, itch, or "burning" in the panty area greatly increased in my practice. When the over-the-counter anti-yeast medications failed to help, these women came to my office for treatment of their "yeast infections." The true diagnosis proved to be **contact irritant reaction**, which means that the skin was damaged by the residue of the bleach and stain removers that are left on the clothes after most ordinary rinse cycles (especially since people tend to add more detergent than is recommended for each load of laundry in order to get the clothes "cleaner than clean"). When those with "infections" rinsed their clothes twice, or switched to a brand without additives, the problem was typically resolved. Sometimes the fabric softeners in the drier must be eliminated too.

One brand of laundry detergent that has a version without bleach, stain removers, perfumes, or dyes—and therefore suggested as safer—is "Arm and Hammer Heavy Duty Detergent: dye and perfume free." You may, however, have to allow the soiled clothes to soak longer.

Complaints of dry, itchy skin, as well as respiratory ailments, are also greatly increased in the colder months of the year, and usually for one reason—dry indoor air.

Drying the Air Virtually Guarantees a Dry Skin Problem

Dry air also affects the skin by increasing evaporative loss of moisture from the skin to the dry air around it. Then, the drier skin is more likely to crack, itch, or peel. That is why I believe the best moisturizer is an evaporative humidifier, which produces neither "warm" mist nor "cool" mist, but mist at room temperature. This mist is "invisible" and leaves no "white deposits" on the surroundings. However, by putting a layer of moisture between the air and the skin, the humidifier prevents evaporative moisture loss from the skin.

In summary, dry air completes the "triple whammy" to the skin, along with hot water and excessive cleansing. The solutions include humidifying the air with the evaporative humidifier, washing and bathing with warm rather than hot water, and avoiding washing products that do harm.

Using Moisturizers: the **Two** Parts of the Skin

(Moisturizers must be applied to the skin when the skin is damp!)

The outer layers of human skin are dead cells that can dry out and thus become less flexible and protective, looking rough, cracked, scaly, wrinkled, and with signs of underlying irritation of the living, self-renewing layers beneath. To stay flexible, soft, and protective, the dead portion, called the "stratum corneum," should be at least ten percent water.

Occlusive moisturizers like petrolatum (**Vaseline**) work somewhat like humidifiers, decreasing evaporative loss. One recommended, available without prescription, is **Moisturel**. This product comes in a **cream or lotion** form and can be used to prevent, protect, or treat chafed, chapped, cracked, or windburned skin. **Moisturel** is often used for minor cuts, burns, sunburn or diaper rash. Since it is occlusive, it can seal out undesirable wetness and irritants, especially under your baby's diaper. (Please note that it is important to use these products that seal water out or seal water in **before** the area of skin involved has been damaged by irritants like stool, urine or blood.

One caution in the use of occlusive **ointments** such as **Vaseline**: they should never be put on the skin folds of moving joints, for example, in the crotch, where the thighs meet the very delicate skin outside the vaginal area. The difference between a cream or lotion and an ointment is critical in those skin areas where two touching surfaces move in opposite directions, since the rubbing together actually grinds the ointment into the skin separations (microscopic) to produce maceration, that is, visible breaks and tears in the skin's surface.

Selecting Water-Seeking, Water-Holding Moisturizers

Other moisturizers counteract dryness a second way. By being **hygroscopic**, which means that they **draw water** from the surrounding skin and air, they can add moisture to the dead layers. So they work best if the air is humidified. Products containing glycerin, or synthetic substitutes for glycerin, work this way.

Most moisturizers use both ingredients: vaseline-like and glycerine-like components. Unfortunately, they often add lanolins, fats, or fragrances that can irritate sensitive skin!

The "AHAs," or alpha-hydroxy acids, are now being added to many cosmetics as moisturizing agents. They are also dead skin peelers, which means they soften the body's natural glue that holds the hardest, oldest, and dullest-looking dead cells together. In prescription-strength concentrations, much higher than those allowed so far in over-the-counter cosmetics, these acids can make the dead cells shed more rapidly and increase the moisture content of the dead cells not peeled, thereby making the skin appear less wrinkled, temporarily. These prescription-strength preparations can thus be very valuable to women. (Unfortunately, this effect is unlikely and unproven in the concentrations used in many of the most expensive and most popular "beauty aids." The money spent on them may be wasted.)

Lac-Hydrin, a prescription moisturizer containing 12% lactic acid (an AHA) is an effective moisturizer combining the water-drawing and skin-peeling AHAs with occlusive ingredients like glycerin. Two cautions: 1) it does contain items like fragrance and parabens that can be irritating to sensitive or damaged skin, and 2)

Lac-Hydrin should not be used by pregnant or nursing mothers, because there is no data to prove it is safe in those conditions for the baby.

For a long time, **Alpha-Keri Bath Oil** has been used successfully to prevent and treat dry skin. Available through your pharmacy or beauty store, regular use in the bath or on a wet wash cloth after washing in the shower can help to avoid the problem. The much cheaper substitute oils are of little benefit.

The various **Eucerin** skin products, which are nonprescription items, might be of value for those with dry or sensitive skin problems that occur despite our three simple suggestions of humidification, avoiding strong washing products, and using warm rather than hot water. These products might save you the time and expense of a visit to a physician.

Let the poor skin alone. What did it ever do to you?

The essential fact to note is that once the natural protective oils in the living layers of the skin have been reduced or removed by detergents or other chemicals, nothing can put the oil back. Therefore, "primum non nocere,"—the basic dictum taught to those who would be physicians—"first do no harm." Do not wreck your skin in the first place.

Picking Soaps, Deodorants, or Detergents to Wash the Skin

We have already mentioned the harm done to the skin by **deodorant** bars, which alter the normal flora of the skin and thereby promote fungus, or in some cases even staph infections. More common, however, the use of **detergent** bars, precisely because they are highly effective in dissolving oils, removes the protective natural oils of the skin, leading to dryness from evaporative loss. This is followed by itching, due to the oil-less skin's contact with airborne or clothes-borne allergens or contact irritants. Finally, rashes and sores can result from the same sources. Thus, those bars that are both deodorant and detergent are potentially the most harmful.

Testing Your Own Washing Bar with the "Glass Test"

The "glass test" is recommended to determine whether you are using a detergent or not. Simply put what you use to wash your skin in a water glass for five minutes, then remove the cleansing bar and immediately dip the water glass for an **instant** in a basin of cold water. If the glass emerges from the basin perfectly clear, it proves the bar is an "effective" cleanser that could be **too strong** to use on your skin. This is especially true if your ancestors were from Northern Europe (including Ireland, England, Scotland, or Wales). The skin of the people from these countries is not only thinner in number of cells and connective tissue but also has fewer oil-producing cells.

Many patients with skin complaints do better by simply switching to a milder **real soap,** such as plain **Neutrogena, Basis, Cashmere Bouquet, Woodbury, Jergens** (not the antibacterial one), or **Sweetheart**. The latter four can be another problem if you are sensitive to the perfumes they contain.

Because most of my own family members have exceptionally sensitive skin, a condition said to be found in twenty percent of the population, we use **Lowila** exclusively. Available through nearly every pharmacy or health and beauty aids store in the world, this bar for cleaning the skin is safe even for a newborn baby with eczema. **Lowila** is three times the cost of most soaps and detergents but well worth every penny if it prevents dryness and itch. Some women smartly save money by using **Lowila** as their shampoo. (I suggest however that a separate bar of Lowila be reserved for that purpose and that you do not use the same piece for body and scalp.)

Using Dove—the Washing Bar Formulated by the Dermatologists

I do advise patients, for reasons of economy, to try **Dove** first, if they have any problems with their present soap; for most people, it is good. However, for many patients with sensitive skin, it has simply not been mild enough for repetitive use. The new **Dove-for-Sensitive-Skin**, without the perfumes and dyes, is a definite improvement.

Looking at the Facts on Wrinkles and "Cellulite"

Wrinkles, the most dramatic visible sign of aging, owe most of their existence to the **sun. Smoking,** which ages every cell in the body, including the ovaries, is a distant second as a cause of wrinkles. Whether one ever lies in the sun or not, a sun screen is certainly a good idea every day. The use of sunscreen decreases the skin's ability to absorb those sun's rays that are needed by the skin cells for the production of Vitamin D. Therefore, extra Vitamin D, available in milk and many breakfast cereals, is advisable whenever sunscreens are used. If your daily vitamin has 400 units of Vitamin D, or you consume dairy products, you should be fine. (Persons over seventy years of age should supplement their diet with 800 units.)

Estrogen, the principal sex hormone of the human female, promotes the production of collagen in the skin and is thus an anti-wrinkle hormone. However, because this hormone has so many other effects on the body, it should **never** be prescribed just for wrinkles.

Cosmetic surgeons can do wonderful things these days, especially if one has an extra ten thousand dollars laying around. For most of us, **Retin-A** cream or lotion, while expensive, is much cheaper. Your public library might have an old copy of *Retin-A and Other Youth Miracles* by Joseph A. Bark, which has been quite helpful in explaining the use of this skin product. The makers of **Retin-A** recommend the simultaneous use of **Purpose,** which is a washing bar or lotion with a sunscreen in it.

Many **cautions** apply to the use of Retin-A, including potential harm during pregnancy and nursing. If a person has any other skin problem besides wrinkles, Retin-A should best be avoided until a dermatologist or other physician knowledgeable and interested in skin problems is consulted. It is, after all, not just another face cream. (In the past, insurance drug plans did not pay for this product, since FDA approval was limited to its use in acne. Now that this agency has approved its use and effectiveness in reducing wrinkles, prescriptions for new formulations like **Renova** may be reimbursed by some health insurance drug plans.)

"Cellulite," a nonmedical but popular term introduced in 1975, refers to the ridged, uneven outer parts of the thighs, hips, and buttocks. These pockets of fat are a very natural development in women and can rarely, if ever, be totally or permanently eliminated. Exercising to tone the muscles in those areas, avoiding obesity, or losing excess weight can only improve the problem a little. The extent of the "affliction" is nearly totally genetic and very feminine, since it is only women who have, by nature, a thick layer of fat under the skin. As with all these bodily differences from the Hollywood or Madison Avenue model, **it is O.K.**, as well as very wise, to decide that it is O.K. **to be less than perfect!** Besides, as Jane R. Hirschmann and Carol H. Munter say, in *When Women Stop Hating Their Bodies*, "Who says buttocks and thighs should be thin?"[2] (More on that topic in Chapter Eight and throughout the second section of the book.)

It is not without good reasons that the **first active health choice** I have proposed concerns the ways to be kind to your skin, namely: avoiding hot water, or products that do harm, and excessive washing, as well as humidifying excessively dry indoor air. By allowing you to reap benefits from **less** effort rather than more, it is unique among the choices in the book. (You will be delighted, of course, to learn that **all the others** invite you to do **more** to control your life.)

2

Attending to Five Other Little Things That Can Mean a Lot

1. Keeping Winter Colds and Sore Throats Away

Ear, nose, throat, and upper respiratory infections are the leading cause of **nonfatal** illness in women at all ages! So how do you reduce or eliminate some of these respiratory problems.

Before I learned the secret of humidification, my office would be filled with the "respiratory sick," year after year, from mid-November to mid-April. This coincided exactly with the time that their heating systems were keeping the relative humidity of the indoor air at seven percent. This very low level of moisture means the air is actually twice as dry as the Sahara desert! However, when a patient ran a humidifier for at least six hours a day in her bedroom, these illnesses typically disappeared entirely.

The problem can be year-round in those areas where low humidity is not limited to the months of indoor living. For example, during the year I was practicing medicine in an area with very low relative humidity, around El Paso, Texas, I was witness to an incredibly large number of men, women, and children who came to the clinics in every month, for treatment of skin and respiratory problems. Thirty physicians in all, we saw nearly a thousand cases every day.

Dispelling the Myth that Colds and Sore Throats Are Due to Cold, Wet Weather

Most people think that getting a chill or wet feet is a common cause of colds and sore throats. Clinical experiments at the University of Pennsylvania Medical School showed quite clearly that this was not true. The researchers could not get their student subjects to contract a cold or a sore throat when they soaked them with cold water and then let them sit in chilled chambers with their feet under water. They concluded that cold and wetness are not the culprits.

Another somewhat amusing but revealing experiment, fifteen years later, showed that eating hot chicken soup prevented transmission of cold viruses to the subjects, but only during the time they were actually eating the soup. So why would soup be helpful only while it is being eaten? It seems the warm moisture from the soup was bathing their upper respiratory tract. I guess mothers always knew that it was the soup **vapor** that saves!

Keeping Yourself Sick All Winter

Looking to get off work? Make sure you stay in dry, unhumidified air and thus turn your membranes into a dry potato chip! The potato chip process occurs when dry air hits the respiratory tract, which includes the nasal passages, throat, larynx, bronchi, and lungs. These areas are lined with a special membrane with hairlike projections called **cilia,** which reject or prevent germs from invading, multiplying, or moving down the respiratory tract. These cilia actually wave, like a wheat field in the wind, in the opposite direction to the air we inhale. The cilia must be moist to do their job. When these membranes are dry, the integrity of the surface membrane cells are impaired, and the cilia cannot work. If this occurs, we are literally at the mercy of the "strep" and other bacteria, the flu and other viruses, and, in fact, all the other hundreds or thousands of dangerous airborne agents. The sinuses do not have cilia, but they still need moisture to keep their membranes intact and their secretions in a liquid and flowing state.

Getting the **Right** Humidifier

If you buy a **warm-**mist humidifier, the mist will condense as water on any cooler structure it touches. Since everything is ordinarily at a lower temperature than **steam**, virtually all the vapor becomes water and is thus removed from the air. Not only will the mist quickly leave the air and therefore be of no benefit to the skin, but the water that is thus formed will damage your furnishings. Warm mist, however, can be very helpful in the bathroom or shower if there is no wallpaper or wood to be water-damaged. Even better, one can now buy a "personal" warm-mist vaporizer, which has a plastic face connection so that the steam goes directly to the nose and throat.

Some humidifiers can look "swampy" quickly, if you do not clean them thoroughly and regularly. By conscientious cleaning you can avoid the **one serious potential problem** from using them, that of spreading **water-borne organisms** of all types that can multiply in standing water. The state-of-the-art humidifiers are no longer the "cool mist" humidifiers in which the vapors (being **colder** and thus heavier than air) tend to deposit faster on the floor and furniture, leaving wet spots on the surrounding carpet and "white dust" on the furniture. The "evaporative" humidifiers put out "invisible" mist at room temperature that tends to disperse evenly and not deposit white dust. The best ones have good filters and run silently. (Recommended: **DeVibiss-Hankscraft, Kaz,** and **Bemis.**)

Some believe that a central humidifier, like **April Air**, especially with an electrostatic air cleaner, provides optimal indoor air, but sometimes even these very expensive units have to be supplemented with bedroom units to get the desired level of moisture. (See the segment, "Cleaning Indoor Air," below.)

Moisture should be added to indoor air not only when it is being heated. For those spending over half their time in **air-conditioned** rooms, the problems from dry air may appear and require the same remedy.

Incidentally, your house plants will also do 200% better when the humidity is increased!

Simply Cooling the Bedroom Does *Not* Make the Air Humid Enough

Some dismiss what I say about humidification since "they sleep with the bedroom window open." But cooling indoor air in that manner does not necessarily moisten it. Because air expands when it is warmed, the volume of outside air at 35 degrees, for example, will perhaps double or triple in volume in the 65 degree temperature of our bedroom. But the total amount of water vapor does not change when that outside air is warmed. As a result, the water vapor, which constituted sixty percent of the total amount that the outside volume of colder air could contain, now constitutes only ten percent of the much larger volume of room air. Thus, an open window usually increases the humidity only marginally. (Many men and women find this physical chemistry too complicated. If you are among that group, please take my word for it and use the humidifier.)

If the dry air problem is severe enough to cause nosebleeds or chronic postnasal drip, one can add more moisture (besides using an evaporative humidifier the entire time the home heater is on) by putting five drops of salt water into the nostrils three or four times a day. Fill a 25-cent dropper bottle from the local pharmacy with salt water made by adding one-half teaspoon of salt to a pint of water. (Over-the-counter commercial salt water nose drops are available.)

Cleaning Indoor Air

Many respected scientists and clinicians claim half of all our pain and suffering is due to the toxins in the air we breathe. Obviously, anyone with respiratory allergies or lung conditions should benefit dramatically if even the bedroom air were pure. Excellent air purifiers are now available, including many that remove particles, especially the smallest viruses, even smaller than those removed by the High Efficiency Particulate Air or HEPA filters, which by definition will remove 99.97% of the air-borne dust, dander, pollens, bacteria and most viruses. Prices average about $250.00 for single-room units and $500-600 for units that clean 2500 square feet.[1]

For those of us who are not fortunate enough to have centralized vacuum cleaning systems to remove most of the dust, getting the

most thorough vacuum cleaner can prove to be a valuable investment in your respiratory health. In addition to strong suction the
vacuum should also have a HEPA filter. A marked improvement in
"allergies" will be noted immediately. (The very best vacuum for
cleaning the air may be a **Rainbow** vacuum, which has a water filter.
Cost about $1600!)

Remember, however, that all the various filtration devices mentioned do not humidify the air.

Selecting the Right Cold Remedy

When a cold is contracted, it is important not to buy cold remedies that will do more harm than good.

Such a product for potential harm would be one that has a **drying**
agent such as an antihistamine when the main problem is not a **runny**
nose, but a congested or **stuffy** nose. **Vicks** has a cold preparation just
for a "stuffy nose." Decongestants such as **pseudoephedrine HCL**,
which is found in over one-hundred "cold remedies," or **phenyl-
propanolamine** which is found in at least thirty-five, are effective for
congestion when used alone, but they can keep you awake.

It is also *inadvisable* to buy a cough remedy that combines a
cough **suppressant** like **dextromethorphan** with ingredients like
guiacol or **guiafenesin** which **induce** coughing by liquefying the
phlegm in the bronchi. Two very popular examples of this *unfortunate* combination of ingredients are **Robitussin-DM** or **Benylin
Expectorant**. A famous example from the past was the so-called **G.I.
gin**, containing an **elixir of terpine hydrate** to induce coughing and
codeine to suppress it. Fortunately, the **Robitussin** can now be
obtained with either only the guiafenesin **or** the dextromethorphan.

Representing another useless combination of ingredients are all
the remedies that combine an ingredient like **guiacol** to **liquefy
secretions** and an antihistamine like **benadryl** to **dry** secretions.

Asking the Pharmacist for Help if You Forget

What should you buy? Tell the pharmacist you want something
like plain **Robitussin** having only the guiafenesin,when you have a

productive cough, to keep the phlegm liquid and therefore loose. When a cough is non-productive and you therefore want to stop it and perhaps get some natural sleep, get **Robitussin** (Pediatric or Maximum Strength) or **Benylin-DM**, both labeled as cough suppressants, containing only dextromethorphan. (If Americans are goung to spend $380,000,000 on cold remedies, they may as well get the correct ones.) Plain **Benylin** contains only an antihistamine and is rarely a good idea, except perhaps for a simple runny nose in young children, whose sinuses are not yet developed sufficiently for secretions dried by an antihistamine to pool there, get stuck, and cause sinus infection.

As the first of the **five little things** suggested in this chapter, the measures suggested for preventing respiratory problems share something in common with the proposals of Chapter One for the skin and the suggestions to follow in the very next part of this chapter. What is similar in each? The answer is that eliminating harmful indoor airborne respiratory agents and keeping the respiratory tract humidified (like the suggestions for the skin in the last chapter and those for the bowel in the next segment) are health interventions that will equally **benefit the male** as well as the female of the species. The happy result that may occur if you heed this segment is that your **husband's** sore throat every November or his winter cold or cough that lasts three months may become only a memory.

2. *Preventing* the Problem No One Talks About

Mark Twain's famous comment about the weather as something everyone talks about but no one ever does anything about hardly applies to the problems that most of us at one time or another will have with our bowels. In fact, eyebrows are often raised when a patient is told that the **most important single bit of advice** I can give them is to make sure they never have a **hard** bowel movement!

Whether the visit is brief or comprehensive, the information is imparted that the patient should decide, for her best health, to use whatever is necessary to prevent constipation, which I define as a **hard** or **difficult** bowel movement. (If their problem is the opposite—too many bowel movements—the suggested intervention is essentially the same, but without the **insoluble** fiber.)

To achieve the elusive goal of **normal** bowel movements **without any gaps,** I try to convince each patient that fiber, not just their favorite beverage, can be truly their personal "elixir of the gods!"

Fiber is, by definition, that part of a plant that cannot be digested, or broken down and absorbed into the blood stream.

Lack of adequate fiber on a daily basis has been implicated as a very significant factor in many unwanted conditions, such as:

(1) **cancer of the colon,** the most common cancer in our country. Tests for it on a regular basis should begin at least by age fifty if a person has no symptoms or bowel complaints and no history of occurrence in a "first-degree relative," referring to your parent, child, or siblings. If there is a family history, routine testing of asymptomatic individuals should begin at age forty. Testing should start sooner if someone has symptoms.[2]

(2) **diverticulitis,** which is the most common reason for emergency admission and subsequent surgery in our American hospitals. This condition occurs in more Americans than any other single serious chronic health problem.

(3) **rectal, anal, or hemorrhoidal problems,** especially pain and bleeding.

(4) **hernias,** which occur in men in the groin area, and in women in the groin or in the vagina, where it can involve the uterus, vagina, bladder, or bowel.

Noting the Real Difference Between *Soluble* and *Insoluble* Fiber

Doctors used to tell patients who had problems of chronic diarrhea, or an irritable and spastic colon, to "avoid roughage." More correctly, the patients might have been told to *avoid or reduce their intake* of **insoluble** fiber, which is contained in wheat and barley brans, seeds, and skins, but *not to stop their intake* of **soluble** fiber, such as oat bran. The distinction can be very important for some, especially for those with too many stools, whose diarrhea might be aggravated by insoluble fiber.

Insoluble fiber primarily acts as a **laxative**, while **soluble** fiber produces bulk by absorbing water and acting as a **bowel normalizer**. By absorbing water, soluble fiber gives the stool form and softness, which often prevents or corrects diarrhea.

Unfortunately for the fifteen million Americans who experience real physical, social, and emotional difficulties from too many trips to the restroom or bathroom, the "nutrition facts" now listed on most American processed foods usually list only "dietary fiber," without distinguishing the solubility. However, the recommended cereals listed below list separate values for the "total dietary fiber" and "insoluble fiber," which will alert you to a possible diarrhea-producing affect.

Fortunately for most people, thirty grams of varied dietary fiber per day seems to work very well, because most people need both types. This need for both types is the reason it is ordinarily suggested that people get their daily fiber from at least several different sources.

Since the average American diet supplies less than half of the recommended twenty-five to thirty grams of fiber per day, and since knowing the type of fiber can be critical for some of us, we shall be very specific about a few natural and a few supplemental sources of fiber.

Getting Bran and *Complex* Carbohydrates from *Natural* Sources

The only **bran** that is soluble is **oat** bran. The breakfast cereals I recommend as the best sources of soluble fiber also contain no salt or sugar. They are **Nabisco** or **Quaker Oat Bran** Cereals. If **constipation** is a problem despite adequate soluble fiber, we recommend cereals with insoluble fiber too, such as **Nabisco Shredded Wheat** in the yellow box, or **Nabisco Shredded Wheat N' Bran** in the small brown box. Both also are without salt or sugar. All the whole grain cereals and fresh vegetables and fruits, especially when the skins are included, are the best sources of combined soluble and insoluble fiber. They are also the best source of **complex** carbohydrates. Carbohydrates should supply fifty-five to sixty percent of our calories, most of it complex carbohydrates, especially if we have any trouble handling simple sugars.

Such a diet, high in complex carbohydrates, tends to produce or maintain, for a variety of known and unknown reasons, normal food cravings and normal utilization of calories, leading to a healthier body weight.

Using Fiber from "Over-the Counter" Sources

It is important to remember that **you should increase the amount of fiber in your diet gradually, so as not to produce gas pains or diarrhea**, especially when using one of the many over-the-counter preparations containing **psyllium**. These products include the **Metamucil** powders, **Fiberall** wafers, and **Konsyl** powders.

Generally, less gas is produced by two other groups of soluble, safe, nonirritating, and therefore non-diarrheal-producing fiber products. The first group are available in the more aesthetically pleasing **tablet form** and contain a man-made fiber product called **calcium polycarbophil**. Brand names include **Fiberall** tablets, **Fibercon** tablets, and **Konsyl** tablets. The second type of bulk-producing soluble fiber, methylcellulose, is the active ingredient in **Citrucel**.

Almost always, the product with the least calories in each group is generally best, provided that you are not sensitive to the artificial sweetener that some of the low calorie preparations contain, or that you do not get too much of it. If one type of preparation doesn't normalize the bowels, try another, or try combinations. Allow yourself plenty of time to get the right combination for you. (**Diaries** or **journals** have been and will be recommended throughout this book for solving various problems and abetting assorted initiatives. Keeping a record of the fibers you have tried and the amounts, at least in the beginning, will definitely help you achieve success faster.)

Heading Off Hemorrhoidal Hassles

The hemorrhoidal veins are most likely to fill with fluid and be a problem from two specific situations: 1) when an individual is forced to strain with a hard stool, or 2) when a person has retained excess salt and fluid (which in women is usually due to a lack of rest in the presence of normal or high levels of the female hormone **estrogen**—an antidiuretic. This hormone has a natural salt-retaining effect on the kidneys, as will be detailed in Chapter Four.)

The most effective immediate treatment for fluid retention in the hemorrhoidal vessels includes both rest, with the lower half of the bed elevated 15 degrees, and the simultaneous application of moist, warm compresses to the painful, itchy, and swollen area. A small "face" or "baby" hot water bottle wrapped in a wet washcloth works fine, if it is applied to the area affected by pain while you are lying face down, with the hip-buttock area elevated. Small "moist heating pads," which can be warmed in minutes in the microwave, are now available and work well for this purpose. **Sitz baths are never recommended for this problem**. The hot water wrecks the skin, and the sitting position used to apply the heat only increases the size of the hemorrhoids.

Tucks, or any preparation containing alcohol, removes the body's protective oils and thus dehydrates the tissues and should not ever be used in this area on a regular basis! (One further **caution**: the typical American recliner, which places the buttocks in a position lower than the rest of the body, can actually **increase** the problems with hemorrhoids, because all the excess fluids in the body will tend to "pool" in that part of the body, which is kept lowest.)

Distinguishing a Problem of "Gas" from "A Change in Bowel Habits"

One of the most commonly expressed complaints is excessive gas. Rarely is it more than a social problem, even if it is accompanied by mild cramps or pains. Air swallowing, sometimes from smoking, often plays a part, especially in thin women, as does the ingestion of carbonated beverages or high fiber foods such as beans, peas, and cabbage (or a lot of other foods that most people eventually, by a process of trial and error, begin to identify). Many people insist that "Beano" helps their gas problem.

In contrast to day-to-day variability in the amount of gas we experience, an unexplained change to constipation or diarrhea that persists for more than two weeks should be reported to a health care professional and tests should be performed.

Surely you will discover that taking responsibility for normalizing your bowel function is not only "easy" but incredibly rewarding over a lifetime.

For my part, when I am falling asleep, I occasionally feel proud that "somewhere out there" live at least a hundred women who will never need surgery or a pessary to keep their bladder, uterus, vagina, or bowel from falling out, because they had a doctor who (as one patient once remarked) "has a thing about bowels."

This segment marks the last of the three **active choices** that should provide equal benefit to men. While my male readers can learn a lot in the remainder of **Section One** about **female physiology** and the **health problems that affect women exclusively** (and in Chapter Seven he can learn those body-mind exercises that will benefit **his** mental and physical health), my suggestions that might require **men to do something** to better control or improve their lives in some way do not resume until **Section Two.** There, the **challenge is issued to *everyone* to heal their relationships.**

3. Dealing with Painful Breasts

Fifty percent of women who go the doctor complain of some kind of pain in the breasts. Fortunately, **breast pain is not a risk factor for breast cancer.**

Despite the lack of any connection between pain in the breast and cancer, since breast cancer affects one in every eight American women, according to the most recent figures, the sudden onset of pain gets a woman's immediate attention. Because of the patient's anxiety about cancer, the wise physician will ask for an immediate exam, as well as check that her periodic mammograms are current.

The reality is that cancer of the breast very rarely first appears as pain. Since painful breasts and breast cancer are both so common, it is possible to have both simultaneously, even if they are not related.

(A related concern regarding the breasts is **soreness**. It has been reported that soreness is much more common in the **left** breast. In my practice, pain on the left is about nine times more frequent than on the right side. That the left breast is 22% larger in most women may be a partial reason but not the whole answer.)

Any lump, dimpling, puckering, thickening, hardening, or rash, however, should be checked by a physician. Bleeding, discharge, rash, peeling, or retraction of the nipple should also be evaluated. Since, in the past, ninety percent of the lumps have been found by self-examination, this practice should not be abandoned. Mammograms can miss even large tumors, although the number missed is decreasing as more and more radiologists are backing up their readings with independent second observer analysis of the films. The amount of radiation received from a mammogram equals the amount received on any 1000-mile airplane flight, which is to say, negligible.

Breast self-examination (BSE) is still important and is best done a week after the period **starts**. The American College of Obstetricians and Gynecologists gives the following suggestions for this exam:

(1) Lying flat on your back, place a pillow under your left shoulder and use the flat portions of the right-hand fingers, held together, to very gently feel and press the left breast, starting from the outer edges, and proceeding, in a spiral direction, to the nipple. The nipple should be gently squeezed as part of the exam.

(2) Switch the pillow to the back of the right shoulder, and, using the left hand, repeat the process. Include the area **below** the armpits, which contains breast tissue.

(3) Repeat as much of this process as you can in the shower, while your fingers and the breast are wet.

(4) Inspect and compare your breasts, looking in the mirror. Look for any of the changes in the skin cited above, or any nipple discharge that results from gentle squeezing.[3]

Regular mammograms, according to the guidelines of the American Cancer Society, should be obtained, even though now, in many cases, the insurance companies, including Medicare, do not pay for all of them.[4] Already, a thirty percent improvement in survival has been demonstrated as a result of yearly mammograms after age fifty, and this figure should steadily improve. Equally important, a fifteen percent improvement in survival rates and a twenty-five percent increase in the ratio of early versus late-stage tumors has been demonstrated from regular one-to-two-year mammograms for women ages forty to forty-nine. (Some recent reports by radiologists maintain it is even more important to get yearly x-rays between forty and fifty because the cancers grow faster in that decade.) It is well to remember that **eighty percent of breast cancers occur in women with no family history.** (Despite the cries about a breast cancer "epidemic," the **overall mortality from breast cancer has not increased** in the past forty years, **nor has the incidence of cancer in women under fifty-six increased since 1950.**) However, **smoking** has been shown in several recent studies to **increase the risk of getting breast cancer**—not decrease the risk, as was formerly believed.

Eliminating **Stimulation** *to End the Pain or Soreness*

Stimulation of the breasts is the usual cause of pain or soreness, whether the stimulation is a result of **massage** by a partner, **hot water** in the shower or bath, or, most commonly, by **excessive movement** of the breast tissue itself because of a poorly fitting bra. As bras have become designed to be more glamorous but less supportive or restraining of movement of the breast tissues, the incidence of breast discomfort has increased dramatically. Spending some money on a **well-fitting bra** at a girdle shop makes good sense. Fortunately, a few such specialty shops still exist. When soreness starts, wear the bra to bed, make sure it is high and tight, and avoid any hot water or massage to the breast. The claim that decreasing caffeine or taking vitamin E (400 I.U. should be enough) helps the situation is probably correct.

Phytoestrogens, which are very weak estrogens found in soy products, cashews, peanuts, wheat, corn, apples, red sage, almonds, and a host of other vegetables, are acclaimed as helpful. Four 500 mg capsules per day of **oil of evening primrose** or one Tbsp. of ground flaxseed, which you can sprinkle over other foods, salads, or soups, are suggested as effective for this problem. The **antioxidants** Selenium and Beta-Carotene are also said to be effective, especially in their natural form in fruits and vegetables. As with so many things in medicine, the doctors and science can often lag behind what experience has already taught you. If you find that those things help, you should follow that experience.[5] (**Caution:** Excess Vitamin A can be dangerous to your health, and quite harmful to your baby, should you get pregnant while taking an excess.)

Saying Good-bye to the "Cystic" Breast/Cancer Connection

Fibrocystic breast disease (FBD) is a **meaningless** umbrella term, a wastebasket into which health care professionals throw every breast condition that isn't cancer. It is no diagnosis at all, as well as being an inappropriate choice of words, since these breasts so described are not really cystic and not at all fibrous. They hurt and feel lumpy and swollen, perhaps even leak a little, because the cells grow and accumulate fluid during the menstrual cycle, and this can produce lumpiness and pain. Ninety percent of women, at some times in their lives, will experience this pain, swelling, and lumpiness, though only half will ever report it.

Patients understandably get concerned when their health care professionals make it a point to pronounce that their breasts are "cystic." The examiners are usually trying to say that the breasts are harder to examine because they are firmer and denser. Numerous studies have shown that there are no more cysts in cancerous breasts than in noncancerous breasts when examined at biopsy.[6] Breast biopsies done at past autopsies showed that more than half of the breasts without cancer had "fibrocystic disease," but that only twenty-six percent of the cancerous breasts had cysts.

Many times the diagnosis of cystic breasts is based on a physical examination, during which the doctor finds firm nodular changes throughout one or both breasts, or "cystic breasts" are mentioned as a routine comment on a mammogram report. The **main importance**, and a very crucial one, is **not that subsequent breast cancer is at all more likely, but that firm and generally lumpy breasts can make both self-examination and physician examinations of the breast much more difficult. There is no other relationship of this condition to cancer.** Recent studies reported from several medical groups have claimed greater success in detecting **breast lesions (but only in women with dense breasts) by** *routinely* **adding an ultrasound** exam of the breast at the same diagnostic visit.

Describiing a *Typical* Clinical Scenario

When Carolyn Z. came in last week, hysterical because her breasts were "on fire" and "it had to be cancer," it was necessary to examine her breasts, which were very full and "lumpy," as they have been for the twenty years I have been checking them. Since I found no **dominant lump**, I suggested symptomatic treatment, that is, no stimulation from massage or hot water and the use of a tight bra around the clock. The pain vanished in three days. Since her last mammogram was over a year ago, a repeat was ordered and was negative. Carolyn now has returned to a state of relative calm.

Interestingly enough, use of birth control pills for at least a few years, or taking regimens of continuous hormone replacement after the ovaries have declined, markedly improves, or often eliminates entirely, this "lumpiness."

Are Cystic Breasts Due to Hormones? Getting Your Facts Straight

Many older women avoid hormones in the last half of their life because they have "cystic" breasts. Sadly, in some cases, their physicians have told them as much. The American College of Obstetricians and Gynecologists, as well as many other similar professional groups around the world, have officially stated that no breast condition, except cancer itself, precludes the use of hormones.

4. Taking the Pain Out of Your Periods

When a teenager is living in fear, waiting for the horrible pain of her next menstrual period, it is easy to say she should be examined by a gynecologist. Easy advice, and good, unless the teen does not want to undergo a gynecological exam. If this reluctance exists, it is probably better not to insist on an exam as the initial step in management, but rather to try the simple remedies suggested below.

Painful periods usually mean the ovaries are working well. In someone who has never been pregnant, pain of some sort in the mid-lower abdomen or lower back on the first day of her period (or sometimes starting just before) is very common.

Physiologically, such discomfort is a sign that the teenager has now reached her "fertile" years. This means she is now ovulating, or releasing an ovum, or egg, from the ovary. Thus, most often it is a proof that her ovaries are functioning as they should be. The pain is due to the fact that the uterus, or womb, has not yet been "matured" by carrying a pregnancy to normal delivery. The cure of this condition as a permanent result of having a baby is dramatic. In someone who has delivered in the distant past, which means more than five to eight years previously, cramps can return, since the opening of the womb, called the cervix, tends to return eventually to its smaller, adolescent or "pre-pregnancies" condition.

A great benefit of a regular exercise program is that such activity lessens the pain of the periods. The **relaxation exercises** discussed in Chapter Seven are especially recommended. Other **natural** suggestions are the **phytoestrogens** just recommended for breast pain. A diet with decreased meats, diary products and fat, with increased complex carbohydrates, B-vitamins (especially B6), and Magnesium is also recommended.[7]

Knowing When to See a Doctor for Painful Periods

Perhaps only a visit to the dentist is dreaded more than a visit for a gynecologic exam. In many cases, even the dental visit is less abhorrent. This unfortunate attitude is at least partly due to a woman's acquired shame about her body, shame that has no basis in fact. As several of the prominent female gynecologists have written, when a woman asks her gynecologist how he or she can endure such "disgusting" work, she is demonstrating quite clearly that she does not **esteem her womanhood or her uniqueness.** This is sad.

The major reason to get professional help for period pain is if the pain each cycle starts to get progressively worse or to last longer. If the pain is severe or lasts more than forty-eight hours, a doctor should definitely be consulted. Most often, physicians are consulted when over-the-counter medications fail to relieve the pain. The best medications are not truly pain pills but are called more correctly anti-spasmodic or anti-inflammatory drugs. The safest and most commonly recommended class are the **ibuprofens,** available in **Motrin, Advil, Nuprin, Metiprin,** or **Pamprin-IB.** The failure of these drugs is usually due to taking the meds too late, that is, after the inflammation or spasm has occurred, or using an inadequate dose.

Ideally, the recommended single initial dose is 600, or even 800 mg, to be taken as soon as one knows a period may be starting, or preferably, before any pain has begun, then repeating one-half that dose, as needed, in four-to-six-hour intervals.

Being Aware of "Endometriosis" as a Cause of Period Pain

The failure of **ibuprofen-type** drugs, used correctly, to relieve the pain is most assuredly a reason to seek a gynecologic evaluation. The first sign of a condition called "endometriosis" is usually periods in which the pain lasts several days, with the severity of the pain increasing every year. It is estimated that five million American women suffer from this condition. Physically, this is a disease in which bleeding and inflammation occur on a regular basis in "uterine-type" tissue inside the abdomen that is not located where it should be found, which is within the lining of the womb. Besides the pain produced, this affliction can destroy fertility and increase the risk of **ectopic** pregnancies, or pregnancies in which the embryo or fetus is not contained within the womb cavity. Endometriosis can eventually even destroy the ovaries, resulting in an early "change."

Treatment can be **surgical** or **medical.** All the natural remedies just suggested for ordinary menstrual pain should be included in any treatment. The **body-mind relaxation techniques** explained in Chapter Seven can substantially alter pain perception and ease much of the despair that those afflicted with endometriosis experience.

Most formal treatment decisions depend on age, the wishes for child-bearing, and the patient's symptoms. Most important, however, treatment should also depend on the extent of the abnormalities found by thorough evaluation of the internal lesions at the time of **laparoscopy**. (This is an outpatient procedure that involves looking into the abdomen and pelvis via a small incision at the naval area, using a special telescope-like instrument called, appropriately enough, a laparoscope). Except for the treatment with oral contraceptives, the **medical** treatments can have undesirable side effects, besides being very expensive. Neither the diagnostic tests, when the condition is suspected, nor the treatment, if the diagnosis is confirmed, should be delayed.

Dr. John Lee, who is a fervent advocate for **natural** progesterone, recommends its use in treating endometriosis.[8]

5. Keeping Your Bladder Forever Young

To the billions spent for skin care, exercise programs and equipment, and diet remedies, plus the staggering cost of heart disease, arthritis, osteoporosis, and smoking, let us not forget to add the cost of surgery, antibiotics, prostheses, and doctor visits that are required by women attempting to preserve or restore bladder function, especially the ability to hold their urine.

Many years before men have trouble in **initiating** bladder emptying, women can begin having problems from the involuntary loss of urine. American women spend over six hundred million dollars every year on incontinence pads alone! Obviously, this remains for women a very common and annoying social problem. The frequency of the problem is such that one-third of **nulliparous** (never had a child) white college women experience problems with urinary stress incontinence.

Spotting the Causes of Bladder Malfunctions

Childbirth, constipation, heavy lifting, obesity, the inevitable estrogen deficiency of the last decades of life, asthma, nerve injuries, or chronic cough (most often caused by smoking) can all play a role in causing or aggravating bladder problems. **Inherited bladder anatomy** can incline a person toward incontinence. Bad bladder habits, such as **incomplete** or **too frequent** emptying, or **holding the urine too long,** can be factors also.

Good bladder practices can never be adopted too soon, especially the faithful daily performance of bladder or perineal exercises that try to keep the bladder, vaginal, and anal sphincter muscles strong. Exercise of the vaginal muscles helps bladder control enormously (at the same time probably increasing success in achieving vaginal orgasm, a not insignificant benefit to most women). The name **Kegel** is usually applied to these exercises of the muscles that close the bladder, vaginal, and anal openings.[9]

Mild incontinence, such as loss of urine only when one coughs or sneezes, can probably be improved or even eliminated by daily bladder exercises. These are often best performed first thing in the

morning, in bed. The bladder should be emptied first. But any time of
the day is good. When done properly, no one should be aware that
you are doing these exercises.

Severe incontinence, or involuntary loss while dancing, walking
up or down steps, laughing, or even from simple walking is a much
more difficult problem to treat. Surgery is often required, though
bladder exercises and estrogenic hormones are usually insisted upon
by the surgeon before surgery. The exercises and estrogen should be
used permanently thereafter in order to increase the degree and
duration of success.

Learning Through Biofeedback Therapy or By Using Vaginal "Cones" at Home

Weighted vaginal cones of graduated weights are now available
to help an individual ensure that she is doing the Kegel exercises
correctly, and to measure the degree of progress. But even these
prostheses work better if the person with incontinence has partici-
pated in a biofeedback bladder exercise training program. This
outpatient training is available at nearly every major hospital center.
The cones now cost about fifty dollars, but could be well worth that
price if they can teach a woman which muscles she needs to contract
to maintain continence.

Often, the same conditions listed above that contribute to the
development of stress incontinence, can produce **herniation**, or a
prolapse or **droppage** of the bladder, womb, or rectum so that any or
all of these structures can fall to the level of the vaginal opening or
beyond. Individuals with a prolapse of the bladder tend not to be
significantly incontinent until the hernia or prolapse, called a **cysto-
cele** is corrected. It is unfortunate but true that attempts to keep the
bladder from falling down can sometimes aggravate the incontinence. Either a **pessary,** which is a diaphragm-like prosthesis that
will support and elevate the bladder so that it doesn't protrude
through the vaginal opening, or regretfully, **surgery** that is not
complete in **that it fails to correct the bladder-sphincter muscles,
can make incontinence worse.** The bladder may be replaced into its
proper position effectively enough, but because the weaknesses of
the pelvic muscles are not also corrected, the new funnel-shaped

configuration of the bladder that the pessary or incomplete surgery creates actually increases the likelihood of incontinence.

As is the case with all of the health care suggestions in this book, the emphasis is on **prevention now**, so that there is less of a problem ten to fifty years from now.

Summarizing the best preventive measures a woman can adopt:

(1) Lift nothing heavier than 30 lbs.

(2) Control coughing or asthmatic wheezing.

(3) Normalize the bowels by taking adequate fiber or softeners, so that there is never any straining.

(4) Reduce excess weight.

(5) Treat the **permanent** estrogen deficiency that begins at age fifty (or sooner) with some form of estrogen supplement. See page 92 for some options.

(6) Start the bladder exercises early.

The most important thing for you to remember is to share the problem with your health care provider because, with very rare exceptions, **something** can be done about it.

The **five little health initiatives** with which you have been challenged in this chapter are not at all examples of health "fads" that come and go in the media on a daily basis. Except for the suggestion of humidification, which might be contraindicated in a person with respiratory problems due to molds or other water-borne harmful agents (unless something like the "Enviracaire" air purifier with the HEPA filter were used), the suggestions presented should be as safe as they are effective. However, despite this factor of safety, anyone with ailments requiring the care of a health professional should best discuss each health suggestion with him or her before starting any of the items in our program. This caution applies equally to the "problems with the ovaries" to be presented next. Incidentally, at **your next office visit, give the doctor a list of all your immunizations. You may need new ones or some boosters.**

3

Handling the Problems
Your Ovaries Hand You

Many women are now quite capable of recognizing the earliest signs of their car's engine malfunction. Unfortunately, the same cannot be said for their early recognition of problems with those two "golf ball-sized" **ovaries** located within the pelvis. In an effort to fill that communication gap, three common clinical situations produced by malfunctioning ovaries will be discussed, namely, the scenario that can be seen in declining or **low estrogen states**, the **menstrual** signs of **hormonal imbalance**, and the three different **patterns of pain** arising from events in the ovaries.

Knowing When Your Estrogen Level Is Not Right

The term "menopause" should be totally interchangeable with "times of estrogen decline or deficiency," whether thirty years before or forty years after the so-called "mid-life crisis." When looked at in this way, young people and their physicians will be less likely to consider menopause as something they need not worry about until later in life, and older women and their physicians will not be so inclined to believe it is something that has passed, and that now there is nothing anyone could, or should, do about it!

My list of "menopausal" signs and symptoms is previewed here to emphasize the point that hormonal problems of too little, too much, fluctuations, and imbalance can occur from the second decade to the last decade of life, affecting the individual not only at that time, but also, and more important, permanently impacting her quality of life for many, or all, of her ensuing years. This is especially clear in the increased risk of osteoporosis that is found in thin women who are much more likely than those of normal weight or above to have intervals of estrogen deficiency. The difference is explained by the fact that **adipose or "fat" tissue** can store, produce, and release the estrogenic hormones that prevent thinning of the bones.

Another example of this "delayed effect" is presented by a recently reported study on breast cancer, which asserted that weight gain in the twenties and thirties increased the risk of breast cancer in the fifties and sixties, at least for the patients in this study. The possible explanation: excess weight increases the amount of estrogen in the body and also then tends to produce a deficiency of the second female hormone, namely, progesterone. There are considerable clinical indications that progesterone deficiency can be **one** of the factors increasing the risk of breast cancer. This is discussed in Chapter Five. (For additional information on a possible connection between breast cancer risk and prolonged progesterone deficiency, please refer to "Breast cancer, hormone connection, progesterone in subject index.)

Many would argue that you cannot blame all the signs and symptoms which follow, on hormonal defects. Perhaps this is true. Surely in some instances during the "change," symptoms that were previously ignored or accepted may now be noticed, and may be no longer tolerated because the problems that are specifically the result of hormone loss are so debilitating. However, in no way are these problems limited to those years around age fifty. My list is as follows: Extreme fatigue,[1] anxiety or panic attacks, flushes, flashes, night sweats, insomnia, palpitations, irritability, depression, mood swings, confusion, increasing absentmindedness or even total inability to focus on a goal, weight gain, increased hairiness, vaginal dryness and painful intercourse, or the onset of bladder irritability, frequency, or recurrent infections. Headaches on the top of the head or over the eyes indicate **low or no** estrogen, while migraine headaches, those headaches that are one-sided, accompanied by nausea, and sometimes preceded by visual warnings, indicate marked **falls** or dips in the hormone level.

Certainly, all these problems can be hormone-related, they can be independent of the will or will-power, and they can often be helped by medical interventions. The best time to institute preventive or corrective measures is as early as possible, though it is rarely, if ever, too late.

As explained in Chapters Four, Five, and Six, there are three main categories of women who are at high risk for estrogen deficiency: 1) very thin women, 2) new mothers, and 3) women whose periods have stopped but who are now totally without symptoms.

Recognizing Abnormal Menstrual Bleeding

When your ovaries are malfunctioning, **abnormal periods** are usually the result. The definition of abnormal bleeding, besides the obvious one of bleeding that is so heavy that the person affected cannot leave her home, might be remembered more easily by using what has been designated as the "one week, three week, five week rule." The following are abnormal: 1) any vaginal bleeding lasting **longer than** _one_ **week**, 2) any vaginal bleeding occurring **closer in onset than** _three_ **weeks**, counting from the first day of the first period to the first day of the next, or 3) any vaginal bleeding that occurs **less often than** _five_ **weeks**, counting from the first day of the first period to the first day of the next period.

If an individual is forty years of age or more, an office "dilatation and curettage" (D & C), or a biopsy of the lining of the womb is definitely advisable, if **two or more episodes** of abnormal bleeding occur between her check-ups. **Spotting,** which is defined as a pad of blood or less per day, should be noted, and mentioned at the next check-up. It should never be included in the one-, three-, five-week rule. Spotting at **mid-cycle** is common, and almost always normal, as is spotting immediately before menstruation. **(Exception:** When a patient has been taking birth control pills for over three months without any spotting and then starts spotting regularly at mid-cycle, she should notify her physician to arrange an exam and pap test) **Post-coital bleeding,** defined as bleeding after intercourse, of any amount, especially if it happens twice, merits at least a phone call.

An excellent habit is to keep a gyn diary, one that records the days of bleeding, spotting, or discharge; unusual symptoms like aches, cramps, or pain; as well as the timing of sexual intercourse relative to any abnormal signs or symptoms. Not only will such a diary maximize your awareness of what is happening in your own body, but it will also provide your physician with much valuable information.

Managing the Most Threatening Ovarian Problem—Pain

Most pain in the lower abdomen, apart from "gas" pains and menstrual cramps, is caused by four common but very different events in the pelvis. Three of these experiences, in which pain is generally the chief or only feature, are due to ovarian changes, are nearly never serious, and do not require surgery or even a rush to the emergency room. The fourth, in which pain is secondary to nausea and fever, is due to the appendix, and is serious. Surgery is the treatment required. Of the three ovarian causes, two involve the normal release of an "ovum" at mid-cycle, an event called **ovulation**. The third cause of ovarian pain occurs later in the cycle or after a period is overdue. In this last instance, the failure of a normal ovulation to occur at mid-cycle results in the formation of a larger and more fluid-filled cyst that eventually bursts or "ruptures." This event typically produces sudden, severe, and widespread lower abdominal pain.

Recognizing When *Sudden* and *Severe Pain* Is Caused by *Ovulation*

Ovulation, defined as the rupture of a mature follicle, or egg-containing cyst of the ovary, twelve to sixteen days before a period, is a regular and normal event in the major portion of the menstrual life of a woman. This egg-and-fluid-release is usually accompanied by a dull ache at or below the level of the belt-line, generally on the right side. Ovulation can mimic appendicitis. The main difference in symptoms between ovulation and appendicitis is in the **order in which the symptoms occur:**

1. In ovulation, the **first symptom** is almost always pain.

2. In appendicitis, the **first symptom is nausea or fever**, then, some hours after, **pain**. This pain typically begins **above** the belt-line, often in the area just below the breastbone. Only after some hours does it typically go down to the right lower abdomen.

Sometimes ovulation can be very painful. Even then, while fever and nausea can be present, these arise hours after the onset of pain. Unlike the nausea of appendicitis, in which vomiting is often a result and the idea of food is repulsive, the nausea of ovulation seems to be directly related to the severity of the pain, and the patient will often be hungry!

Countless emergency-room visits are made daily for the natural event of ovulation. Much time could be saved and much suffering prevented if these few simple points about what is happening at ovulation were more widely appreciated. Definitely, what is needed at the first sign of pain is not a hectic rush to the hospital but rather to stay home, for a few hours at least, in bed, with the legs and chest elevated on pillows, placing a moist heating pad over the lower abdomen, and taking two extra strength **Tylenol**, perhaps with some **Mylanta II** (or any other antacid that **doesn't** contain **calcium carbonate,** which often produces gas and bloating, and which could really create diagnostic confusion).

One very important **caution: If fever or nausea precedes the onset of pain, an emergency evaluation should be sought.**

Getting Quick Relief From Ovulation Pain

The pain produced by ovulation should begin to respond within an hour to the symptomatic treatment just listed. If the symptoms get worse after a few hours of treatment or if, after ten or twelve hours, the signs and symptoms are not much improved, a call to the physician is in order. A few well-chosen questions, and he or she should be able to tell if an immediate exam is needed.

Summarizing:

Ovulatory pain is the almost certain diagnosis if severe pain is the first symptom, especially if it awakens you from a sound sleep.

The diagnosis is virtually certain if your next period is also due in two weeks. Also favoring a diagnosis of ovulation is being hungry, despite any nausea.

Appendicitis is the almost certain diagnosis if fever or nausea occurs first, before the pain starts. The diagnosis of appendicitis is also more likely if the pain that follows the nausea or fever starts in the **upper abdomen** and then descends to the lower right.

Remember, in the common clinical presentation of **sudden pain at the time of the mid-cycle** produced by ovulation, the most important suggestion is: Stop all but essential activity until the pain is relieved.

Learning the Two Other Types of Ovarian Pain

An equally common presentation of pain from the ovaries is the onset of a mild **ache**, also starting at **mid-cycle**, and also due to ovulation. The big difference from the previously-described, sudden and severe, knife-like pain is that the initial mild ache, instead of disappearing within an hour or two, **gets gradually worse** over the subsequent day or days. In these patients, one usually finds that the individual in question, despite the ache, proceeded immediately to a job or activity that required much physical movement. Jogging, playing tennis, or engaging in aerobics would be examples of excessive movement, since all these types of activities result in the "swinging of the ovaries," one of which is now leaking fluid from the site of cyst rupture. If one pictures the leaking ovary hanging in space on a string connected to a fixed structure above it, then the increased leakage produced by shaking that ovary by body movements can be better appreciated.

Thus, in the moments or hours subsequent to ovulation, any unnecessary movement of the lower abdomen should cease, so that the rupture in the follicle or sac can seal, and the leakage of the irritating fluid from the ruptured sac can be kept to a minimum. Unless the ovary is swung by active body movement, the total escaped fluid usually measures less than a teaspoon, and so the symptoms are minimal and short-lived.

A somewhat more exaggerated clinical picture is seen when ovulation does not occur at mid-cycle and the normal monthly ovarian cyst continues to enlarge, even to three or four times the normal size and volume. When this enlarging cyst eventually does rupture, it usually produces symptoms that are not minimal and are not short-lived. Typically, in those cases in which the cyst gets very large, the period does not come until the cyst breaks! This is because the intact cyst continuously produces large amounts of the female hormone estrogen, which prevents the period. Then, when the cyst does rupture, estrogen production ceases immediately and this withdrawal of estrogen produces a period. The picture the patient presents in the emergency room is **sudden severe pain all over the lower abdomen,** in many cases radiating into the rectum, upper abdomen, and/or inner thigh, often followed by slight fever and nausea. All this occurs **late in her menstrual cycle,** or, more typically, when the period is overdue. In virtually every case, her period occurs within hours, either before or after the sudden onset of pain. (If pregnancy is a possibility, tests to rule out a pregnancy complication must be started.)

Getting a Laparoscopy ("to look") Not a Laparotomy ("to cut open")

If surgery, which is rarely needed, is decided upon for various reasons, it should usually be done by **laparoscopy, not laparotomy.** A laparoscopy means introducing a tubular, telescope-like instrument, called a laparoscope, through a very **small one-quarter-inch incision at the navel,** and performing the surgery through that area. A laparotomy involves a much larger incision and thus involves an in-patient stay and prolonged convalescence. The laparoscope was introduced into this country in the early 1970s, by gynecologists, but the technique involved took nearly two decades to find widespread application in other surgical areas. Now, the principles of what is called "minimally-invasive surgery" are revolutionizing diagnosis and treatment of nearly every surgical condition in medicine.

Summarizing what to do when the first symptom is right or left-sided pain at the beltline or slightly below:

(1) Stop exercise and all strenuous activity.

(2) Try to rest with chest and legs elevated. This keeps the fluid from the ovaries from irritating nerves going to the thighs, or those

nerves on the surface of other abdominal organs. Such spread of fluid usually produces nausea and low-grade fever.

(3) Employ "moist" heat. For example, either a hot water bottle wrapped in a wet wash cloth or a moist heating pad may be applied to the lower abdomen. A hot water bottle without the wet cloth under it will warm only the skin, but not the internal irritated areas, so it will not help the pain.

(4) Avoid using **Ibuprofens,** or any so-called **"non-steroidal anti-inflammatory drugs"** (referred to as NSAIDS) for this condition. Rather, I suggest the use of **Extra-strength Tylenol.** The NSAIDS are not only more likely to produce nausea in these situations and complicate the picture, but they can also theoretically interfere with the healing and sealing of the ovarian cyst leakage area, and thus increase or prolong the pain.

(5) If the pain is not greatly improved within twelve hours, if nausea is still present, or if there is, **at any time,** fever over 99.6 degrees Fahrenheit, arrange to see a physician quickly.

The challenge to understand what is happening with your ovaries is the most difficult health choice presented to you thus far. In terms of the hassle your ovaries produce in your life (nearly every women has several life- or at least vacation-threatening incidents to talk about), becoming aware of functions and malfunctions of these organs has much more importance to your daily health and happiness than becoming the expert automobile mechanic alluded to in the opening paragraph of this chapter.

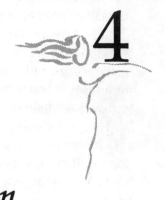

Coping with Premenstrual Tension

> *". . . the mass of men lead lives of quiet desperation"*
> —Thoreau

> *". . . (or) noisy desperation"*
> —Thurber

Perhaps no medical subject, whether discussed in the professional literature or in the everyday media, generates more controversy than the condition popularly called **premenstrual tension syndrome, or PMS** for short. Though it affects millions, in fact ninety percent of all American women at some times and to some degree, less than ten percent of women are ever so severely affected that they alienate their families, do violence to property, children, or spouses, or miss work.

Many symptoms have been inappropriately included under the heading of **PMS,** a term that was first used in 1931. The **most characteristic complaints** are anxiety, irritability, tension, confusion, and marked insomnia to the point of being wide-awake all night. However, **the symptom necessary for making the diagnosis is uncontrollable anger, or what we usually refer to as rage**. Some physicians may not require this type of anger to make the diagnosis of PMS, but for me it is essential. **Mood swings** are often included in the list of PMS symptoms, but should not be.[1]

Premenstrually, many women who do **not** have PMS experience bloating, breast tenderness, fluid retention with temporary weight gain, cravings for sweets or food in general, dizziness, palpitations, fatigue, and headache. These complaints should not be the basis for making the diagnosis of premenstrual tension. Depression or crying spells are definitely not typical PMS complaints.

The psychiatrists consider PMS a psychiatric illness and give it the label of **late luteal phase dysphoric disorder**. (The **luteal phase** of the menstrual cycle is the two weeks after ovulation). By making it a "mental" illness, psychiatry offends some feminists, who see it as yet another put-down of something that is extremely common and uniquely female. When the pain or dysfunction is **uniquely** a women's problem, the individual involved frequently feels helpless, insecure, and ashamed. She often considers herself a "bother" or even "odd" or "weak." A compassionate and affirmative outlook on the problem by those in relationship to a woman regarding any of these "female" ailments will be quite beneficial to her in handling the problem. Of course, this need for understanding includes her physician.

Believing that PMS Definitely Exists

Unbelievably, many people claim this affliction does not even exist except in the imagination of immature, self-centered, or neurotic females. Having lived from infancy with **ten** unselfish, mature, intelligent, other-oriented, and morally strong women, namely, my mother and my sisters, I have had first-hand evidence that the condition is indeed real. Probably a large part of the reason that PMS gets labeled a **neurosis** is that success in treating it has been elusive.

Although one does not have to understand the effects of the **two female sex hormones, namely estrogen and progesterone**, to employ our program for treating PMS, a little basic knowledge of what these hormones normally do to your mind and body can lead you toward valuable insights into your own unique condition. I will defer a discussion of progesterone until the segment "Taking Progesterone for PMS If You Really Need It," at the end of this chapter.

Estrogen, the most important female hormone, is produced by the **follicles of the ovary**—the little nests of cells that can make hormones—located in the outer layer of the ovary. Production occurs from the average age of ten to fifty or sixty. This hormone powers, modifies, preserves, renews, or in some way affects virtually every system in the body, including the brain. **Temporary** and **slight falls** in estrogen production typically occur twice in every menstrual cycle, and these falls can cause crying spells, tiredness, mild depression or the "blues," anxiety, panic attacks, headaches, insomnia, irritability, or any other of the other symptoms described in the very first part of Chapter Three. (In Chapters Five through Eight, the relationship between a woman's weight, or more precisely, her percent body fat, and her moods and symptoms, are discussed in detail. One important fact: **Adipose tissue is a site for storage and conversion of estrogen**. Consequently, **thin** women have **wider** daily variations in estrogen levels because they have fewer fat cells to produce, to convert, or to release estrogen when ovarian production is low, and no place to store it when the level is too high. The bottom line is that very thin and very heavy people suffer the most from hormone-related problems.)

Estrogen's actions on the brain are also evident typically in the premenopausal, menopausal, and the immediate postmenopausal years, when the production of estrogen by the ovaries changes forever. At permanent menopause, ovarian production of estrogen first declines and then totally ceases, producing the classic symptoms that were outlined in Chapter Three. It is **the decline of estrogen** that produces the symptoms. **Once estrogen is gone, the symptoms of the change vanish.** Even a lifelong problem with migraine headaches typically disappears when all estrogen is gone.[2]

(**Note:** If the decline is very gradual, as can happen in thin individuals, there may never be any symptoms of the "change." In marked contrast, during each menstrual cycle, it is the very thin women whose temperament and emotions are most likely to be affected by the **wide changes** in the blood estrogen levels from week-to-week.)

Diagnosing PMS by the Anger

No one in our present society is a stranger to violent outbursts of temper, a condition more often seen in men than women, often for very trivial reasons. Moreover, the fact of women's frustration and sense of powerlessness, which Mary Valentis and Anne Devane claim, in their book *Female Rage,* is a result of "an inauthentic sense of self," produced by an unrelenting requirement to be feminine, can certainly be a source of **free-floating rage** in any woman, at any time, given a triggering set of circumstances.[3] However, despite the fact that uncontrollable or unreasonable anger can have multiple causes, the diagnosis of PMS is not justified without it.

When the clinicians who are researching the treatment of PMS do not limit the patients in their studies to those patients who exhibit extreme anger or rage as one of their symptoms, such clinicians invariably fail to find consistent benefit from any of their interventions. By including symptoms that can have assorted hormonal and nonhormonal etiologies, they assemble in their studies patients with several different and distinct conditions. (As one might expect, using one treatment for several different conditions has not been very successful).

By way of illustrating the essential concept that a specific treatment should be applied to a specific abnormality, when Betty T. came to my office recently for "terrible PMS," she did not mark "yes" to any of the typical PMS symptoms on the patient questionnaire. She never became violent, never hit anyone or threw anything in anger, and never really had the strong **urge** to do so. In addition, she never felt "out of control," never felt like she was "losing her mind," and never evidenced to the family any totally irrational behavior. Because none of these symptoms were present, my diagnosis could not be PMS, and I would never treat her as I would treat someone with PMS.

If you would like to kill **yourself**, it could reflect a serious depression. If it only happens, and happens recurrently, during the days of the period, and not the week before the period, it could be very easily due to **low estrogen that might require estrogen supplementation.** You certainly should not be treated as PMS. (As it turned out as a result of further questioning, Betty T. had **mood swings,** not PMS, and needed to attune herself to the effects of her **markedly varying estrogen levels** throughout each menstrual cycle.)

However, if you would like to kill **someone else,** or feel the uncontrollable anger to which I have been referring—and if this feeling is also very temporary, recurrent, and limited to the premenstrual interval—especially if that someone else is a person or persons who usually mean the most to you (and about whom you, in fact, care very much)—then your condition could well be diagnosed as PMS. Again, **the distinction is important, because treating the wrong disease is akin to treating the wrong patient**.

According to my understanding of the hormonal problems that form the basis for **PMS, the problem is never due to lack of estrogen**, which is **the** essential female sex hormone. Rather, the hormonal imbalance, when indeed there is one, is an **excess of estrogen relative to the amount of progesterone**.[4] If my diagnosis in any given case is incorrect and the condition is not due to **estrogen excess** in the presence of falling progesterone, then treatment with progesterone will very likely make the problem worse. (More on this point under the segment on treatment, later in this chapter.)

Progesterone is produced by those ovarian cells that are left around the ruptured cyst **after** it has just released an "egg." Unlike estrogen, which is produced every day, progesterone is produced only for an interval of two weeks, after ovulation. Thus, **a very important point to remember is that if ovulation does not occur, no progesterone is produced, and there can be no "true" PMS!**

If the egg released at ovulation is not fertilized, that is, if conception does not take place, the rise in progesterone production is soon reversed and then stopped. This relatively sudden loss of progesterone induces a period that tends to be "neat," defined as a good menstrual flow that lasts only a few days. When ovulation does not occur, and therefore no progesterone is produced, menstruation is usually irregular, with periods that are often too light or too heavy, too long or too short, too close together, or too far apart. Ironically, cramps with the period are generally a proof that progesterone was produced in that cycle.

Working on Your Weight Can Affect Your PMS

Since your percent body fat affects hormonal balance, mainly because fat cells store, produce, and release estrogen, the occurrence of PMS is affected by your percent of body fat. The number of fat cells affects hormone-related events. It is a fact that simply being too skinny can prevent **ovulation** from starting its regular monthly occurrence in early adolescence and that excessive weight loss through dieting can cause you to stop getting periods.[5] Being too heavy can also prevent **ovulation**, or stop its regular occurrence once it has begun, even though the periods continue. However, excessive weight only rarely stops the periods, and then only when obesity is prolonged or excessive, or when the woman has been subjected to severe stress.

A prescription for progesterone will be of little or no benefit, and may even do some **slight** harm, such as producing or exaggerating menopause-like symptoms, if estrogen excess is not present. The timing of the progesterone treatment must also be exact. Unless progesterone use is limited precisely to the exact days of estrogen excess, the condition that **is** present is very likely to be made worse by its use. Recall that when progesterone is not produced at all, the predominant clinical manifestations are typically "mood-swings," which can be extreme if you are thin. You might experience days of aggression or **hyperactivity**, described as "jumping out of your skin," or "climbing the walls," or even in some cases, "being euphoric." These effects correspond to days of **high estrogen production.** On the days of low estrogen production, you might find yourself tired, depressed, teary, anxious, confused, perhaps even a little "headachy." These different emotional pictures have elements of PMS to be sure, especially the anxiousness and confusion. The essential difference from PMS is that all these potentially devastating symptoms are not limited to the week before the period and will not be helped by giving progesterone. They are, in fact, often made worse. Most important, rage is not present.

Those **very overweight** individuals who have **no** progesterone, seem never to get as hyper or as depressed as those who are **very thin**—though, admittedly, some have an underlying element of aggression, frustration, or hostility. However, all symptoms seem to surface unpredictably, not just premenstrually. These heavy individuals with no progesterone can sometimes benefit from progesterone replacement therapy, but the absence of progesterone should be established first. (A basal thermometer to show the absence of the two-week temperature elevation after ovulation is recommended to document the lack of progesterone.)

Summarizing: In mild to moderately overweight individuals, those women over thirty-five, and any woman subjected to severe stress on a regular basis, the excess estrogen, relative to progesterone, produces PMS, with anger, aggression, or rage predominating. It is in this situation that brief intervals of progesterone treatment usually works best, especially if combined with other important interventions, to be outlined in the following segments.

Using Other Weapons to Attack PMS

> "I think that the majority of PMS cases would disappear
> if every modern woman retreated from her duties
> for three or four days each month and had her meals
> brought to her by someone else."
> —Christiane Northrup,
> Women's Bodies, Women's Wisdom

It is important to emphasize in the beginning that, despite all that we have said up to this point, the thirteen million American women with severe PMS at some time in their lives cannot expect a cure, or even significant improvement, by simply correcting their weight and taking some hormones. Many have emotional problems not due to hormones at all, but rather caused by unremitting stress, inherited or acquired temperamental deficiencies, a foolish diet, excesses of exercise or lack of any exercise, or a lot of misfortune and bad luck. Even Aristotle (who, incidentally, dismissed women as inferior beings) admitted that good fortune could contribute as much to our happiness as everything else combined.[6] The lack of good luck might mean being born into abject poverty, having a very dysfunctional family, or having other physical disabilities that make life very stressful. Losing a good job, illness in the family, or any number of other "bad breaks" can cause a person to "lose it." Choosing a bad marriage partner can obviously be a factor! Personal motivation, education, insight, or being in an authentic love relationship are all factors that can overcome the effects of PMS to some extent. Rarely, however, do these gifts eliminate the symptoms entirely.

If there was one treatment effective in the treatment of PMS, everyone would surely know it. There simply is no single effective treatment. However, in addition to correcting hormonal status, when that is proven necessary, and improving weight, a wide variety of relatively simple health initiatives, especially when used in combination, can reduce the symptoms significantly.

Starting with Exercise and Rest

A program of physical exercise is absolutely fundamental to the effective control of PMS. Exercise has an immediate effect of raising the level in the brain of **endorphins**, which are the body's **natural opiates**. These natural chemicals elevate the mood. (**Hard work**—probably because it is compulsory and not voluntary—is generally, **but not always,** a counterproductive substitute for planned exercise and does not often relieve the inward feelings of aggression and rage, although it does allow the emotional energy that these feelings generate, a socially acceptable outlet.)

A **thirty minute brisk walk**—preferably sometime between 2:00 p.m. and 7:00 p.m., outdoors (or indoors on the **Power-Walker, Walk-Fit, Nordic Track, Nordic Sport**, or the **Fast-Track,** as recommended in Chapter Seven), followed by a **forty minute lie-down,** flat, with legs slightly elevated—is the ideal and best investment in well-being that any woman can make, but especially one in the throes of a PMS episode. Even a twenty minute walk and a twenty minute rest may be enough. Besides all the other acknowledged benefits of exercise, the walking pumps the salt water, which leaks into the body tissues from the veins, due to hydrostatic pressure that increases when women sit or stand, **back into the veins.** Once returned to the veins, the fluid can be **carried to the kidneys** and eliminated. The **retention of saltwater**, mainly in the lower two-thirds of the body, below the kidneys, which occurs in women as an **estrogen effect**, is normally markedly increased during the week before the menses. **Recumbency,** or lying down, especially on your side, markedly **speeds up salt water** elimination by the kidneys. (In Chapter Two, when the subject of hemorrhoids was being discussed, it was pointed out that any recliner that doesn't allow the kidneys to be at the same or lower level than the lower half of the body will interfere to a degree with fluid transfer to the kidneys.)

Walking in a pool, with the water at least to the waist, is another and very efficient way to eliminate fluids, as any woman who uses a pool regularly will attest. The pressure of the water on the tissues increases as the depth increases. Thus the water functions as a perfectly designed "pressure-gradient" support stocking and enables the walking to act as a pump to force fluid back up to the heart and then to the kidneys.

It must be noted that without a **premenstrual** program of exercise and rest, any PMS treatment is much more difficult, because fluid retention definitely increases symptoms. Naturally, doing away with the salt shaker and salty foods premenstrually will lessen the amount of fluid retained in the first place and diminish the problems that the excessive fluid creates. Such problems include:

(1) **Swelling of the brain**, which does a lot to "mess up" the thinking processes and create irritability and a sense of "unease."

(2) **Swelling of hemorrhoidal and other pelvic veins.**

(3) **Retention of fluid in the body's other most "dependent" tissues,** such as in the feet, ankles, or legs, during the day and evening, and the hands and eyelids during the night. After the hours of sleep, the fluid transferred to the hands or face might still be present there when the women arises. For example, during sleep, gravity stores the excess fluid for a time in the tissues under your eyelids. If one gets up early, "puffiness" is seen. If one so affected stays in bed long enough for the fluid under the eyes to be transported from the area under the eyes to the kidneys, and thus eliminated, the area under the eyes is left dark and sunken. Certainly, the **true beauty rest** is the one that eliminates the extra fluid accumulated during the first half of the day. Thus an **afternoon walk and lie-**

down gets the fluid to the kidneys where it is eliminated, thus avoiding the **excess fluid problem.**

Avoiding with Diligence the Sugar "Binges"

The consumption of **refined** carbohydrates, generally referred to as "sweets" and desserts, can produce the same emotional highs and lows as estrogen does. Thus they can make PMS worse. On the other hand, **complex** carbohydrates (pasta, whole-grain cereals and bread, some fruits, vegetables, and the new food product available as a liquid shake called "**PMS ESCAPE**") directly raise the level of serotonin, a natural mood-elevating brain chemical.[7]

Chocolates remain the **number one home remedy** for PMS. They are, in fact, the **food most preferred by women** under any circumstances, **period!** Chocolates definitely can help PMS since they are usually one-half fat, which contains mood-elevating tryptophane and phenylalanine, and one-half refined sugar, which quickly restores blood sugar levels to normal, thus calming the nerves. If a woman would stop at one piece and add a complex carbohydrate to keep the blood sugar from falling sharply later, I would encourage its use. (See also page 117.)

Thus chocolates are not necessarily bad, and may even be good in some instances. (As will be explained in Chapter Eight, it is a **big mistake** to make any food "forbidden.")

Christiane Northrup, an ob-gyn herself, asks if "taking a long (mindful) bath (might not) feel as good as eating that hot fudge sunday?"[8] (This suggestion is one of the many **relaxation exercises** or techniques discussed in Chapter Seven.)

Letting Your *Stomach Hunger* Be Your Guide

The scourge of overeating is fundamentally the result of using food for comfort. Learning the practice of eating only to satisfy "stomach" or **biologic** hunger is a worthwhile goal for almost anyone, but especially a woman subject to PMS. Biologic hunger, unlike "psychic" or **emotional** hunger, intensifies with time and does not go away until some food is eaten. Taking a glass of water or plunging into a distracting activity does not help at all to relieve the physical feelings of true hunger, as it often does with nervous hunger. Because of their variable hormonal levels day-to-day, and even hour-to-hour, women would do much better **eating more often,** and in **smaller amounts**, especially during the most stressful days. While cutting back on total calories is often a good idea, anyone with an "eating problem" should avoid **both** overeating and fasting.

Adding a Nutritional Supplement That "Works"

Many patients through the years have reported less anxiety, depression, and headaches when they take vitamin B6, especially the week before their period. Vitamin B6 speeds up the production of two of the best known natural brain chemicals, serotonin and dopamine. Magnesium is also necessary in this process, so you should include this element as well as trace minerals like manganese and zinc. There are herbal products with helpful ingredients from dong quai, peony, licorice, peppermint, and ginger sources that could help. **L-Tryptophan**, which was intended to combat the depression that can occur premenstrually, was in vogue for a long time. This very effective central nervous system stimulant was abandoned about ten years ago because of contaminated capsules from one Japanese supplier which produced serious and painful blood and muscle problems. While Tryptophan products are slowly returning, I caution against their use.

Advice: mixing/matching your own vitamin or mineral preparations is not as good as asking a health provider who is knowledgable about herbs, vitamins, and minerals. He/she might solve your problem. As a member of the Scientific Advisory Board of **Nature's Wealth,** a company devoted to finding natural answers to health problems, I have the ongoing opportunity to actively participate in formulating several products exclusively for women, especially "SYNERGY 3000 WOMEN," which adds the most successful plant estrogens to the company's basis nutritional supplement, "SYNERGY VI 2000." This company welcomes questions and suggestions for its products. Some of your questions are also forwarded to me. Call 800-77-NATURE (800-776-2887).

Testing the Benefit of **Tranquilizers** in PMS

Ativan, a mild tranquilizer, can help, as has been shown in double blind cross-over studies of PMS. (Such studies are required before we can assert efficacy of any drug treatment for a particular condition.) This success has been achieved without producing the physical dependence that drugs in this class can produce if they are taken every day, and especially if taken several times a day for more than a few weeks. A prescription is required for this medication and, for your safety, a maximum of twenty-one doses per cycle, or three per day for the week of symptoms, should be prescribed. (No one should drive a motor vehicle after taking any mood- or mind-altering drug.) **I confess that I have rarely prescribed tranquilizers for anything in the last fifteen years, seeing them as just one more way to avoid the self-awareness that is the first step toward justifiable self-respect. Besides, regular exercise, a healthy diet, and proper supplements work better!**

Taking Progesterone for PMS—*If You Need It*

If the diagnosis of true PMS is correct, treatment with a graduated dose of **natural, not artificial, progesterone** works very well.

A few years ago, an investigative medical reporter for *McCall's* magazine wrote, "Natural progesterone works—it's cheap, and it's harmless—why don't all doctors use it?"[9] She was absolutely on target as now more and more physicians are prescribing it, especially for treatment of the menopause. This is evidenced by the millions of prescriptions for it filled by one pharmacy alone, namely the **Women's Pharmacy** in Wisconsin. Natural progesterone is now available in most pharmacies under the trade name *"PROME-TRIUM."* The only caution is that it contains peanut oil, so anyone allergic to that cannot use it. Progesterone skin cream or gel, under the trade name **Pro-Gest**, is also available.[10] **Never use progesterone by any route without medical supervision because too much could make you estrogen deficient.**

Progesterone now available in capsules is extracted from **yams.** It is "micronized," or made into very small molecules that are not destroyed by the stomach acids. **Unprocessed wild yam is of no proven benefit for anything. The several active ingredients must be extracted first and chemically modified.**

Natural progesterone usually produces serenity, but the higher doses sometimes needed can cause drowsiness. That is why the fractionated, or divided, dose should be squeezed into the last six or seven hours of the day. If it seems to produce anxiety or other menopausal symptoms in some patients, the diagnosis of PMS is called into question, as this should not happen if excess estrogen is present. If menopausal symptoms result when progesterone is taken, these suggest that a previously undetected estrogen deficiency exists. (The mechanism is that the patient's borderline low estrogen levels are, in effect, lowered further by the anti-estrogen effect of progesterone, at the brain level, and the deficiency becomes clinically evident. Thus, oral progesterone can also be used in the premenopausal years as a test to detect a hidden estrogen deficiency.)

Synthetic progesterone's chemical name, which may appear on the prescription, is **medroxyprogesterone.** It has several different brand names, the most common of which are **Provera**, **Cycrin**, or **Amen**. Medroxyprogesterone is often seen as identical, or at least equivalent to, natural progesterone, both being included under the term **progestin**. However, natural and artificial progesterone are **NOT** identical. They are not only different, but are, in fact, often totally opposite in their effects.[11]

Artificial progesterone makes ovarian dysfunction worse during the reproductive years, because it prevents progesterone production by the ovary. It is precisely this effect on the ovary, not its potent effect on the uterine lining or the cervical mucus, that makes it, when given by injection every three months, the most effective method of birth control, short of actual removal of the ovaries. In contrast, natural progesterone, taken in one menstrual cycle, increases ovarian production of progesterone in the next cycle and eventually makes the ovary function better.

Synthetic progesterone has had great usefulness in management of menopause and post-menopause, but in these instances also, care must be taken to use it in the new lower doses that are less likely to produce the previously seen undesirable side effects such as weight gain, skin rash, migraines, depression, or "malaise," which means a feeling of not being well.

The last suggestion to all patients, those with PMS or those without it, is to use a simple, one-page diary sheet, divided into 365 blocks to record bleeding, spotting, symptoms, and hormone intake. With this technique, the success or failure of any treatment can be monitored, and both the patient and doctor can be alerted quickly to problems and changes. **The menopause**—the onset of permanent estrogen deficiency—might be detected earlier by a diary.

In the next two chapters, I share my thoughts about the onset of a woman's permanently low estrogen production. The decrease or loss of estrogen affects virtually every cell of a woman's body and can impact her health and her relationships.

In the last decade and especially in the last few years, there has been extensive world research in the area of oxidation and free radical damage. Oxidation, which most simply could be thought of as "internal rusting," occurs in our bodies every day. Many experts now believe that the vast majority of known degenerative disorders, including cancer, arteriosclerosis, Alzheimer's, macular degeneration, osteoarthritis and others, are in large measure a result of oxidative damage. There are nutrients in nature including vitamin E, vitamin C, carotenoids, green tea, red wine, grape seed, coenzyme Q10, isoflavones, selenium and others that function as antioxidants to block free radical damage. Our diet (no matter how well we eat) is clearly deficient in many of these important nutrients. In the last several years there have been multiple studies published in highly respected medical journals indicating that getting the right forms and amounts of the antioxidants can lower stroke incidence by 73%, heart attack rate by 77%, macular degeneration by 43% and cancer mortality by a whopping 50%. If these results are correct, women have new options: estrogen, nutritional supplements (including those with plant estrogens), "designer" estrogens or SERMS (see page 94), and several drugs to treat or prevent osteoporosis.

The question is **obviously "What** should I do for the menopause?"** not **"Should** I do something for the menopause?

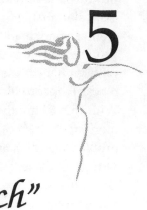

Selecting Your Own Menopausal "Approach"

"Whatever . . . hormone replacement therapy may or may not do, isn't our real need now to forge deep new purposes and bonds and nourish old ones, with man, woman, and child?"
—Betty Friedan, *The Fountain of Age*

Being Part of the Solution, Not Adding to the Problem

Before getting into a detailed discussion of hormones, menopausal signs, and menopausal symptoms, I suggest (as I have already suggested and will continue to suggest throughout this book) that you keep a record of your thoughts, feelings, emotions, pains, or symptoms in a **written journal**. For this particular passage in your life, however, why not especially stress your menopausal **goals**. Christiane Northrup, whose recent book was quoted several times in Chapter Four, has written, "the very process of writing down (your feelings, emotions . . .) and thinking about them sets something magical in motion. That magical **something** is the power of intent—**the power of our thoughts to create.**"[1] In fact, everyone of us, at any age, should **spend some time every day focusing on what we do want** for that day and **how it would feel to have it.** Concentrate in all these exercises on what is positive and good for you—what "works."

Make it a point to express your appreciation for all the happenings in your life that are good. By focusing your attention on them, you make them more powerful positive influences on your subsequent thoughts and feelings. Another good idea: try avoiding TV and the newspapers (with all their "sad" news) for awhile, so that this positive approach to your life can get rolling.

"Why do physicians, especially gynecologists, make a big deal about the change? My mother and my older friends, even my family doctor, says it's no big deal!"

At least one patient will assert an idea along these lines during virtually every one of my sessions at the office. Everyone has an opinion about menopause. Few have the facts! **The biggest obstacle to rational discussion of the menopause is misinformation.** Even the word itself, "menopause," is misleading. The word refers to a single event in a woman's life—the specific date of that period which subsequently proves to be her last. (The average age for the last period in the USA is 51.4 years of age. It is often later in nonsmokers and heavier individuals.) This definition is unfortunate. Because of it, most women thus think of the "change of life" as a mid-life event and often ignore or simply fail to notice the symptoms that occur, sometimes for many years, before this "last" menstrual period. What is even worse, *women without symptoms* never consider asking for tests, especially before their periods have stopped completely—tests that could detect a fall in hormones or the onset of bodily degenerative changes. These latter changes in the body, whether they begin at forty or many years later, are totally undetectable without tests.

The **scientific community itself can also be a source of misinformation**. Frequently, an article on the menopause will appear in a medical publication, including both journals and books, that is misleading or not totally factual. In many cases this occurs because of the author's simple repetition of "well-known" (but erroneous) facts. **Three simple illustrations**:

Misinformation # 1: "In 1900, the average life expectancy was 50 years, and very few women lived much beyond the menopause."

The **average** age part is true, but the second point is not! While the number of postmenopausal women living now is equal to one-half of the postmenopausal women who ever lived, that stills leaves room for a large number of postmenopausal women in previous generations (at least in the 18th and 19th centuries) to experience the problems of prolonged estrogen deprivation. The **average** life expectancy remained low because of the large number of deaths from childhood diseases and obstetrical and gynecological complications.

Perhaps it is no accident that **feminism** in the western world, especially in the United States and Great Britain, **was born in the same generation—the middle decades of the 19th century—that saw the introduction of procedures for more effectively treating women's gynecologic and obstetric problems**. For women who lived before that time, death from a "malfunction" of the ovaries or womb was a constant threat. Childbirth, a simple miscarriage, hemorrhage from the womb due to cancer, benign uterine tumors, blood disorders like hemophilia, or even simple hormonal imbalance, could all prove fatal. The earlier centuries were another matter. Though precise figures do not exist, it is probably accurate to say that **in the 17th century fewer than thirty percent of women reached menopause, and only five percent reached the age of seventy-five.**

Men's historically paternalistic attitude toward women was surely due, at least partly, to women's past vulnerability to early death.

Misinformation # 2: "If a woman reaches the age of 50, she can expect to live until she is 82."

Again, this statistic is misleading! This figure is an average of all women at age fifty, not often a valid prediction for the particular woman who happens to be in my office and who wants to know **her** true life-expectancy. In fact, a nonsmoking fifty-year-old woman, who makes an average attempt to take care of herself, who is not obese or an untreated diabetic or hypertensive, and who is not a substance abuser, can expect **forty-two**, not thirty-two, more birthdays! A fifty-five year-old, under the same conditions, can also expect at least that many.

Why do I give such importance to these distinctions? Precisely because, by stressing a woman's inevitable longevity, I might convince her to prepare for it. Unfortunately, without good health habits, the possibility is increased that many of the last years will be lived with pain or serious disabilities requiring custodial care.

Twenty million elderly Americans, at least two-thirds of them women, are presently unable to take care of themselves. The two chief reasons: (1) **dementia**, defined as the inability to relate to reality, and (2) **arthritis**, which makes walking impossible. While there are two-and-one-half times as many women as men surviving past age eighty-five, these two conditions of arthritis and dementia, plus women's higher incidence of strokes, heart attacks, and most chronic diseases after age sixty-five, put a disproportionate number of **women** in need of custodial care. (Estrogen therapy, among other new interventions, should change all this.) Fortunately for the patient and the costs to society, ninety-five percent of that care is still being provided by unpaid family members or loved ones.

Misinformation # 3: "You cannot have hormones because . . . you have a bad heart . . . a previous heart attack . . . high blood pressure . . . diabetes . . . you smoke . . . you had phlebitis . . . you had a reaction to the "pill" . . . you have gall stones . . . you have cystic disease of the breast. . . ."

Fact one: The number one present indication for hormone replacement therapy is **cardiac** risk.

Those women at greatest cardiac risk include:

(1) those who have a low level of "good" or HDL cholesterol,

(2) those who have **high blood pressure—which must be totally controlled before hormones** are given. (**Nearly one of every four** women in their forties has high blood pressure, that is, a pressure of 140/90 or higher. The percentages rise to seventy percent at age sixty-five. In fact, **twenty million American women have high blood pressure!**),

(3) smokers, even those who smoke "only" three cigarettes a day,

(4) diabetics, and

(5) those who have known coronary artery disease.

Fact two: The presence of gallstones might prohibit **oral** estrogen, but **not transdermal estrogen** (the **skin patch,** skin cream, or gels), which do not increase the amount of cholesterol in the bile.

Fact three: The blood-clot-producing effect of the birth control pill is due to a potent and **artificial estrogen** component, **estinyl**, which is essentially unrelated to the **naturally**-occurring estrogens.

Fact four: **Cystic breasts**, or in fact any condition of the breast that is not cancer, is **not a contraindication** to the use of hormones. This is an explicit statement of the Committee on Therapeutics of the American College of Obstetrics and Gynecology.

Eighty-five percent of the female population have cystic breasts! This is a fact that physicians should stress when they tell a patient that her breasts are cystic. My own experience agrees with the textbooks' claims that, after several years of the pill or balanced uninterrupted menopausal hormones, the cystic breasts typically improve, or the "cystic disease" actually disappears.

Judith Reichman, a gynecologist herself, writes in *I'm Too Young to Get Old: Health Care for Women Over Forty*, "We are never 'too sick' or 'too fat' or 'too old' to benefit from estrogen. . . . (B)e wary of doctors who dismiss you as being too **high risk** for estrogen replacement."[2]

Getting Your Health Information from the Media Can Be Dangerous

The **mass media** should not be forgotten as the **major source of information that is incorrect or misleading**, especially with "information" calculated to scare you about hormones (and prompt you to listen to or read what they provide—the principle being "Good news is no news!"). Television, women's magazines, and the newspapers all make their daily contribution to the **pool of anxiety and confusion**. Susan Faludi, in *Backlash*, shares my lack of confidence in the media's ability to get their facts straight. In fact, she exhaustively documents the media's use of its influence to create trends, or **make** the news, rather than **to report** it.[3]

Several examples of media bias in reporting medical data are familiar to nearly everyone. Besides appearing regularly in print, they are expressed daily in my office:

*Media Myth # 1: "Hormones **Cause** Breast Cancer"*

The Facts: No organization charged with the safety of drugs, including but not limited to the World Health Organization, the Food and Drug Administration, the British Council on Drugs and Therapeutics, or the American College of Obstetrics and Gynecology, **has ever stated** that estrogen therapy causes breast cancer. Betty Friedan, admitting that the doctors in her own family attack her and other nonprofessionals on health for writing negatively about initiatives taken by the health professionals, nevertheless continues to view hormones as the culprit in the rising incidence of breast cancer. She maintains this belief even though **no study has, in the fifty-five years that estrogen has been prescribed, established that fact. Though the overall incidence of breast cancer keeps rising (except for women under fifty-six), the mortality rate from breast cancer has not changed since 1950!**

In fact, when the blame for breast cancer is placed on the hormones used to treat the change, a woman is less likely to face the truth that a significant breast cancer risk (one that is indisputable) arises from excess fat at the waist! **Apple obesity**, which describes the condition in which the waist circumference is more than eighty percent of the circumference at the hip, correlates quite consistently with the increased risk for breast cancer. Therefore, your concern about weight should be directed toward removing the fat at the waist (and not so much the extra pounds at the hips, buttocks, and thighs, which is referred to as **pear obesity**. Of course, if there is so much fat **below** the waist that the ankle, knee, or hip joints are traumatized by it, then you should go to work on those areas as well.[4])

Several of the countries of the world that use little of the birth control pills or hormonal treatment of the menopause, including Ireland and Czechoslovakia, have had a higher incidence of breast cancer than the USA, which has generally ranked fifth among the industrialized nations of the world. The **countries with the highest incidence of breast cancer also have the highest per-capita intake of animal fat**. This is yet another reason, along with the risk for heart disease, strokes, high blood pressure, diabetes, and other cancers, for getting a fat counter and limiting your daily fat intake to thirty percent or less of your daily calories. (Sixty grams of fat is typically about the maximum amount of daily fat that anyone should ingest.) On the other hand, **orientals** who consume a diet high in weak estrogens (referred to in Chapters Three and Four as **phytoestrogens, or plant estrogens,** which are found in soy products in high quantities and also to a varying extent in 300 other vegetables) have a much lower risk of breast cancer. Selenium and other antioxidant substances found naturally in many fruits and vegetables are also postulated to reduce the risk of breast cancer. I do not recommend megadoses of antioxidants, especially randomly selected. Studies have shown contradictory effects on the incidence of cancer in persons taking antioxidant vitamin supplements in a mix-and-match fashion.

Media Myth #2: The "Swedish Study" Showed That Hormones Cause Breast Cancer

The facts: First reported in the United States in 1989 in the **New England Journal of Medicine**, one study from Sweden has been repeatedly quoted as "showing that estrogens cause breast cancer!" The article proved no such thing.[5]

First of all, it was only an eight-year study and it is generally accepted that breast cancer requires eight to ten years to be detectable after its beginning as a mutation or abnormal change in a single cell.

Like the many studies on estrogen's relation to **heart disease** that produced "results" totally opposite to what is now nearly universally accepted (for example, the original studies were so poorly done that they "found" that estrogen **doubled** the risk of a heart attack (sic), though we now know that estrogen can **cut the risk fifty to eighty percent**), the Swedish study also failed to take into sufficient account the reasons that hormones were given in the first place. For example, the same pre-existing hormone **deficiencies** that were overlooked in the poorly-done heart studies could have accounted for the apparent bad results in the breast cancer studies. After all, physicians presumably try to limit all medications to those people who need them and the women who were most likely to have been given the hormones were the ones who lacked them.

Despite these and other serious flaws, **the "Swedish study" explicitly concluded that the most commonly prescribed estrogen in the world did not increase the risk of breast cancer**.

The one wonderful undisputed real finding of the Swedish study that is rarely emphasized in the scientific or lay press, appeared at the same time in the *Journal of Epidemiology*.[6] The same authors, using data from the same patients, compared the number of women who **died** in the two groups of 27,000 each. Indeed, death is an end-point, or bottom line, about which there can be no argument. What they discovered from their statistical research should have been proclaimed from the housetops, especially since it agreed with the findings in twenty other studies previously reported. **Most of the studies show that death is more likely (in the Swedish study twice as likely) in the *untreated* women than in the group of women taking hormones!**[7]

The greatest single risk factor for breast cancer is age! It is three times more likely at age ninety, when estrogen has been essentially absent for decades, than at age sixty, when estrogen has been present for most of the preceding fifty years! Other cancers **decline** in incidence after a certain age.

One thing everyone on both sides of the question must admit: no one yet has the final answer to the hormonal connection, if any, to breast cancer. The nine-to-fourteen year national "Postmenopausal Estrogen-Progesterone Intervention Study"—PEPI, for short— should provide firm answers to that question. This study was started in 1992 under the aegis of the National Institutes of Health (NIH). It is following 163,000 women prospectively (not twenty years after the fact, like the other breast cancer studies we keep hearing about in the media). The cost of the study, which is also measuring the effectiveness of other treatment interventions affecting women, is a staggering $600 million. At least we have been assured that the statisticians and the clinicians who have planned the study have taken every precaution to provide us with meaningful and valid results.

Media Myth #3: *"Hormones Cause Other Cancers"*

The facts: The vague and scary insinuation that hormone replacement somehow reawakens or feeds a myriad other cancers within the body permeates the thinking of millions of women at all levels of intelligence and education. **The fact is, that is simply not true.**

Only cancer of the womb is connected to excess estrogen, but the risk of developing this cancer can actually be **reduced** by the proper regimen of hormone replacement.

Markedly excess estrogen over a long period of time, a situation that is most likely to happen in women who are obese, hypertensive, diabetic, or those given estrogen therapy without progesterone, can increase the risk of developing uterine cancer. Three-quarters of the cases occur in women who have had no pregnancies or one pregnancy. Deficiency of progesterone relative to estrogen over a long period of time is universally accepted as the major factor in the development of uterine cancer. (This same long term deficiency of progesterone relative to the amount of estrogen is proposed by some experts as a major factor in those **breast** cancers not due directly to genetic inheritance, that is, in about eighty-five percent of all the breast cancers.)

No clinician would give estrogen without balancing it with progesterone or synthetic progesterone in the patient with a uterus. Rather than increasing the risk of uterine cancer, such treatment decreases it. Many of us feel the same way about the breast benefit and therefore include natural progesterone in our treatment with estrogen, even for those without a uterus.

Media Myth #4: *"Hormones Make You Gain Weight or Become Hairy or Bald"*

The facts: Only **synthetic** progesterones, for example, **Provera, Amen, Aygestin, Cycrin, Micronor, Nor-Q-D,** or **Norlutate,** can occasionally do those things. This is why they are never my first choice for hormonal replacement therapy. In fact, I seldom use them unless I **want** the patient to gain weight or I want to stop her menopausal bleeding more quickly.

However, **weight gain is the usual result of estrogen** *decline.* **Estrogen, in fact, helps to** *prevent* **male-type obesity or fat around the middle.**

Women gain some weight in mid-life for the same reasons men do—reasons like lack of exercise, more free time, boredom, sexual frustration, anxiety, depression, or simply more time and interest for cooking and eating—with one very important difference. The body's natural "solution" to failing ovaries is to change the way food energy is used and stored, producing weight gain from that change alone. There could even be a direct relationship between estrogen and a fat-reducing hormone, such as the one recently discovered in laboratory rodent studies and postulated to be present in humans.

Whatever the scientific explanation, we do see often, as an apparent adaptive mechanism in women, that the decline in estrogen production by the ovaries somehow sparks a bodily increase of adipose, or fat tissue. The production of estrogen by this tissue then replaces that of the ovaries. Despite its different origin, this new estrogen protects the individual, for a varying number of years, from many of the degenerative changes of the menopause.

Thus, the scenario of weight gain during the change is a result of the failure to prescribe estrogen or a matter of giving too little estrogen and starting it too late. The same ovarian decline and loss of estrogen that causes weight gain is also responsible for the central bodily hair increase and the thinning of scalp hair. The problems with male-type hair distribution occur after the decline in estrogen because the ovary, the adrenal gland, and receptors in certain areas of the skin still manage to manufacture or convert other hormones to those of the male-type.

Another Very Popular "Point of View": "My mother is eighty-two years of age and she still lives alone and does everything for herself, including driving. She sees the family doctor four times a year for heart and blood pressure checks. Why should I worry about your program, especially since I'm too busy to do any of it anyway?"

My answer to this very common and reasonable statement: "Wonderful. You are so blessed. I'm sure you appreciate her good genes, and I hope that you have inherited most of them. However, your mother's life will not be over until she breathes for the last time, and that could be many years away. Please, at least, get a 'DEXA' scan of her hips to make sure a hip fracture isn't imminent." Unfortunately, Medicare still sometimes refuses to pay for this test, even though a simple, once-a-day pill for osteoporosis is now available.

With women over eighty-five being the fastest growing segment of our population, the likelihood of spending time dependent on society and/or family is very real. Interventions that can decrease this possibility should at least be investigated. Moreover, it has been shown over and over that a women is **never** too old to start estrogen.

My mother lived ninety-eight years, but needed ten years of primary care from my sister Peggy and her husband, Paul. However, mom's last two years were spent in a nursing home because she could not walk and was too heavy to be carried. In her final two years she was totally helpless, physically and mentally.

Recognizing That *You* Are the One Who Ultimately Decides

Of all the choices presented to women requiring them to **do something**, none are as important as the active choices they make during the years of permanent estrogen loss. Undoubtedly, what our parents, friends, and associates think and say, or in some cultures never discuss, can profoundly influence our medical decisions. Nowhere is this more true than in a woman's approach to menopause and aging. Daughters often take their cue from their mother's personal experience. One telling but nonmedical example concerns a story that appears in print periodically, describing a daughter who always cut a sizable piece of perfectly good meat off both ends of her hams before she baked them. One day, a neighbor asked why she cut the ends off. The daughter really didn't know, but she decided that the next time she saw her mother she would ask her. Her mother's answer: "My pan was never large enough to hold an entire ham!" Unfortunately, many of the decisions about menopause seem to be like that.

Knowing the Change When You "Get There"

My answer to the question, "Will I recognize the change of life when it's happening?" is this: You may have "been there" many times—in the sense that women have times of **temporary** hormone deficiency before they "get" to the day when their hormone deficiency is **permanent**. Both situations merit attention. The need for a total health program, based primarily on exercise, diet, good health practices, and **the need for periodic hormonal evaluation, is** clearly not limited to the five or ten symptomatic years around age **fifty**. To ignore this truth is to invite a myriad very real physical and emotional problems in every decade.

The second essential truth about the "change of life" addresses the question at the beginning of this chapter, namely, why do some physicians, hopefully most gynecologists, make a big deal of the menopause, even though most women have "no problem going through it?" **We make a big deal about it because the permanent loss of estrogen initiates or accelerates permanent degenerative changes in virtually every system of the body, and these changes have little correlation with how any woman** *feels*—that is to say, regardless of how many symptoms she has. No one "gets through" these changes; they continue permanently until the end of life.

The impact of waning estrogen production is determined by many factors, some understood and a few still somewhat mystifying. Certainly, much is known about the influence on menopausal disruptions of factors such as (1) self-esteem, (2) the type of culture into which one was born, and (3) the presence or absence of a support group or a knowledgeable or interested friend, especially a loving husband. Finally, the pattern of the estrogen decline itself, usually a function of one's weight, is an extremely important variable determining the type of menopause you experience.

Seeing Menopause a Better Way—as a Glass Still Half-Full

Most physicians would strongly agree with my statement that **expectations** of problems in the menopause can **lead to fear**, anxiety, confusion, and even depression, with all the **physiological prob-**

lems such emotions generate. On the other hand, if a woman can interpret the menopause positively (that is, no more periods, PMS, mood swings, cramps, migraines, pregnancies, teenagers, carpools, or chauffeuring), and perhaps keep a journal of all these good changes and all the new possibilities now available to her, as well as all the good things that are happening already in her life, many of the imagined unpleasant scenarios will fade away.

Dr. Richard H. Helfant, in *Women, Take Heart!*, stresses that it has been his experience as a heart specialist dealing with women that somehow everything in a woman's life is modified by the woman's own expectations and her opinion of herself. Many times, her good and not so good evaluations of herself take on a life of their own as a kind of self-fulfilling prophecy.[8] In fact, cardiologists are unanimous in their assertions that heart disease itself, as well as the outcome of their interventions, are intimately connected to the patient's outlook and emotions, with countless studies having been published relating depression to a worse prognosis and a good mental outlook to a good physical outcome. Family physicians can verify from their own practices the statistics showing that spouses die within the same year much more often than medical conditions can explain.

Cardiologist Bernard Lown, in *The Lost Art of Healing*, cites a medical report entitled "Killed by the Imagination," which early in his career made him forever starkly cognizant of the **mindbody connection:**

"A Hindu physician was authorized by prison authorities to conduct an astonishing experiment on a criminal condemned to death by hanging. The doctor persuaded the prisoner to permit himself to be exsanguinated (bled to death), assuring him that death, though gradual, would be painless. The convict, on agreeing, was strapped to a bed and blindfolded. Vessels filled with water were hung at each of the four bedposts and set up to drip into basins on the floor. The skin on his four extremities was scratched , and the water began to drip into the containers, initially fast, then progressively slowing. By degrees the prisoner grew weaker, a condition reinforced by the physician intoning in a lower and lower voice. Finally, the silence was absolute, as the dripping of water ceased. Although the prisoner was a healthy young man, at the completion of the experiment, when the flow of water stopped, he appeared to have fainted. On examination, however, he was found to be dead, despite not having lost a single drop of blood."[9]

Preselecting Your Response to the Menopause

How a woman feels about herself during this chapter in her life depends on many things. Her race (Caucasians suffer the worst distress from menopause), religion, past achievements, job skills or other talents, success as a parent or spouse, presence or absence of pain or physical ailments, inherited temperament, and formal and informal education, all significantly influence, though they do not totally determine, a woman's confidence and ability to stay in control or adjust to the **bodily changes of menopause,** as well as those changes that are best described as mental and perceptual. While a high personal self-rating can be the most positive advantage a woman has in coping with menopausal changes, many of the most "successful" women have confessed to having problems coping with this phase of their life. Still, if her self-confidence and self-respect is solidly based on self-awareness and self-acceptance, all that needs to be added for her successful adjustment or treatment is accurate information and the willingness to act on that information. (**The possession of high self-esteem in the absence of the correct information can be disastrous**. A case in point: the American educational system has made "increasing self-esteem" its primary goal by providing praise and affirmation to the extent that our high school seniors have the highest self-esteem in the industrialized world but they rate the lowest when academic test scores in math and science are compared. Their subsequent post-high school achievements in the subjects tested generally bear out these test results. In one recent year, only 900 doctorate degrees in mathematics were awarded in the United States, with the majority going to foreign students. Only ninety-seven degrees were awarded to American women, for reasons that are discussed in detail in Chapters Nine and Twelve.)[10]

Though divided on countless issues, **feminists unite in declaring that women tend to have lower self-esteem than men.** This tendency to low self-esteem, feminists claim, is surely the result of a male-dominated society's demand that women be "feminine," that is, that they be passive, dependent, nurturing, and cooperative, as part of their "natural role." But also included as part of the message that women hear from infancy is that women are somehow weak, with imperfect or ailment-prone bodies that constantly need adjust-ments or fixing. Just as experiences like PMS can make such some women feel inadequate and "ashamed," so can the onset of meno-pause.

Unquestionably, **successful management of the real changes of mid-life demands that a woman take charge**—that she know what's going on and get the facts to make prudent decisions that will best preserve her ability to obtain or to retain a life that is as independent and productive as she chooses to make it. A lot of living can be packed into an extra forty or fifty years!

In societies where increased age is a cause for respect or esteem, China being one obvious example, menopause is rarely, if ever, traumatic. Other Asian countries are similar. In most of these coun-tries, when in doubt about a woman's age, it is more diplomatic and respectful to choose a modifier in addressing them that is reserved for an older, rather than a younger, person. In many native cultures, menopause represented the beginning of new wisdom for the woman, as her "wise blood" was now being retained. In addition, in most Oriental cultures, at the age of sixty and beyond, a woman's wisdom is "acknowledged."

In our country, where youth is worshiped, menopause is often seen as the end of attractiveness, or even the end of "usefulness." Thus it is that, after years of being treated as a "sex object" and not as an equal person, such women begin to think that way of themselves. When menopause is seen as the beginning of the end of everything important for happiness, complaints and psychiatric illness are much more likely.

If a marriage has the great asset of open and honest communica-tion, menopause can be, from a symptomatic standpoint, only a brief distraction, for the problem will be shared. Rather than being a source of division, confusion, and alienation, the mid-life changes in such a marriage can bring the couple closer. In fact, in the most typical scenario, when a physician is consulted, it is the husband who suggests the consultation, because he senses "something is wrong." On the other hand, when the marriage has never been "good," the problems of mid-life, whether real or perceived, can end the relationship and often do.

Although it is unfortunate, Gail Sheehy's assertion in *Silent Passage* that many **doctors**, sometimes even gynecologists, are apt to say that nothing much can be done, is true. Some may simply order a few hormones to "tide" the patient over her symptoms.[11] As physicians we can get just as tired, weary, discouraged, or unhappy as the rest of humankind. (This is a fact, not an excuse.) However, perhaps this failed responsiveness on the part of many physicians is the reason why **only two percent** of doctor visits after age sixty-five, and **only four percent** of visits from ages sixty-five to seventy-four, involve a **gynecologic exam or pap test**.[12] In the absence of a sensitive and caring physician, a significant difference in one's coping with the symptoms can be provided by a spouse, other friends or family members, or even a menopausal support group

Letting *Weight* Affect Your Menopausal Experience

It may seem paradoxical perhaps that **thin women**, who lose virtually all their estrogen early and completely (because they have few fat cells to make, store, or release estrogen), often have few, if any, menopausal symptoms. This is probably the result of their having been estrogen deficient a variable portion of each menstrual cycle throughout their lives, and the decline in their forties and fifties is simply a protracted and very gradual extension of this deficiency.

Obese women—defined as those more than twenty percent over their ideal weight—can have **menopausal symptoms** like hot flashes, flushes, night sweats, migraines, or temperature intolerance for twenty years and yet not have a deficiency of estrogen that significantly impacts their physical health.

Clearly, consultation with someone who is experienced in the use of estrogen and progesterone for the menopause and after—whether that primary physician be a gynecologist or a family doctor—could be one of your wisest decisions when you begin the second half of your life.

While books have been written about menopausal symptoms, which, after all, is what everyone talks about, it is the degenerative changes, the **signs of menopause**, sometimes noticed but too often missed, that should be feared. Because these changes can be slowed or reversed, they cry out for treatment.

To prudently manage the menopause, tests should be done to accurately assess the hidden changes occurring in the body. The results of these tests should form the basis for the decisions of treatment.[13] If the hidden effects of estrogen deficiency are not taken into account but are ignored, the result may be suboptimal treatment, or no treatment at all. Though the problems thus caused may not be evidenced for decades, they are no less real. For example, the changes from high cholesterol or the daily loss of calcium, and all the other changes, to be detailed now, will eventually take their toll. For older women, with or without symptoms, testing is still the key to treatment.

Understanding the Changes of the "Change":
The **Permanent Decline** in the "B's": **B**rain and **B**ehavior, **B**lood, **B**ones, **B**owels, and **B**ladder

Changes in the Brain and Behavior

The husband who tells his wife, "I don't know what's wrong, but something is; you are not the same person I've lived with for thirty years!"—is noticing brain and behavioral changes. Anxiety, confusion, loss of memory, panic attacks, inability to focus or concentrate, top-of-the-head or over-the-eyes headaches, one-sided headaches preceded by visual changes and accompanied by nausea (which is a typical migraine headache), dizziness, marked fatigue, lassitude, crying spells, or even depression, can be signs of the effects on the brain of declining or absent estrogen. So much has been written denying estrogen's incredible influence on the brain, but studies in just the last three years on blood flow patterns, as well as brain-glucose utilization in laboratory animals, have provided results consistent with many prior studies and show clearly that estrogen significantly improves brain circulation and metabolism.[14] Psychological testing at times of hormone deprivation nearly unanimously supports widely-accepted lay observations that estrogen is very important to brain function.

From a physiological standpoint, falling estrogen levels should be related to depression, at least temporarily, since as estrogen falls, monoamine oxidase (MAO) is increased in the brain. MAO destroys two powerful neurotransmitters having to do with keeping the brain functioning and the mood elevated. However most of the mild depressions at menopause could be situational or stress related.

(Just as at puberty when the changes are much more obvious for girls than for boys, so also do the more abrupt changes at mid-life tend to be noticeable. In fact, **men might get "depressed" too, if their change of life was as dramatic as it is for some women:** if they incurred pain in attempting sexual relations or if they lost sexual feeling entirely; if their face was getting visibly red at the worst possible times; if they were soaked with perspiration even on the coldest days or cold on the warmest days; if their body was exhausted and crying for rest and yet they could not sleep; if they were having headaches so painful that they wished they could cut off the top of their head; if their heart would intermittently and without warning start pounding at over 150 beats a minute; and if they were living with a chronic sense of impending doom!)

However, **psychotic or clinical depression** of a moderate or severe degree must never be blamed solely or primarily on the menopause, unless the woman involved has had similar psychotic depression at a prior time in her life, and now the menopausal symptoms themselves create the overwhelming stress. Time should not be "wasted" trying hormones while the psychiatric problem goes untreated.

As far as the brain itself is concerned, **estrogen has been shown in recent studies to have the same efficacy in preventing strokes and stroke deaths as it has demonstrated in preventing heart attacks and cardiac deaths.** Several recent studies have indicated that **estrogen may also decrease (by as much as forty percent) the incidence and severity of Alzheimer's disease,** a totally disabling condition that affects three million American women now, with the incidence expected to double in the next ten years.

Having said that hormones are very important to the brain, it is essential to stress that **neither intelligence nor memory itself necessarily decline, whatever the chronological age,** until the individual involved, for whatever reasons, chooses to disengage himself or herself from challenging daily pursuits which require planning, organization, and choices, or decides to discontinue all physical exercise. Happiness and mental health is even more dependent upon mental and physical exercise as we get older. From this truth, it follows that as far as the mind is concerned, **maintaining relationships and keeping the old body moving is much more important than hormones.**

Changes in the Blood

Headaches and dizziness are also the result of changes in the blood vessels themselves. Spasm of the tiniest arteries is an effect of falling estrogen levels. One very common evidence of this spasm is the cold hands and feet, experienced not only at the menopause but many times previously, during the periods.

The May 1994 issue of *Circulation* reported a discovery that the smooth muscles in the coronary blood vessels have estrogen receptors, thus providing one way this hormone could be protective against heart attacks! Another mechanism is ascribed to the fact that estrogen loss causes the level of **fibrinogen** in the blood to rise. (Fibrinogen is the substance in the blood which actually forms the blood clot.)

Since 1990, more women than men die of heart attacks and strokes in this country—500,000 per year. Estrogen decreases the risk an average of fifty percent, but the improvement is as high as eighty-four percent if the cholesterols are abnormal before treatment.

Major changes occur in the cholesterols in the blood as estrogen levels start their chronic decline. This can be a first sign of the start of permanent estrogen decline. In all the ways that increase the risk of heart attacks and strokes, the cholesterols get worse when estrogen levels go down. More women die of heart attacks or strokes than from all other causes put together—one every minute in this country. Since the development of blood vessel blockage is believed to take at least twenty-five years, those women who die of heart attacks and strokes before sixty-five years of age, accounting for thirteen percent of women's cardiovascular deaths, would have had to start their disease by forty years of age, at the latest.

In our own laboratory, since 1988, our patients' blood studies have verified that the early **decline of "good" cholesterol** (the HDL) is an **early measurable sign of the onset of "chronic total estrogen** decline," which, of course, defines the "change of life." The "choles-terol **ratio**," obtained by dividing the total cholesterol by the HDL cholesterol, is now widely accepted as the best predictor of the risk for coronary artery disease—the higher the ratio, the greater the risk. Thus, when checked year to year premenopausally, **a rising ratio provides one of our most reliable clues to the onset of permanent menopausal changes.**

A change in the heart-rate regulatory system also is possible from estrogen declines. Palpitations are often triggered, even in the earlier menstrual years, by even very temporary falls in estrogen.

Certainly, in the last few years of the 20th century, more and more women at risk for cardiovascular disease are being given hormone replacement for this primary indication. Besides the per-sonal devastation of heart problems, there is their staggering annual cost of $88 billion in America.

It is essential to note that whether hormones are taken or not taken to prevent heart attacks, it could be life-saving to quit **smok-ing, which is much more devastating in its effects in women than in men, not only relative to lung and breast cancer, but also to cardiovascular disease**. Lung cancer kills more American women overall now than breast cancer, though breast cancer still kills more women between the ages of forty-six and fifty-five. Despite the increased risk for women, more teenage girls than teenage boys are now smoking. Studies have shown that smoking three cigarettes per day doubles a woman's risk of a heart attack and triples her risk for a stroke, though even nonsmoking women are twice as likely than their male counterparts to die of their first heart attack. Studies have also shown that women have been less likely to survive the operative treatment of a blocked artery. (This decreased survival is due, in part, to the delay in diagnosing the blockage in women because of the fallacious belief that coronary artery disease doesn't occur very often in women. Also contributing to women's problems with heart disease is that some of the tests that are diagnostic in men, for example, the EKG, may not be as clear in women.)

(One **caution in regard to quitting smoking**: any insistence that a patient quit smoking may need to be accompanied, not only by medical assistance in the form of a nicotine skin patch, but some-times also by a psychiatric referral, especially in those patients with a history of either severe depression or other addictions. The medical help is provided in the form of nicotine skin **patches** of progressively lower strength. (The patches have been shown in numerous reports to be more effective than the **gum** because they provide more stable blood levels of nicotine. It is postulated that rising and falling levels of nicotine keep stimulating the "addiction center" in the brain, making withdrawal more difficult.) The American Cancer Society will gladly provide a list of all the local programs available to help you stop smoking. Call 1-800-ACS-2345)

Dealing with Changes in the Bones

Osteoporosis, or thinning of the bones, used to be the primary indication for hormone replacement, since estrogen's efficacy in preventing or markedly delaying this disease is well-proven and universally accepted. Twenty million American women are affected by this condition, with one-and-a-half million suffering fractures every year at a cost of ten billion dollars. In fact, fifty-four percent of women will experience an osteoporotic fracture in their lifetime, and one in every three will fracture a hip by age eighty, after which the risk increases. In the USA a woman, usually white and thin, dies of a broken hip every fifteen minutes! During that same fifteen minutes, three additional women, who do not die from their hip fracture, do require custodial care, one-half of them permanently. However, osteoporosis is not exclusively a postmenopausal concern, since up to fifty percent of the bone that a woman loses in her lifetime can be lost **before** the "last period" occurs. (A surprising recent report out of the Mayo Clinic stated that deciding that a woman is significantly osteoporotic based on "well-known risk factors," like smoking, thinness, inactive life-style, or being of fair skin, results in a misdiagnosis about one-half the time. Thus, anyone could be at risk.)

By the average age of thirty-three, a woman has the highest total bone mass she can ever hope to achieve without the new treatments. Unfortunately, nearly one in five women already have abnormal bone density when they reach this age. While **remodeling** of bone continues for the rest of life, total body calcium cannot be increased without treatment, only lost to "the silent thief" of osteoporosis. By age sixty-five, a woman can lose twenty-five to forty percent of her total original maximum bone mass, mainly from the spine, with the most rapid rate of loss occurring during the few years preceding and following the "last" period.

Several recent studies show that hormones benefit the bones of even those women in their eighties, thus contradicting earlier reports that had claimed lack of benefit after age seventy-five.

Every woman should be tested for osteoporosis by the time of menopause if she chooses not to take estrogen, and treated if necessary for this condition. Therapy consists of a daily nasal spray or tablet form of the drug that stimulates bone formation.

Calcium, in the total absence of estrogen or osteoporosis-treating drugs, is of minimal benefit, as is vitamin D, which would normally promote good bones. Too much calcium, in the absence of treatment, increases the risk of kidney stones. Very thin postmenopausal women, who have no natural source of estrogen, since their fat stores are nonexistent, and who decide **not** to take estrogen or drugs to treat osteoporosis, should be especially careful about getting too much calcium.

However, the recommended daily dose of calcium for all ages keeps being revised upward—the minimum is now one gram per day, with one-and-a half-grams advised in adolescence, pregnancy, while breast-feeding, and after age sixty-five (if not taking estrogen).

Sunscreens increase the need for supplemental Vitamin D, since under ordinary circumstances sunlight causes this vitamin to be produced in the skin cells. Aging doubles the amount of vitamin D required. (For persons over seventy, the requirement doubles to 800 units per day.)

Smoking increases the risks of osteoporosis, just as it increases your chances of heart disease and strokes. It also ages the skin.

Most important, whenever any woman starts losing her estrogen and decides she is not going to replace it, she should be encouraged to get tested for osteoporosis, and if significant osteoporosis is seen, she should be offered one of the other treatments.[15]

Noting Some of the Changes in the Bowels

The bowels are like the blood vessels in their response to declines in estrogen. Like the latter, they also tend to become more spastic, and therefore more sensitive, to emotions as well as to diet. Evidence of this connection is manifest in many women throughout their menstrual years by constipation tendencies most of the time, switching to diarrhea during the periods themselves, when the hormone levels are lowest. These effects are due to the direct action of hormones on the muscles of the bowels, and also indirectly, through the nervous system. Most important, three recent studies have shown **that hormones protect against the development of colon cancer,** the third most prevalent cancer in women after breast and lung cancer.[16] In one study involving more than 400,000 women, a forty-five percent reduction was seen. Several other studies reported through the media have claimed a similar reduction in colon and rectal cancer when a baby aspirin has been taken every day.

Expecting Changes in the Bladder and Vagina

With very rare exceptions, permanent estrogen loss leads to annoying, if not disabling, bladder disorders. Thin women precede heavier women by at least ten years in the development of frequency, urgency, incontinence, or recurrent bladder infections. This is due to the earlier onset of estrogen deficiency in thinner individuals. Estrogen, by any route, will almost always improve the situation, though it may take as long as eighteen months, in long standing cases, and the bladder exercises must be performed daily in order to see significant improvement.

Painful intercourse often begins as the first real menopausal problem, because the vagina, like the bladder, depends on estrogen to provide normal moisture, acidity, thickness, elasticity, and self-renewing ability.

Putting the Main Points Together

Granted that there exists considerable confusion, debate, or disagreement regarding what menopause does or does not do to a woman and her relationships, certainly it must be admitted that the decline in estrogen has the very real potential to wreak havoc psychologically, physically, and also sexually, for all subsequent decades of one's life. However, it is important to note that some women, perceiving a loss of allure or attractiveness at this time, abandon their preoccupation with conformity or with the problems of their children and begin to become more aware of themselves and of their "other" talents. As a result of this new emphasis, they re-embark on the journey they abandoned at the "storm of adolescence," and start living a more authentic life. For some, they literally finally "get a life" of their own.[17]

Attempts to do something medically about the menopause are frequently mocked by those who shout, "If it ain't broke, don't fix it." Betty Friedan states that "making menopause a disease that requires constant care, cure, and treatment, may inadvertently hasten our death, (by preventing us) from facing our own changed needs for intimacy and purpose, diet, sleep, and exercise."[18] Such an accusation should inspire the medical profession to make it eminently clear that when a deficiency of something as important as estrogen exists, a woman is taking control when she has the deficiency corrected!

Certainly those who treat the menopause should first determine that permanent estrogen deficiency has begun. Perhaps if estrogen were not so intimately identified in the public mind with being "feminine," there would not be such a strong rejection of its use by those women who view "femininity" as a man-made set of obligations and the use of estrogen as yet another example of men trying to prolong women's usefulness as sex objects. Sadly, I have personally seen the vigor and health of older patients in their seventies and eighties prematurely lost as a result of this politically-motivated therapeutic nihilism.

Once I suggested to the three women working daily with me in the office that it would be worth a million words to photograph a group of fifty of our patients, putting the hormone-using half on one side and the non-hormone-users on the opposite side. My co-workers quickly added their own suggestion, "Mix them together randomly—there won't be any problem deciding who's who," confirming to me that after a few years, they could tell as well as I could whether a woman was taking hormones or not. (Admittedly, all three women take hormones themselves, so there might be a bit of a bias in their remarks. Still, to me, a blatant rejection of hormones, simply "on principle," can prove to be a very serious mistake. That point is the cornerstone of the next chapter.)

6

Doing Something About Estrogen Loss

> *"Hormone replacement at menopause had its beginnings in the 1960s. . . . In the late 1960s and early 1970s, approximately one-third of women over age fifty were using estrogen."*
> —Mansfield and Voda

> *"Estrogen forever, feminine forever!"*
> —Robert Wilson[1], *Feminine Forever*, 1966

(**Review:** "Menopause" is a misleading term, because it erroneously suggests that hormone deficiencies are limited to a few years around fifty. More important, it implies that the hormone deficiency or loss ceases to be a cause for concern after those few "menopausal" years. In effect, this is the same as saying, "**Nothing is** *permanently* **broken that needs to be permanently fixed.**")

Paying Attention to *Temporary* Estrogen Loss

Hormonal deficiencies, as explained in Chapters Three, Four, and Five, are possible at any age. The **new mother** who suffers from severe postpartum depression or even simple "baby blues" is most likely experiencing a temporary menopause, in the sense that her estrogen level is very low. Dramatic improvement is now being obtained in that condition when estrogen is included in the treatment.[2]

The woman who suffers a migraine headache every month just before or with the onset of her period (as my mother did every month until her "change," due to her excessive thinness) is experiencing a very temporary menopause and can be helped dramatically by simply applying an estrogen skin patch a day or two before the expected onset of her period. The same thing can be said of all the very thin girls who experience headache, depression, anxiety, panic attacks, or marked fatigue during the week of the period. An estrogen skin patch can generally eliminate the problem. (The many intervals of estrogen deficiency experienced by women who are very thin is discussed in Chapters Three through Nine. Obviously, I consider the extreme thinness of American models and movie actresses to be an evil very much to be avoided, especially if the resultant estrogen deficiency is not dealt with by the use of the "pill" or some other remedy.)

Frequently, women who are simply thin (I am not referring here to women who are **very** thin), and who take the birth control pill, often experience symptoms like the "blues" and marked tiredness during the week that they take no hormones, because they lack adequate fat. Without the fat to release estrogen, the pill, which stops much of their own ovarian estrogen production, is their main source of estrogen. Again, a skin patch of estrogen during the non-pill week will usually eliminate most of the symptoms!

(In my discussion of PMS in Chapter Four, I explained how the lack of the body fat, which stores, produces, and releases estrogen, can aggravate a woman's tendency for **mood swings**. Thus, while **mania** and **depression** are **not PMS symptoms**, when either of these conditions are due to a psychosis, they can be confused with simple, hormone-induced mood swings. The distinctions are important, since recent reports claim that forty percent of the population, male and female, are subject to real psychotic depression at some time in their lives, and this serious condition cannot be effectively treated without first being diagnosed. The condition is often denied or hidden by the patient and the family, because of **societal ignorance**

of the fact that psychosis is not self-inflicted. Since the stigma attached to depression promotes secrecy and thus prevents proper treatment, physicians who are not psychiatrists are often the ones who must make the diagnosis and refer the patient for the proper care.[3]

In contrast to psychotic depression (or the **true** *Chronic Fatigue Syndrome*), a woman who is "depressed" primarily because of low or absent estrogen is not "disabled" by her **apparent** sadness. In fact, she gets her work done. She is not even genuinely sad, yet she cries without having any specific reason for the tears. Unlike real depression, the affected individual usually has no difficulty falling asleep.

Although a physician can usually distinguish hormonal problems from psychiatric problems in a woman with mood-swings, mania, or depression by a thorough history, there are some cases when the treatment of choice between "psycho-therapeutic" drugs and estrogen and progesterone (or both) becomes a difficult decision.

Refusing to Accept Permanent Estrogen Deficiency

As Gail Sheehy correctly pointed out in *Silent Passage*, those physicians anxious to manage menopausal problems have been rare indeed.[4] Worse, women over sixty years of age have typically been told, "You are too old now for treatment to do any good." You can easily imagine the attitude that women over seventy or eighty face. Widows especially tend to be written off, as far as needing any type of hormonal replacement.

When we tell women to take charge, our actions as physicians must signal caring, interest, and hope.

While things have improved slightly in the 1990s, the vast majority of postmenopausal women are not being treated at all, except perhaps temporarily and symptomatically. Adequate treatment should include:

(1) A total health examination, with a complete history, physical exam, and tests appropriate for each situation, following the "Guidelines of the American Cancer Society for Routine Testing of Asymptomatic Women."

(2) An exercise program, as absolutely basic at every age, and then dietary adjustment to complement the exercise program if the patient is too thin or too heavy.

(3) Hormones, if needed. (The day of hormone replacement therapy has not yet arrived! Surveys report that fifty percent of those women who do seek care after the onset of permanent estrogen loss never take any hormones. Of those who try hormones, only half persist for more than six months. This means that only one in four of those who actually have access to hormones in the menopausal and postmenopausal ages are actually taking hormones regularly. Compare these figures with those from a generation ago, when one menopausal woman in every three was taking estrogen. What happened to change estrogen use? The answer is that the use of estrogen abruptly stopped when it was found that estrogen could produce uterine cancer. Fortunately, hormonal replacement regimens in which sensible doses of estrogen, taken along with progestins, under the careful supervision of a knowledgeable physician, should make **uterine cancer more rare in treated individuals than in those women who take no hormones.)**

What should be the determining factor in the decision to take hormones? In practice, the severity of symptoms is the biggest determining factor in inducing women to start taking hormones, next to the doctor's suggestion. This statistic is true even though the severity of symptoms is typically greatest in those women whose **need** for hormones is the least. (This is so because the thinnest women, who are most likely to be lacking estrogen, especially those who do not adaptively gain weight at the change, lose estrogen through a steady and unremitting decline and thus often feel no differently than they have all their menstrual life, while the heaviest people, who usually have ample estrogen for many extra years, have **symptoms** into their sixties and seventies due to the daily rises and falls of the level of estrogen. Thus the predominance of complaints in women who are heavier results from the fact that most of the classical menopausal symptoms are due to **changes** in estrogen levels, not to absolute **absence** of estrogen.)

There are, of course, symptoms that are due to loss of estrogen, rather than due to changes in the estrogen level day-to-day. Vaginal dryness, bladder irritability, non-migraine type headaches, and most of the emotional distress are all typically due to persistent, low estrogen levels.

The "percentage-of-use" experience in my own practice is only slightly higher than the national average, despite my explicit commitment to hormonal therapy. Only two-thirds of the patients to whom I suggest hormones actually start our hormone replacement program, with one-third of these dropping out within six months. **Need** is the chief determining factor in my practice for proposing hormones, as part of a total health program, whether this need is perceived by the patient, from symptoms, or discovered by my exam or the clinical tests. The main reason patients stop hormones is the problem of unwanted bleeding. "Nuisance" bleeding, which provides a source of worry to both the patient and her doctor, is the one major drawback of using natural progesterone to treat the menopause over a prolonged interval of years.

The only absolute contra-indications at present to the prescribing of hormone replacement therapy are:

(1) active liver disease,
(2) cancer of the breast or uterus, present or past, and unexplained genital bleeding,
(3) active thrombo-embolic disease, and
(4) uncontrolled high blood pressure.

All four of these conditions can be aggravated by estrogens.

Also, **oral** estrogens should never be used if the individual is taking anticoagulants or has gallstones, because oral estrogens counteract the anticoagulants and can disturb the gallstones by increasing the excretion of cholesterol in the bile.

Determining Your Own Need for Hormones

Helen, a very active working woman of fifty years, asked the very typical question, "Do I need hormones?" at her last semiannual checkup. My first response was also typical: "Please tell me what you think, and then, if it applies, what those around you think." She thought she needed hormones, "and so did everyone else." She "was changing," and, in fact, she "was sure she had already changed" in several obvious ways. She was not sleeping well, was irritable and short-tempered, and had started to feel uncomfortable "when anyone got too close to her." Touch, even by her husband, was often painful. Worst of all, she had started to gain weight, after always being slender.

Before Helen could make an educated decision, or I could make my best recommendation on benefit-versus-risk, I needed information from a battery of blood tests, which would include hormone levels, lipid profiles, diabetes screen, liver enzymes, blood calcium levels, and some other general chemistries. She would also need her annual mammogram, which was now due anyway. A pap test, urinalysis, and stool test for occult blood had been done as part of the gyn exam. I also suggested that she read at least three of our "top ten" recommended recent books on the menopause, in addition to Gale Sheehy's *The Silent Passage* and Betty Friedan's *The Fountain of Age*.[5] Both these books focus on the menopause and beyond, but differ sharply in their conclusions. A videotape on the menopause was also provided. In the event Helen was to choose or accept a trial of hormones, the test results would determine the starting dose and the route of administration.

Before Helen agreed to start hormones, she wanted me to assure her personally that hormones would not give her cancer, make her gain weight, cause her to lose her hair, give her more hair in the wrong places, or "cause migraines like they have done to many of my friends." In reply, I went over the thoughts presented in Chapter Five. I stressed that there are no guarantees in medicine, and that some women have side effects that cause them to stop their pills days, weeks, months, or even years later. I cautioned that if the pills were not taken according to directions, they could actually produce menopausal symptoms and/or problem bleeding. In fact, I warned her that bleeding could be a problem, even if she did everything right.

I suggested that she take estrogen continuously but use progesterone intermittently, at least in the beginning of treatment, in order to continue the periods. By "keeping" the periods and correlating symptoms and bleeding with intervals of progesterone use, much very useful information is quickly available to the physician, which can be used as a guide for future treatment. A daily diary is most valuable for this purpose. Helen was also cautioned that failure to keep a diary—on which she would record symptoms, bleeding, or spotting, if any, and hormone dosages—would increase the possibility of bleeding problems in the future. In fact, she should "probably not take a replacement dose of hormones if the diary was going to be a problem."

For those women who do not desire or need total hormone replacement for treatment of their change, I always recommend a tiny dose of **vaginal hormone cream** several times a week in order to maintain the health of the vagina and bladder. I offered that option to Helen also, in the event she chose to forego hormones at this time. This simple intervention of intravaginal estrogen is best started in thin women at age fifty or when their periods stop—whichever comes first—and in heavier women ten years later. Without it, millions of American women wage an uphill battle with incontinence, frequency, urgency, and bladder infections, generally starting ten years after their estrogen significantly declines.

Helen agreed to keep a diary and to start the hormones, so we again reviewed briefly the most common side effects, especially the **breast soreness and fluid retention**. These are common problems in women at any age, but hormone replacement makes them more likely, at least temporarily. They do, however, usually disappear on their own, even without any specific treatment.

Since Helen had a total cholesterol/good cholesterol ratio slightly above 4.5, the "top normal" value for women, we did not recommend the estrogen **skin patch**, which has no proven effect on restoring a "female level" of good or HDL-cholesterol. Because the cholesterols were only slightly off and the patient had no family history of cardiovascular disease, the minimum effective anti-symptom, anti-osteoporosis dose of oral estrogen was recommended—a 0.625 mg dose of **Premarin**. In various doses, this particular estrogen preparation has been used for nearly fifty-four years and counting, and is now the most prescribed medication in the world.

Since Helen still had her uterus, progesterone was also prescribed. Unlike estrogen, which the body needs daily, natural progesterone would be used for only two weeks per cycle, thus mimicking exactly the situation when the ovaries were functioning normally. Eventually, when this regimen failed to produce periods, the progesterone would be changed to the same dosage every day.

Helping Yourself, Feminism, and Your Country, with Hormones

The major feminist issue of the nineties is surely the medical, social, and political answer to the question, "What should a woman choose to do with the second half of her life?" The medical answer is the easiest: **if estrogen is deficient, replace it!**

The social and political decisions required of a woman at midlife I see as vitally important to the future direction of this country. Unfortunately, bringing about any significant change from the past is surely going to require considerable alterations, of doctors and patients alike, toward the **medical management of these extra fifty years.** Obstacles to the participation of health providers in making clear recommendations for maintaining women's health include their ongoing perception that there is a lack of a certain consensus on all the effects of hormones over several decades of use. The legal profession's "use" of purported dangerous side effects from hormones is a significant obstacle, as is the sensational bent in reporting by T.V., radio, newspapers, and magazines. Connecting serious diseases that occur in a patient taking hormones to her use of hormones always seems to have front-page potential.

Not surprisingly, then, the majority of physicians still would prefer not to be involved in the ongoing process of education and explanation, reassurance and encouragement, and reassessment and adaptation that the hormonal treatment of mature women requires. While "problems" apply to some degree to every medical intervention, with "menopause management," the feelings for and against hormones run high, making the stakes astronomical.

Admittedly, physicians' poor past performance in communicating clear information is responsible for a little of the present confusion, neglect, and controversy, but not most of it. As stressed in Chapter Five, most women have made up their minds about hormones from what they have been seeing and hearing for years, especially from the media, and most of it has been "bad."

Doing Something About the Cholesterol Connection

Presently, in addition to the use of estrogen in women to lower cholesterol, billions of dollars are spent on many different cholesterol-lowering drugs. Some of these medications are very new and have possible adverse short or long term effects, so very frequent blood tests are required. Some have been used for a long time, so that their side effects and dangers are well understood. These medications are prescribed because of the general acceptance of the claims that the correlation between the levels in the blood of the various cholesterol types and the risk of coronary artery disease can be nearly quantitated.

The precise correlation of cholesterol and disease is expressed in the two most commonly seen statements:

"For every one milligram **drop** in **total cholesterol,** there is a two percent drop in mortality. . . . For every one milligram **rise** in **good cholesterol,** there is a four percent drop in mortality."

Each doctor's answer to the medical question, **"Why use other drugs in women when estrogen will do it better, safer, easier, and cheaper, at the same time providing incalculable other general health benefits?"** is of incredible importance. Because more women die of heart attacks and strokes than all other causes put together, and they start doing so about twenty-five years after their clinical histories would suggest that their estrogens began to fall, it is imperative that cholesterol levels be monitored and correlated, and, if the cholesterol problem is due to low estrogen and not to heredity alone, that estrogen be considered as the first drug of choice. (Since 1988, I have been able to correct the abnormal cholesterol fractions in ninety-five percent of the cases in which estrogen deficiency was proven to be present, through using estrogen and natural progesterone alone.)[6]

The thirteen percent of cardiovascular deaths that occur in women before age sixty-five can almost always be traced to a family history of fatal early stroke or heart attack—for example, a father who died between thirty and fifty years of age, and/or a mother who died before age sixty-five. The women in these families often have, at age forty or earlier, the **lower HDL-cholesterol levels** that we do not find in normal women until the post-menopausal years.

Besides estrogen's proven ability to reverse deteriorating lipid values, there are at least seven other explanations for its cardio-protective effects.[7]

The truth that we do not know with scientific certainty how estrogen works, or if more specific protectors against heart disease exist but are yet to be found, in no way diminishes, for me at least, the urgency of the cardiac indications for estrogen replacement therapy.

When I find a lipo-protein abnormality, I attempt to point out that while a heart attack kills one American woman every minute (and we are talking about possibilities that may be thirty or more years in the future), a heart attack that does not result in death, but rather disability, occurs three times as often.

Again, my point is that life should be good until the last breath. What is decided between the ages of fifty to seventy can affect a woman's fate thirty years later.

Happily, the fourteen-year **Postmenopausal Estrogen-Progestin Intervention Study** (**PEPI**), initiated by a National Institutes of Health grant under then-director Dr. Bernadine Healy, and now into its fifth year, recently reported confirmation, after three full years of clinical trials, the same beneficial changes in cholesterol profiles that we have found in our patients from 1988 to 1995.[8]

Women whose blood pressure is normal without treatment and whose lipid profile is still in the premenopausal range, probably do not need **oral** estrogens. While the estrogen **skin patch**, now available in four dosage strengths, is the only non-oral total estrogen therapy preparation presently approved in the USA, the technology is available (and being used on a widespread basis elsewhere in the world) to provide estrogen **skin creams** or other skin preparations, on a regular basis, to do most of the things estrogen can do. Using the skin-route can in some cases be preferable medically or even much safer. For example, the patch is a safe route for patients with gall-stones, those with a significant history of blood clots who are taking anticoagulants, or those whose blood pressure control is causing problems. The "patch" has been shown to be effective in controlling hot flashes and other vasomotor symptoms, keeping the vaginal and bladder function "normal," as well as protecting against postmeno-pausal osteoporosis.

Unfortunately, the patch often produces a temporary "red mark," which can be itchy, especially in warm weather.

Inserting a very small amount of estrogen **vaginal** cream to correct or prevent bladder and vaginal problems caused by estrogen loss is very effective for that very limited purpose and has been used for decades. **An easier and better way** to get the tiny dose of estrogen necessary to maintain normal bladder and vaginal tissues, without stimulating the lining of the uterus, producing bleeding, or adding the risk of inducing uterine cancer, is with the new vaginal ring ("Estring"), which is about one-inch in diameter and one-quarter-inch thick. Most users can easily insert it. It is replaced every ninety days. **Note:** The package insert for the cream or the ring frightens many patients or their caregivers, since it lists the same two hundred possible side effects that are listed for the birth control pill. This listing of serious side effects is unfortunate because the small amount of estrogen involved is **extremely safe.** (In over three decades, I have never seen a case of uterine cancer in a woman using vaginal cream, nor have I seen any published reports of any, and biopsies of the womb lining in users of the ring have failed to show any estrogen stimulation.)

Recall that the **adrenal** hormones, produced in response to stress, and the **non-estrogenic hormones** from the postmenopausal **ovaries,** can be converted to estrogen, especially by the adipose areas of the middle and lower abdomen. Since menopausal symptoms are due to hormonal fluctuations, heavier women thus have more menopausal symptoms, and for many more years.

Getting rid of symptoms is much easier if you can share a record of symptoms/bleeding/interventions on a regular basis with the one treating you for them. Since awareness is the essential first step in self-improvement, it will never be more important to have a private journal of daily feelings and emotions, as well as a record of the "thinking out" of your plans, fears, goals, and possibilities.

However compelling the evidence that the benefits of estrogen outweigh the risks, **the majority of women reject hormones** as unproven or, at least, as potentially unsafe. It is imperative, therefore, to stress that **because you reject hormones does not mean there is *nothing* else you can take to delay aging.** The journals of

Allopathic medicine are now filled with studies demonstrating the benefits of much larger doses of vitamins and minerals, and of long known foods and herbs from Native American, Chinese traditional medicine, Indian (or Ayurvedic) medicine, as well as from European (especially German) traditions.

Checking Out **Non-Hormonal** Treatments

Keep a diary for your healthcare provider, and a personal journal as explained on the previous page.

Since exercise is the key to both health and happiness, set up a "no excuses" program. Set aside three hours per week for aerobic exercise (or do assorted daily chores and activities at the same pace as a brisk walk for short intervals that add up to a total of thirty minutes.) Exercise often decreases hot flashes quite well. Be sure to include some yoga or t'ai chi. Check out a few books on the **Relaxation Exercises** described in Chapter Seven. (The references are there, too.)

Cut down on stimulants containing caffeine (which give the liver a lot of extra work to do). Limit depressants like alcohol to red wine, or eliminate alcohol entirely. Drink green herbal tea, which is incredibly good for you. Avoid excessively warm clothes and environments. Clothing should be layered for easier additions and subtractions as needed.

Stop smoking. (Call 1-800-ACS-2345 for assistance.)

Try to adopt a diet low in saturated or animal fats (use a fat counter and stop at fifty). A new butter substitute, "Smart Balance" has no trans fatty acids (which are never good) and plenty of mono-unsaturated fatty acids **which are good for you** if you can handle the calories. Use olive, canola, peanut, and walnut oils, and never use ordinary vegetable oils, palm oil, or coconut oils. Seek out complex carbohydrates and get 30-40 grams of mostly soluble fiber every day. Check out the phytoestrogens in vegetables like cohosh, squaw root, or red sage at the local health food store, especially if hot flashes are a big nuisance, or simply splurge every day on vegetables, especially soy products. (Try soy milk; it is incredibly delicious.) Almonds, oats, cherries, peas, garlic, parsley, onions, and numerous other vegetables have these weak estrogens too, and will help. Better yet, ask your health care provider to find you a reputable "nutriceutical" company that has plant estrogen products for the "change" and beyond. (See page 54 for reference to "my" company.)

Besides getting some form of replacement if you are in an estrogen-deficiency situation, you should supplement your diet with up to 800 mg. of selenium, 200 **mcg.** of chromium, 2-10 units of boron, 200 mg. of zinc, some manganese, 400-800 units of vitamins E and D, up to 25,000 units of the precursor of vitamin A, beta-carotene (which seems to be work best if obtained naturally in yellow or orange fruits and vegetables), 400 **mcg.** of Folic acid, 1500 mg. of calcium, 2000 mg. of linoleic acid, available in one tablespoon of crushed flax seed or four 500 mg. capsules of Evening Primrose Oil, and no more than 200 mg. of vitamin B6. A complete listing of herbs helpful for any of the symptoms of the menopause and post-menopause is available.[9]

Acupuncture has also been shown to help menopausal symptoms, and there is now much evidence to suggest that the benefits are not at all imaginary. In fact, it has been shown that acupuncture generates the production of substances of great benefit to the nervous system.[10]

The male hormone testosterone sometimes helps when a woman has a problem with libido, but I never use it without estrogen and progesterone and only when they do not help **and** the woman is willing to accept some masculinizing effects, like weight gain, slight hair problem increase, and some slight deepening of the voice.

Some new, over-the-counter drugs for the menopause and beyond (the weak natural estrogen **estriol** and DHEA) are definitely experimental. I would never substitute them for the hormones proven effective over fifty years, until such time as their benefit to heart, bone, and other systems were thoroughly documented.[11] DHEA has been repeatedly linked with an increased risk of cancers, including those of the ovary, prostate, and pancreas.

"EVISTA," the first **selective estrogen receptor modulator (or SERM),** is now an **alternative for estrogen in preventing osteoporosis.** It may decrease a woman's risk for heart attacks (unproven). It does not stimulate the lining of the uterus, so there are no periods. Avoid it if you have had phlebitis.

Getting With the Program Immediately After Surgery

Everything that has been stressed in this and previous chapters about prompt diagnosis and treatment of permanent estrogen loss applies with even more urgency when functioning ovaries have been removed suddenly by surgery. Besides the dramatic termination of estrogen production, all the other **anabolic steroids** produced by the ovary are suddenly also lost. This loss can decrease appetite and sex drive, as well as muscle mass, strength, and energy level. Hopefully, your surgeon will be knowledgeable in the comprehensive requirements for managing the changes such surgery has initiated. You should certainly ask your doctor **before the operation** if he or she plans to assume responsibility for managing the surgical menopause.

One very significant bonus of the removal of the womb, besides preventing future cancers, is the resulting freedom from the "nuisance" bleeding or sudden heavy periods that can accompany even the most carefully followed hormone-replacement regimens, even into the eighties or nineties.

Major pelvic surgery has often resulted in temporary problems in sexual relationships. However, after performing over 1000 hysterectomies, I cannot recall one instance of a woman reporting any permanent substantive change in sexual performance. In a few cases where a change was first alleged, further questioning led to an admission that the problem had pre-existed.

Being Reasonable and Unbiased in Your Approach

Many women oppose the "management" of permanent hormonal deficiency on the grounds that hormone therapy is just another instance of male exploitation. They persist in this view despite the fact that several studies in the early nineties showed that, compared to male physicians, **female health care providers were nineteen times more likely** to prescribe hormone replacement. Claiming that male physicians and the drug companies preach the need for treatment in order to make money, without sufficient regard for the long term risks, a considerable number of women see "Hormone Replacement Therapy" (HRT) as a "feminist issue," not a health issue.

Unfortunately, the proven changes from permanent failure of the ovaries, that have been discussed in these last two chapters, clearly demonstrate that management of such changes **is a medical issue**. As stated earlier (page 57), the **medical** question for every woman who cares about her body and her well-being at the time permanent estrogen deficiency begins is **"which of the many options for doing something about the change am I going to choose?" Certainly a decision to do nothing is inexplicable!** If a woman doesn't want HRT, she would be wise to seek a medical provider knowledgable in matters of nutrition and supplements. (Vitamin E probably would have prevented my two heart attacks in 1991, but I had refused to follow the advice from my patients on that antioxidant.)

There are now so many studies published in major journals suggesting or proving the benefits of herbal medicines, antioxidants, vitamins, minerals, probiotics, and fiber, that any professional in health care who doesn't investigate them should have to explain his/her decision to those seeking his/her advice.

At a time when she no longer is overwhelmed with the responsibility of nurturing everyone else in her family (often being frustrated and angry from the response), she can, by finally giving top priority to nurturing herself, begin the full use and development of her own talents.

"Staying fit" is one of the best ways to be good to yourself. What you eat and how often you exercise have a tremendous impact on how you think, feel, cope, and function. So, before exploring the ways to create or heal your relationships, which is the challenge of Section Two, an exhortation is needed for embracing the final, and **most important** requirements for staying healthy: following a regular program of safe exercise (Chapter Seven) and treating food as a friend, not an adversary (Chapter Eight). The potential rewards are incalculable.

It is not at all hyperbole to predict that, as the pieces of the health challenge are seen clearly and accepted by more and more women, those of us who have taken a male-dominated society for granted may well live to see the next century become the "Century of the Woman." "One can resist an invasion of armies," Victor Hugo wrote, "but not an idea whose time has come."

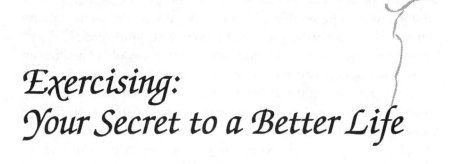

Exercising:
Your Secret to a Better Life

"What really matters is what you do with what you have."
—Shirley Lord

A pediatrician friend, whenever he refers someone to me for care, generally warns them that "Doctor Schaller will give you a hell of a lot of things to do. Listen to his explanations, accept his printed handouts, and in fact take them home and read them carefully before deciding which of his suggestions you can accept."

The **hardest fact for patients to accept is the absolute importance of a planned program of exercise**. Unfortunately, without exercise, nothing works.

Surprisingly, even the monks who founded the contemplative religious orders—those devoted not to social acts of charity but to prayer—wrote into their rules more time for moving the muscles than anything else, including praying. Showing wisdom and insight, they were, in effect, recognizing the very real human tendency for laziness, and that laziness of the body leads almost inevitably to all kinds of sloth, including the spiritual kind. "Temple maintenance" requires stamina!

Common sense and our experience teaches us that we develop positive attitudes, more self-respect, and more energy, in proportion to the priority we give to formal exercise. Unlike hard work, which can be anything from simple wear and tear to a form of slavery, sensible exercise is both restorative and liberating for the total person, especially because we choose freely to do it.

Scott Peck, in *The Road Less Traveled*, states that real loving, even of ourselves, is impossible without work.[1] While he was not talking about exercise specifically in that instance, the quintessential "work" for most of us could be planned exercise, which would constitute an authentic "loving of ourselves." Indeed, no other human activity can provide more physical and mental benefits—**when you "wake up" your body, you "wake up" your mind. The spiritual benefits are extra.**

Not every exercise is recommended for everyone, though virtually any exercise at any age can be helpful, provided it is done willingly and does not produce pain. Calisthenics or weight-lifting, even and especially at age ninety, can markedly improve one's quality of life. (This type of exercise is called **anaerobic,** since the energy used is taken directly from the breakdown of sugar in the muscle or blood. Alternating twenty percent of this type of exercise with eighty percent aerobic exercise, which requires large amounts of oxygen, is the **best** way to replace fat with muscle (which weighs more but burns up more calories). It takes fifty calories a day just to keep one gram of muscle alive. Fat requires much less. But not all exercises are good, or even safe, as a basis for a regular exercise program. This statement applies especially to women, as I will explain.

Fortunes have been made in the business of exercise, by self-interested and well-intentioned persons alike, at the expense of the health of many women, especially their long term health.

Frequently, a patient will announce proudly that she has just bought a stationary bike on which she intends to "get back in shape." I did the same thing twenty-two years ago. Fortunately, for me at least, I soon switched to brisk walking. Any exercise that stresses the knee cartilage should be avoided. Nothing is going to undermine the quality of a woman's life, especially after age sixty, more than "knee-wearing" exercises, like stationary bikes, step-climbers, and rowing machines. They will, admittedly, strengthen the muscles and bones, but eventually they will wear down the cartilage in each knee joint.

Eliminating Jogging from Your Exercise Program

For women, jogging is not at all as beneficial as it has been purported to be. I never recommend jogging for a woman with functioning ovaries. Besides the high possibility of producing eventual damage of one sort or another to the joints of the lower extremities, jogging is never recommended for women for many other reasons as well. (**It is especially important not to use exercises like jogging as an addiction, that is, as a way to run away from the stress or pain in our lives.** No one can run away. To attempt to distract yourself from, to bury, or to deny any negative or painful thoughts, feelings, or emotions—as will be stressed repeatedly in the last two sections of this book—succeeds only in making the problem more difficult to handle later and also makes it a more potent present and hidden motivator of your actions.)

To list a few adverse effects to women as a consequence of jogging:

(1) Running on a day the ovary is actively leaking fluid (for example, the day of ovulation) can result in pain, nausea, and fever that can exactly mimic the signs and symptoms of appendicitis. Any exercise on ovulation day that results in "swinging of the ovaries" has the potential to intensify ovulation pain to the extent that the woman ends up in the emergency room. For two decades it was common, when taking a medical history of a woman at the first gynecological exam, to learn that her appendix had been removed in her teens (with the added comments that the appendix was "removed before it burst and a ruptured ovarian cyst was taken care of at the same time"). In the last thirty years or so, we have been able, because of better antibiotics and many other safeguards, to be much more confident about waiting to allow ovarian events to correct themselves without surgery.

(2) The euphoria from running, or any high-intensity exercise or workout, can be addictive, just like chocolate, and for some of the same reasons. Besides the mood-elevating release of brain chemicals called endorphins, which vigorous exercise causes, there is an initial mobilization of all the body sugar, from the liver and the voluntary muscles, which produces a temporary "high." However, a mental "low" typically follows, due to the fall in blood sugar produced by

the body's insulin response to high sugar levels in the blood. This "letdown" can be disturbing psychologically at times, to say the least, especially if the estrogen level is also falling or is low at the same time. Thus, symptoms like the "blues," tiredness, dizziness, and marked hunger can be exaggerated by the wrong exercise routine, faulty diet, or a problem with hormones.

(3) Women who are "into running" are often markedly below the twenty-two percent body fat that they should have for best health. As repeatedly stressed in Chapters Three through Nine, excessive thinness translates to lower estrogen, which in turn leads to an increased risk of osteoporosis. Thus, joggers are not necessarily strengthening their bones as they believe, but rather in some cases may be actually increasing their risk for osteoporosis later.

Picking the Best Exercises For a Lifetime

Brisk walking is the best exercise. It is more aerobic than jogging, so that two of the usual purposes of an exercise program, namely, cardiovascular fitness and weight control, are achieved more easily. A twelve-minute mile, or walking at a speed of five miles per hour, is the ideal, but a twenty-minute mile is a good initial goal to work toward. More calories are expended, and the exercise is more aerobic, if upper body movement is included.

The **Nordic Track** concept is good because upper body movement is included and little or no impact is involved, but the original machines were too big and bulky for most people, and hard to learn, to move, and to store. They were also expensive. Recently introduced modifications, however, have solved most of these difficulties. They include the **Walk-Fit**, the **Power-Walker**, the **Fast-Track**, or the **Nordic-Sport**. All these models, which provide an upper body workout along with the lower body exercise, can shorten significantly the length of the workout needed to make the session aerobic—or of benefit to the heart and circulation. But, as outlined below, even with this equipment, the minimum length of time to have the body **begin** to mobilize fat stores is generally given as twenty minutes.

People unable to walk must of necessity substitute other activities. Swimming, or walking and otherwise using muscles and joints in a pool, can be a wonderful substitute for walking. Pool activities, however, are not weight bearing, and therefore they are not nearly as protective against osteoporosis, the "thinning of the bones," which for over four decades was the primary indication for hormone replacement in women. (Now, of course, the primary indication for hormone replacement therapy is the prevention of strokes and heart attacks.)

Learning and Observing the Fundamentals of a Planned Program

The world's oldest system of health-related knowledge, namely, the Indian system of **Ayurveda** (the "science of life"), has many principles regarding exercise. For example, no matter what "body type" you are according to their criteria, the time between 6:00 a.m. and 10:00 a.m. is the best time to exercise. One is cautioned "never to exercise after the sun has gone down."

No exercise should be done that produces pain. The original **Callanetics** video was, for a long time, the largest selling exercise video of any kind, and for a very good reason—it was an excellent program for persons with back problems.

We have all seen people whom we knew exercised too strenuously or too long. **Addiction to exercise** is nearly always the cause of exercising excessively, not ignorance. Unfortunately, excessive exercise can eliminate many of the benefits achieved by a regular program for fitness, besides preventing the person involved from bringing their real problems into awareness. Too much exercise can be harmful in the same way that overwork can. Exhaustion, wear and tear of the cartilage or other articulating surfaces, pain, stiffness, and depletion of normal energy reserves, with resultant chemical imbalances, are never desirable. In fact, one cannot admonish enough—"No regular exercise technique should be adopted without some professional consultation (usually your physician), and nothing continued that causes pain!"

Three hours per week is the recommended total time for the aerobic portion of a planned exercise program when simple brisk walking is chosen. The duration of each session should be a **minimum of twenty minutes and a maximum of sixty minutes**. The duration should be selected that will best achieve or maintain our most important health goal—a body fat composition of twenty-two percent. This goal will be discussed at length in the chapter on diet. If we wish to reduce our total body fat, we must exercise longer than twenty minutes, since all the energy in the first twenty minutes comes from the sugar stored in the blood, the muscles, and the liver. To mobilize fat stores maximally, the session should last sixty minutes. Not only does this aid removal of unwanted fat from the right places first (the waist and lower abdomen, for example), but the use of adipose tissue for energy results in a desirable, mild acid-base change in the blood, which takes away the appetite for a few hours. A woman who has **more than thirty percent** total body fat can reduce that percentage by workouts lasting **one hour, three times per week.** On the other hand, **a woman who is less than twenty-two percent body fat**, and therefore does not want to reduce her total body fat, should exercise a **maximum of thirty minutes six times a week**.

The President's Council on Physical Fitness and Sports recommends a forty-five minute/three-mile walk as a goal for a moderate exercise program. This time interval is, of course, perfectly fine for the average woman who doesn't mind losing a little weight. If this length of walking is selected, it should be done four times a week, so as to maintain the same ideal of three hours per week of brisk walking.

For those who cannot set time aside for brisk walking, wonderful news was proclaimed by a 1995 Joint Committee of the Center for Disease Control and the American College of Sports Medicine. Their report stated that it was O.K. to get the required thirty minutes a day "in spurts," eight to ten minutes at a time, as long as what we were doing—walking, calisthenics, going up stairs, gardening, running the vacuum, or other physically demanding housework—was done at a "brisk pace." This should be heartwarming news to the seventy percent of us who "don't have time for a formal exercise program." (Unfortunately, in their 1996 follow-up report, the same Joint Committee acknowledged that for best results, thirty minutes of vigorous activity is necessary every day.)

For optimal cardiovascular benefit, a monitor for the pulse should be worn when working out to ensure that, in some part of the workout, one achieves sixty-five to eighty-five percent of one's maximum heart rate. The maximum rate is calculated by subtracting your age from 220. The training range for a sixty year old would thus be 220-60 x 0.65 to 0.85 = 104 to 136. Keeping the heart in the training range for twenty minutes or longer will produce an aerobic workout that improves heart and circulatory fitness. A study of 18,000 women for nearly two decades showed an eleven-fold difference in cardio-vascular events—strokes and heart attacks—between those who maintained a regular exercise program and those who did not exercise.

Exercise is even more important in women who smoke, since smoking just three cigarettes a day will double a woman's risk for a heart attack.

The most important value of sustained exercise sessions is the maintenance of a normal metabolic rate, a benefit appreciated by those fighting a battle against obesity. By a mechanism poorly understood but easily demonstrated, regular intervals of exercise provide the principle means of achieving the main physical health goal for women—a body composition that contains twenty to thirty percent body fat. In fact, for the seventy-two hours following a sustained aerobic workout, the body is "disinclined" to store calories as fat. Recall also that in each of the previous four chapters, I have stressed the relationship of your percent body fat to your health and emotions.

Adding Another Kind of Exercise for the *Body/Mind*

While there is no question that exercise in moderation can be a very effective antidote for mild anxiety/depressive states, there are bodymind exercises that can produce relaxation without perspiration. The suggestion is made that you devote at least twenty minutes every day to one or another of the various "relaxation exercises." A detailed explanation of these exercises can be found in: *Healthy Mind, Healthy Woman: Using the Mind-Body Connection to Manage Stress and Take Control of Your Life* by Alice D. Domar and Henry Dreher, *The Relaxation Response* by Herbert Benson, and (for excellent illustrations of the yoga neuromuscular and neurorespiratory stretching exercises) *Boundless Energy: The Complete Mind/Body Program for Overcoming Chronic Fatigue* by Deepak Chopra.

Following are eight different approaches to the **relaxation response**, presented in brief outline. (It is suggested that a quiet, private place be selected, where you won't be interrupted by anything or anyone, that you try to set aside at least twenty minutes for the exercise at about the same time every day, and that you select a comfortable position that is not, however, conducive to your falling asleep.)

1) **Breath Focus.** The key to the relaxation response is to shift from the shallow chest breathing most of us use (especially when we are tense or harried) to **abdominal or diaphragmatic breathing**, which is eminently more oxygenating and physiologically normalizing. It may take considerable practice (at least it did for me) to have the lower abdomen **go out with inspiration and in with expiration**, indicating that the diaphragm has moved down to aerate the entire lung (including the lowest half), and then up, to cleanse the lung of carbon dioxide.

The various other mental and physical processes that are suggested to accompany this type of breathing distinguish the **other approaches** to relaxation that are to follow. However, simply doing this type of breathing without adding anything else can be gloriously relaxing. (Even doing diaphragmatic breathing for a few minutes frequently throughout the day, an exercise referred to as a "mini," can keep you calm in the most trying of circumstances, including before and during your visit to a gynecologist.

2) **Body Scan.** After using diaphragmatic breathing to get focused and to begin to relax, proceed to conscious awareness, one at a time, of all the various parts of the body **as you breathe in**, and the **letting go of tension in each part as you breathe out.**

3) **Progressive Muscle Relaxation (PMR).** This exercise is essentially the same as the body scan above, with one addition. Instead of simply noticing the tension in each particular body area or part as you inhale, you actually **increase the degree of muscular tension** in that area before you allow the muscle to relax as you exhale. This is one of the best approaches, if your mind tends to be "too active."

4) **Meditation.** This approach is essentially **breath focus** but adding awareness of a simple word, phrase, or very brief prayer as

you breathe. Some people have minds that are too active to meditate, at least when they begin to employ these techniques. If it doesn't work for you at first, try it later, but in the meantime move on to something else.

5) **Prayer.** The practice of prayer is just like a meditation but with a heartfelt spiritual meaning or belief attached to the word or phrase you select to focus on and the allowing of some gaps in **your** mental verbalizing, to **listen**.

6) **Mindfulness.** This approach carries our minds and especially our senses into the present moment. Everyone should do one thing every day with mindfulness, whether it be taking a stroll, bath or shower, or peeling the potatoes. The key is to bring in awareness of the tastes, smells, sounds, feels, and looks (colors, shapes, contrasts, beauty) of the scene or situation. Joy and fulfillment can only be experienced in the present moment, and mindfulness is a way to more clearly see, experience, and accept the present moment.

7) **Guided Imagery**. This technique is a wonderful way to recapture the rapture you felt as a child when you believed in magic carpets and good fairies, and when animals and dolls and virtually all of nature was friendly and "human." While using focused breathing to start, let your mind imagine scenes, places, or experiences that are pleasant and nonthreatening. You can imagine a walk on the beach or along a beautiful mountain stream, or a breathtaking vista overlooking a lake or beautiful valley. Be sure to focus on the smells, colors, shapes, and sounds present in those scenes. If you want, you can use your own magic carpet to take you to the place of your dreams. (A few years ago, I imagined I was able, along with a companion, to fly to anywhere in the universe I wanted, entirely on my own power. So I did. The experience was so real and exhilarating that I still often think about "my trip.")

8) **Yoga**. Yoga exercises can be very beneficial in many ways, especially as a supplement to the other recommended exercises. However, they do not belong in the category of aerobic exercise or calisthenics. Though there are many different systems and different emphases in yoga, they all involve stretching, moving, and breathing in coordinated ways. Most systems add one or another form of meditation or other relaxation techniques. Yoga exercises are not competitive or strenuous, but they can provide a wonderful way to

relax both mind and body. When you are anxious and confused, yoga can get you out of your head and into your body. Many women have attested to the fact that many of the yoga positions or movements can help PMS, menstrual cramps, or menopausal symptoms. Books or diagrams are usually not adequate to teach you yoga. Some personal training first is strongly recommended.

Letting the *Exercise Message* Sink In

The **Talmud** (the study of which remains central to orthodox Jewish religious life) declares that there are three things a person must do before he/she dies—have a child, plant a tree, and write a book.[2] Perhaps you will forgive me when, in my enthusiasm, I presume to add one last thing to the list—aerobic and anaerobic exercises, and some relaxation exercises, as follows:

1. Three hours **maximum** for the **aerobic** exercise, if you use a treadmill. A maximum of one hour at a time, if you wish to lose fat—spaced at 48- to 72-hour intervals. Otherwise, use a minimum of twenty minutes each time.
2. **Anaerobic** exercise, even very briefly, as often as you can.
3. The easiest **relaxation exercise**—the breath focus—should be done whenever you perceive stress, and the others when you have the time.

In the next chapter, we have to consider a topic that for too many women is a source of unhappiness, shame, stress, anger, or frustration. In keeping with the principles set forth in the introduction to this book, **weight or any other physical attribute is never a measure of the person.** Therefore, the tips for getting closer to your ideal weight goal are presented strictly for the purpose of better health, and a forceful exhortation is included to decriminalize food and to avoid formal "diets" of any kind. The only explicit dietary suggestion, as you will find, is to pick up a **fat counter** at your neighborhood supermarket and keep track for a few weeks of how many fat calories you are getting. I will tell you in the next chapter what you might do with that information (if you wish).

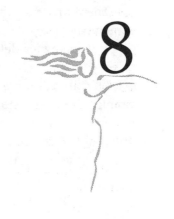

Throwing Away All Your Diets

"At some time in our life, we have to stop being someone's neglected baby. . . . Victims stop being victims the moment they recognize their power to choose."
—Geneen Roth, *When Food is Love*

"H.A.L.T.—Don't get too hungry, angry, lonely, or tired."
—Slogan of Overeaters Anonymous

Diets are not only physiologically counterproductive, which means they do not work, but they are also, and much more importantly, psychologically disabling. By keeping us focused outside ourselves, they make an external guide responsible for our well-being and self-worth. We thereby refuse to accept the truth that while many things in our lives are beyond our control, even our physical shape, our eating habits are not one of them. Because we can control or choose what and how much we eat, why should we foolishly pretend that such decisions are controlled by a diet, so that when the diet does not get us to the weight we desire, we excuse ourselves by insisting it was the diet that "didn't work?"

I promise in this chapter to omit the scientific details, which are virtually impossible to understand, and which keep changing anyway. My intent is to eliminate any notion of guilt, which should **never** be part of your approach to food.

There are only three basic concepts that I would like you to remember:

1) Your genes determine how much fat your body is going to store.

2) You will increase the amount of fat your genes have programmed you to store by "fasting," or by failing to perform a sufficiently stressful exercise every two to three days. You can safely and easily maintain your genetic weight, or even reduce it a little, for as long as you continue periodic exercise, and eat every time you are "stomach" hungry.

3) However, you should not eat more than is necessary to satisfy stomach hunger, when it occurs, since **the fat you eat can become the fat you wear.**

A *Glamour Magazine* survey of 33,000 women showed ninety-eight percent of them believed that weight affected how they felt about themselves, with over one-half saying it was the most important thing in their lives.[1]

In 1951, Miss Sweden was 5 feet, 7 inches tall and weighed 151 pounds! In 1983, Miss Sweden was 5 feet 9 inches tall and 109 pounds. The same dramatic change in dimensions, in fact even more extreme, occurred in the White Rock Mineral Girl, whom the older women would remember. Our Miss Americas of the past generation have been the slimmest in the competition, so that the "fairest" in the land have also been the slimmest.[2]

Conforming to the Culture Can Be Dangerous to Your Health

Unfortunately, what I refer to as **thinness envy** can induce at adolescence a horrible obsession to conform to a cultural ideal that is absurdly unhealthy. Unnatural thinness defines "attractive," and this criteria causes women to do unnatural things to be thin. Mental health therapists confess to never having met a woman who was happy with her body. Not just disliking their bodies, women often loathe their fatty thighs or flabby stomachs. The obese especially are the lepers of our society—rejected with much more thoroughness than are the bullies, the handicapped, or foreigners.

As Peggy Claude-Pierre demonstrates convincingly in *The Secret Language of Eating Disorders,* to say all eating disorders, or most of them, are the result of a cultural imperative to be thin, ignores a vast amount of recent evidence indicating that those with eating disorders are often the best persons among us. Those children who, from very young ages, manifest hypersensitivity to the needs or problems of other persons, animals, the environment, or whatever, often develop serious eating problems later on. In such cases, blaming the victim or her family would be blatantly wrong.

Whatever the basic cause of eating disorders, there seems to be no doubt that by adolescence many have caught the thinness message to the point that it can even control their lives. In the case of compulsive eaters, as described by Claudio Bepko and Jo-Ann Krestan in *Singing at the Top of Our Lungs*,[3] there is a rebellion, for a variety of reasons, against "the indoctrination into the code of goodness" that adolescents must adopt in order to be more feminine. The title refers to their rejection of the "ideal," not by passive silence, but rather "singing," that is, making apparent their rebellion by their daily harmful dietary choices.

There are, of course, other reasons why perhaps as many as **twenty million women in America have eating disorders**. When people lived in small towns, where people knew each other enough to credit and appreciate other talents, appearance was not the only criterion available for rating people. But today it is almost the only one.

In the subconscious mind of the compulsive eater, the longing to be loved is translated into an overwhelming need to be thin, and that is a major, life-altering mistake, since obsessing about food dooms the individual to weight disorders, guilt, shame, and anger. Those who work with eating compulsions teach that painful experiences from earliest childhood on, which were "put away and forgotten," affect the way you "eat" and the way you "love" or otherwise relate to people in the present. Thus, it is claimed, before we can be healed, we need an understanding of our earliest patterns of dealing with love and with food. For example, **do we use food that we can give to ourself, which won't reject us or punish us, and which will always be there for us, as a substitute for love, which always seemed to be withheld because we were not lovable (thin?) enough?** Is our desire to be heavy ("unattractive") an attempt to escape further sexual abuse? Is our compulsion to make ourselves as small as possible due to an exceptional awareness of the needs of others and shame at admitting any needs of our own? In fact, were we "mothering" our parents as we sensed their needs instead of enjoying a normal childhood?

Whatever the causes, those with eating compulsions require outside "guidance." The food-addicted person seeks love, "connectedness," or "intimacy." Quoting Geneen Roth, "I am not speaking of friends or lovers. I am speaking of Intimacy . . . (which requires) surrender, trust, and a willingness to face, rather than run from, the worst of myself."[4] Some people seem to become compulsive eaters because they believe they have something to hide that is worse than being fat. To face the truth might take them back in time to those moments when they learned not to face or speak the truth, but rather to hide it, even from themselves. Now they protect themselves from discovery by rejecting intimacy, especially having "learned" instead that the only way to get what they want is to give it to themselves, and that they are not "worthy" of any gift from someone else.

Unfortunately, people with eating disorders are typically not consciously in touch with their thoughts, feelings, and emotions. They feel "bad" or "down" but usually are not consciously aware of the reason, nor do they even distinguish such things as physical pain, anger, sadness, or loneliness. They simply "take action" to eliminate their marked "unease," by eating or not eating. **Anger is cited by nearly every observer as the most frequent "unconscious" emotion released by overeating.**

While anorexia is primarily a condition seen in adolescents of the middle class, compulsive eating is found in all classes, and at every age. Bulimia is also an equal opportunity disease.

Anorexia nervosa typically presents or is aggravated by stresses surrounding the entrance into adolescence. The anorexic's thinness can, in fact, prevent both the development of secondary sexual characteristics and the onset of periods. Bulimia nervosa, on the other hand, typically seems to manifest itself as a problem later in adolescence and early adulthood. The major stresses are apparently produced by a reluctance to emerge from adolescence into adulthood.

Whatever the causes, eating disorders are self-destructive. The weapons of starvation or prolonged fasting, bingeing, or purging, are not sufficient to win this war against one's own genetic inherit-ance. Besides the psychic trauma produced by starvation, there is physical trauma to many different organ systems, including the body's defenses against various diseases. Perhaps most frustrating of all to the individual's attempts to gain or lose weight is the body's incredible ability to adjust to excesses in diet or in exercise. As a result of this adaptive tendency, replacing either a very low calorie diet or an excessive exercise regimen with a "normal" diet or exercise program usually produces a surge in weight!

Building a Healthier Body by Battling Bulimia

Bulimia is the most common eating disorder in young women, occurring nine to ten times more frequently than in men. It is three times more frequent than anorexia, though the precise number of cases is disputed. For example, the incidence reported for college-age women varies in the literature from three percent, which is probably too low, to twenty percent, which is definitely too high. Binge eating is not a psychiatric disorder unless it is combined with purging or "emptying," that is the misuse of laxatives, diuretics, enemas, medications, induction of vomiting, fasting, or excessive exercise. The corresponding incidence of anorexia is disputed, though the three-to-one ratio for bulimia compared to anorexia is generally accepted.

Nearly one-third of bulimics are previous anorexics, but while anorexics refuse to maintain a minimal normal weight, most buli-mics are in the normal weight range.

Bulimics are typically the ultimate people pleasers: the straight-A student, the special child, the cheerleader, the class president, or, as in the case of Jane Fonda, a person whose figure needed to be "perfect." The late Princess Diana was a bulimic in adolescence as a result of childhood trauma, but her discovery on her honeymoon of Prince Charles' continuing intimacy with Mrs. Camilla Parker-Bowles was the first of many enraging experiences in her marriage. His continuation of that affair, among other humiliations, worsened Diana's bulimia and eventually led to self-mutilations and suicide threats.

Bulimia undoubtedly can serve many unconscious functions, for example, as an "acceptable" way of releasing anger. On a conscious level, it may start simply as a result of fasting as a way to control weight. As with many such attempts to change the weight that is normal for us, the body adapts to the decreased caloric intake so that normal eating then produces weight gain. (See page 116.) The preoccupation with weight leads to a preoccupation with eating, increasing the tendency to binge. Since even the normal amounts of food are too much for our altered needs, purging becomes a necessity. Eventually, control of eating, bingeing, and purging is lost entirely, since bulimia, like all addictions, or self-destructive compulsions, becomes more and more powerful. Eventually, bulimic victims end up sacrificing everything in their lives for the perfect figure.

Actress Tracy Gold of the TV sitcom "Growing Pains," Pat Boone's daughter Cherry Boone O'Neill, Karen Carpenter, and Jane Fonda are but a few of thousands of celebrities who have had the bulimic addiction. Besides other serious physical problems, including sudden death, that can occur, the teeth enamel are often seriously damaged from repeated exposure to the stomach acids from the induced vomiting.

Avoiding the Epidemic of Anorexia

Anorexia, whatever the basic cause in any given individual, is often sustained by the cultural imperative that women must be very thin to be beautiful. Like bulimia, this obsession starts out as a dietary challenge, but one that eventually requires all the unfortunate victim's talents. Anorexics are typically the brightest and most talented young women in their families or groups. They are, however, typically too compliant in their approach to life, too eager to fulfill parental expectations, or, in some instances, to relive their parents' lives.

Extremely difficult to treat, anorexia, once recognized, should be considered a serious physical and psychiatric problem, one that kills directly at least 100-1000 adolescents every year in our country.[5]

The association of eating addictions, mutilations, and suicide attempts is well recognized. The mutilations, which include "delicate" self-cutting, usually with a razor blade, and burning, are common at all levels of society, although they are seldom discussed. These hidden "punishments" are a result of a perceived "unworthiness" by the victims. Girls are four or five times more likely than boys to attempt suicide. Boys, however, are more likely to die in the attempt. (Note: Teenagers are now, more than any other group, intolerant of homosexuals to the extent that gays account for one-third of all the teenage suicide attempts. Parents of children who consider themselves to be homosexual have to be especially kind, understanding, and supportive.)

Admittedly, the tremendous increase in all eating disorders, which continues to the present day, is potent testimony to the cultural forces driving our young people in many unfortunate directions.[6]

Mary Pipher, in *Reviving Ophelia: Saving the Selves of Adolescent Daughters,* writes that a health department survey in her midwestern town showed that forty percent of all the teenage girls in the town had considered suicide the previous year! No similar epidemic was seen in older or younger females, or in adolescent boys.[7] Such seem to be the pains of conformity!

Eating Sensibly for the Right Reason—Your Health!

While these issues are basic to my prescriptions for your happiness and personal fulfillment, **in the specific matter of what is your best weight, the issues of feminism or femininity should not be applied to the calculation**.

If the amount of money spent for dieting could be applied to the national debt, our country would be solvent in one generation, since Americans now spend thirty-three billion dollars per year on diets alone. If "diets" actually worked, there would be, obviously, no diet industry. Despite all this money, the number of adult Americans who are more than twenty percent overweight—by definition, "obese"—has increased from twenty-five percent in 1960 to one in every three adults in 1995. While the lasting value of "weight-loss" diets is widely debated, ranging from the most optimistic reports of twenty-five percent permanent success to the most commonly reported five percent or less, few would argue that sensible eating, as described at the beginning of this chapter, and exercise must go together, and be continuous, if continuous success is to be achieved.

Ironically, for most of human history, people, especially women, who were not at least a little plump were judged to be either too poor to afford adequate nourishment or in poor health. The bodies and faces of the women painted by Peter Paul Rubens (1577-1640) epitomized the ideal of seventeenth century beauty. In fact, in many quarters of western society up to 1920, a suggestion of a double chin was a definite beauty asset. "Thin" was definitely not "in."

By contrast, the past three generations have worshiped and sought thinness to the point that, for many women, their success at achieving their weight goals has been, in fact, destructive to their long- and short-term health. The Duchess of Windsor was quoted as saying, "A woman cannot be too rich or too thin."

Focusing on the Simple Reasons We Watch Our Weight

When ninety-eight percent of women say they are not happy with their weight, even those who are obviously skinny to everyone else, what they are really saying is that they are unhappy with their figures. According to one recent national study, sixty percent of fourth grade girls were dieting. The overwhelming number of women wish to remove at least six pounds from their lower abdomen and thighs. In the preface to their book, *When Women Stop Hating Their Bodies: Freeing Yourself from Food and Weight Obsession,* Jane R. Hirschmann and Carol H. Munter **see hatred of your body as central to your oppression as a woman**, in much the same way as Naomi Wolf stated it, in *The Beauty Myth.* Susie Orbach's book title says it all in that regard—*Fat Is a Feminist Issue.*

Never allow anyone to give you the message that "you are not enough." Give yourself credit for everything you are and do, including your thoughts and your body size. (If you don't, who will? Recall our earlier suggestion that you keep a daily journal to acknowledge your strengths, gifts, talents, and accomplishments, no matter how slight they may appear to you.)

Beware of dieting so that your husband will love you more or someone (your mother?) will be pleased. (If this statement seems somehow strange or unloving, it is probably time for you to reread the segment, **Understanding the Message . . .** beginning on page xvii.)

As they did in their earlier best-seller, *Overcoming Overeating,* Jane Hirschman and Carol H. Munter urge women to accept and love their bodies as authentically their own, and to speak to themselves about their dietary practices with both forgiveness and admiration.[8] I support wholeheartedly their basic suggestions—that you develop the ability to know when you are eating to satisfy "stomach" hunger, and when you are eating to satisfy emotional needs. Equally important is the ability to select in each instance the food or foods that will best provide you with what you really want. The authors also urge that you maintain a constant and authentic dialogue with yourself and with others if at all possible, regarding all your activities relating to food and figure. Self-loathing, self-contempt, or other uncharitable remarks are discouraged, since self-acceptance is necessary if we are ever going to accept others.

Checking Out Your "Ideal Weight"

My weight prescriptions have little or nothing to do with beauty and everything to do with health. The healthiest weight for women, when hundreds of statistical variables on disease and survival are computed, is given as that which provides them with twenty-two percent body fat. Studies have shown that this level of body fat best ensures sustained ovulation. A percent body fat of seventeen percent is said to be necessary before periods can begin in adolescence. For these and many other reasons, having mostly to do with your risk for injury or illness, achieving your ideal weight, or a little more, is seen as a very worthwhile health goal. But **throw away the diets (and your scale, as explained below)!**

I provide each patient who wishes to know her "ideal" weight with her precise weight goal, using a method for the calculation that is over 99.5% accurate and requires just three easily obtained measurements—height, waist, and hip circumference. (See page 246 of the Appendix.)[9] A physician wishing to make his directive even simpler to follow, can provide the patient with only an ideal waist measurement goal. Progress in fitness can then be followed using one variable—the belt size. Concentrating on **the only area that directly correlates to health, namely, the waist,** helps to de-emphasize all the other body-image concerns as well as making it easy to monitor progress. **So keep your tape measure!**

Body mass index tables, calculations obtained by dividing weight by the height squared, or the commonly used life insurance tables with broad ranges for small, medium, and large frames, are usually **quite inaccurate** in providing guidelines for your ideal weight. Since they do not take into account where the weight is distributed, such tables should be discarded. For your present and future health, it is of utmost importance, as we will explain further on pages 117 and 118, to know **where** your body fat is located.[10]

A very low calorie diet, or fasting, is never a good dieting technique. And it never works. Whenever a person decreases the carbohydrate intake, the metabolic rate, or the speed at which calories are used by the body, is decreased. Weight can be lost initially quite rapidly, but generally from most of the wrong places. Most unhappily, the loss is not permanent. If or when normal eating is resumed, the weight **gain** is greater and faster than the initial weight **loss**. You could bet the ranch on that. **For the same reasons, drugs like Fenfluoramine and Dexafenfluoramine ("REDUX") never did provide** *permanent* **weight loss. Both were dangerous and are now off the market.**

Scientists can argue about the existence of a "set point," or caloric management thermostat in the brain, but few people in nutritional management dispute that some center or centers in the brain, or some hormone not yet discovered, not only controls appetite but also regulates caloric absorption, utilization, and storage.

Something is wrong in our emphasis on carbohydrates as the principle components of our diet. One-third more Americans are now obese compared to the last generation. Apparently the so-called "complex carbohydrates" in fresh fruits and vegetables, whole grain breads, pasta and cereals are often converted very quickly to "simple sugars" which stimulate insulin release and therefore fat storage. Thus it may be true to say "the **pasta** you eat is the fat you store."

If properly understood and all the principles followed, the "Zone Diet" of Dr. Barry Sears seems quite reasonable—30% fat and protein, and 40% carbohydrate, and no meals greater than 500 calories (Sears, Barry, 1997, *Mastering the Zone*, Regan Books: New York).

For sure, candy, cakes, pies, and other foods high in sugar, seem to have enormous effects on the brain centers involved with mood and temperament, especially in women. Chocolate itself can be a potent and habit-forming food, since it has mood-elevating central nervous system effects. (**Thus, I am admitting that *what* you choose to eat *can have* some bearing on your problems with weight**.) A diet containing more complex carbohydrates, as opposed to refined sugars and flours, should keep the changes in blood sugar to a minimum—thereby causing less feelings of hunger, euphoria, and depression that result from swings in the blood sugar. They also allow the body to achieve or maintain a more consistent metabolic rate. Apparently it has been found that the fewer the fluctuations in this metabolic rate, the less likely it is that you will store fat.

In addition to avoiding alcohol and "simple" sugars, daily exercise is a must.

The American Heart Association (AHA) and the National Institutes of Health (NIH) recommend that thirty percent or less of our dietary calories come from fat. Most people in America eat much more. Since each gram of fat contains nine calories, compared to seven for alcohol and four for a gram of carbohydrates and protein, a person who gets about 1800-2000 calories a day should get only 540 to 600 calories from fat, which means eating sixty to sixty-four grams of fat. (Don't reduce fat intake too much or your body itself will make more of the "bad" kind, and your body won't be able to assimilate from the bowel the antioxidants in your food and supplements.)

However, one very important caution about making any food forbidden: if a particular food is "not allowed," say, for example, chocolate-covered macadamia nuts (to select Judi Hollis' favorite "downfall"), then eating them is going to produce guilt. Feeling guilty produces the same kind of pain that causes us to eat more than we need in the first place. A plan for sensible eating must include permission to eat anything that will satisfy our stomach hunger effectively. **Nothing outside of us is the problem.** The problem is **our decisions** to eat beyond our physiologic needs in any given instance.

Shifting Your Weight to Help You to Be Healthier and to Feel Better

Only the excess fat around the waist correlates directly with an **increased risk of diabetes, high blood pressure, strokes, heart**

disease, and breast cancer. So, when you start an excellent exercise program with walking as eighty percent of it and weight lifting as twenty percent and you find that after many weeks there has been little change in your weight, you should not be discouraged. Your goal is not to look like a supermodel but to increase fitness, well-being, and life-expectancy by simply getting rid of the "spare tire" around your middle. Muscle weighs more than fat so you must monitor your success with a tape measure or belt size and throw away the scale (Apple vs. Pear Obesity. **Notes 5, 4**). Unfortunately, the amount of fat does determine the production, storage, and distribution of the two essential female hormones, estrogen and progesterone.

Women who are thin are often emotionally labile. Their diaries would probably reveal that they are "shot out of a gun," "climbing the walls," or "euphoric" about one-third of the time, very tired or "weepy" one-third of the time, and "normal" in between. Because estrogen has such a marked effect on energy, this sharp contrast in moods mirrors large estrogen fluctuations, due to the lack of fat tissue to store excess estrogen or release any when the level is too low. As a consequence of repeated low levels of estrogen, during which time she may or may not be depressed, blue, anxious, or confused (typically with periods and just before ovulation), she will lose calcium from her bones and thus become osteoporotic much earlier and much more severely than her heavier counterparts.

Most thin women, however, **do *not* manifest or are, at least, not aware of extremes in mood or activity, being productive, hard working, and too busy to be anxious or depressed.** Many will admit, however, that "some weeks are much better than others." Some women do share the masculine tendency to deny or block out the awareness of such negative personal feelings. Others may consciously choose to spare everyone the vagaries in emotions resulting from being a normal, thin female.

Being *Overweight* Can Be a Hormonal *Drag, Too*

In contrast to the women we have just been describing, heavy women generally have too much total body estrogen most of the time, which often interferes with ovulation, fertility, menstrual cycle control, and progesterone production. The woman who is more than twenty-eight percent body fat is probably producing too much estrogen. Despite this excess, she often experiences "menopausal" symptoms, due to sudden, brief **fluctuations** in estrogen levels.

It is important to remember that increased anxiety, flushes, flashes, sweats, headaches, confusion, or memory disturbances are characteristic of a large temporary **decrease** in the level of circulating estrogen and are **not typically seen with persistent low levels, or even total absence of estrogen**.

The heavy woman is also much more likely to be **progesterone deficient**. Since progesterone tends to produce serenity, the syndrome of premenstrual tension tends to be more common and more severe in **moderately** overweight individuals whose extra fat tissue provides too much estrogen for the amount of progesterone available. The hostility and aggression in this condition seem to be aggravated in our culture, where heavy women tend to have less self-esteem. Progesterone deficiency or absence, caused by **marked** obesity, is commonly associated with infertility, as well as all kinds of menstrual bleeding disturbances.

Using Weight as a Way to Predict How Your *Change* Will Be

The percent body fat impacts significantly not only on the **timing** but also on the **extent** of mid-life changes. Thin women tend to have few, if any, symptoms during mid-life, while heavy women are often overwhelmed. Thin women are "used to" estrogen deficiency, due to their lack of fat cells to store or make the hormone. Also, in thin women, the estrogen level goes down to zero very gradually over many years. When the loss is complete, generally by age fifty-five at the latest, the level stays very low, and the woman is essentially free of "menopausal symptoms."

On the other hand, it is the great abundance of fat cells in the heavy woman that supplies a considerable amount of estrogen for years, though in **very changing and unpredictable amounts.** Unfortunately, it is the changing levels in the blood that produce practically all of the symptoms. Adipose tissue produces estrogenic hormones by conversion of potentially male-type hormones from the adrenal glands (the body's stress glands) and from the post-menopausal ovaries. This is why **the heavy woman may have twenty years** of the flushes, flashes, and other symptoms.

Fortunately, the majority of thin women acquire fat stores at mid-life by gaining weight, usually in the lower abdomen. This added fat, by converting other hormones to estrogen, provides a natural replacement for the ovaries' falling production of estrogen. If these thin women are given sufficient hormone replacement, and given it soon enough, they will not gain as much.

However, in order to further minimize the risk of **excess weight gain** in heavier women concerned about their weight, **natural progesterone should be the hormone of choice** to be tried first, along with estrogen, in the hormonal treatment of menopause. This is so because **synthetic progesterone can cause weight gain as one of its side effects**. On the other hand, if the woman needs to add a few pounds, a synthetic progesterone like **Provera** might be a good idea.

Summarizing What Is Most Important About Food

Virtually anyone can meet the very important challenges issued in these two chapters, namely, eating and exercising in such a way as to begin to approach their ideal weight. Remember, this weight goal bears no relationship to the demands of fashion or slenderness but rather to the demands of health.

Unless medical conditions require that certain foods be avoided, we can eat anything we want. No single food is forbidden. Fat grams should be counted for awhile, as we attempt to learn how to keep our fat grams under sixty per day. Substituting bagels for muffins and skim milk for whole milk (or better yet, soy milk with calcium added) are good ways to start.

What we want most to remember are **the three factors besides heredity that determine how much fat the body is going to store**: 1) a sustained aerobic workout at least every two or three days signals the body not to store fat; 2) the same thing happens when we avoid the "fasting" which increases fat storage when normal eating is resumed; and finally, 3) when we respond immediately to stomach hunger, we must not eat any more than is necessary to stop the feeling of hunger. Like so many skinny people we know, we might find ourselves eating something quite often, but never being hungry when it's "time" to eat. Avoiding "simple sugars" whenever you can is also a very good idea, because it avoids high swings in the blood sugar level, which, in turn, avoids high swings in the insulin level. It is high insulin levels that increase fat deposition. (A fifth reason to gain weight is specific to **the "change"** and seems to be an evolutionary adaptation to falling estrogen levels. The fat tissue that is added at the change of life will make estrogen, replacing the ovarian production.)

What *should* **be your personal weight goal?** The answer to that question begins with the confident assertion that the Freudians had it all wrong when they concluded that little girls had "penis envy" (as we shall see clearly in Part Two). While men have the problem with penis envy, women have a far greater problem, namely, "thinness envy." So much money is spent on being thin and attractive that, were every women to decide today to forego these goals, the economy might collapse within a week.

Lee Hakala, who won the Nike Fitness Innovation Award in 1995, and who has never weighed much under 200 pounds, got it totally right in her book, *Thin Is Just a Four-Letter Word: Living Fit—for All Shapes and Sizes* (Little, Brown & Co.: Boston, 1997). Everyone's primary thought should always be fitness, not figure.

Pledge to yourself that within a year you will be able to walk at least three-and-a-half miles in one hour and do it three times every week of your life. You will never again have to be concerned or ashamed about your fitness, weight, or figure. And be sure to use your speed and the tape measure, never the scale, to chart your improvement.

By taking the guilt and the stupid dictates of fashion out of our approach to food, we are well on our way to greater health and happiness.

In Chapter Nine, the final chapter of this **section on "Staying Healthy,"** four of the most common health questions of adolescence will each be introduced by a very brief individual case history. The fifth and final case presented prompts a commentary on an important social issue concerning the parenting of adolescents—facing the very common question of what to do when your unmarried teenage daughters are sexually active or plan to be.

9

Facing the Health Problems of Adolescence

"How might it have been different for you if, on your first menstrual day, your mother had given you a bouquet of roses and taken you to lunch, and then the two of you had gone to meet your father at the jewelers, where your ears were pierced, and your father bought you your first pair of earrings. . . ."
—Judith Duerk, in *Circle of Stones*

It is the profound emotional and psychological changes of adolescence, rather than the physical changes, that can most determine the course of a woman's life. An understanding of these former changes can provide the key to an understanding of the woman, and of her struggle for happiness.

Mary Pipher's study of adolescence, *Reviving Ophelia: Saving the Selves of Adolescent Daughters*, was written out of the author's sudden realization, missed during her twenty previous years as a clinical psychologist for teenage girls, that American culture of the 1990s had become "girl poisoning" to an extent undreamed of a generation before. Adolescent girls were now like "saplings in a storm." The gains of feminism were seen as having done nothing to slow the increasingly traumatic and disruptive demands of a more dangerous, more sexual, and more media-directed culture. (The lyrics of the

music which reaches more adolescents than any other type of "information" sends one powerful message to the boys, namely, **dominance (or sadism),** and one powerful message to the girls, namely,
submission.)[1]

The great power of the media to control adolescent behavior is all
the more reason why teenage girls should be acknowledged as they
are, and honored, cherished, and praised for their every good intention and honest effort. They should also be encouraged to speak their
minds, taken seriously, and encouraged to follow their dreams. *Above
all, never stop telling them what you think is right and what you expect of
them, even if you are sure they are going to ignore your advice.*

(The relational aspects of adolescence will be discussed at
greater length in Chapter Twelve.)

Choosing the Time for the First Gynecological Exam

Betty T., trying to be a responsible mother, inquired, "When
should I bring my daughters in for a pelvic exam?" I had delivered
her last three children, all boys. Her three oldest children were girls,
ages eighteen, seventeen, and thirteen. My response was that each
daughter would ultimately decide whether she would accept a gyn
exam, but that now was the time to begin the education process for
good health practices, especially those involving exercise and diet.
Adequate calcium was a must—a gram-and-a-half every day.
Weight extremes should be avoided, and adequate fiber needed to be
an important part of their eating program.

A general, non-gynecologic, physical "check-up"—including an
evaluation of sight and hearing, routine blood tests and urine analysis, and a skin test for Tuberculosis—was imperative. They should be
checked for immunity to Rubella, or German measles, and the vac-
cine given as necessary, because once a pregnancy has occurred, no
immunization can be given to those found susceptible to that disease
until the pregnancy is completed. Acquiring a rubella infection in
pregnancy can result in fetal damage. All other immunizations
should be brought up-to-date, including regular measles, mumps,
diptheria, polio, and tetanus.

A one-page diary was provided, on which all bleeding, pains, headaches, and other specified symptoms possibly related to hormones were to be noted. Any such information from the past, which could be remembered, was also requested.

A daily charting, on a graph, of "basal body temperatures" for a few months—to be taken by mouth each morning, upon arising, using an easily read digital thermometer—was suggested as the single most effective way to check for normal hormonal production by the ovaries. If this temperature chart (called a BBT) was "biphasic"—that is, showing at least a one-half degree rise, when the average temperature the two weeks before the period was compared with the average of the other days—it would be a proof that the ovaries were fully functioning.

A gynecologic exam would be advised, if any problem was revealed from the foregoing surveys. Problems might be:

(1) Any bleeding or pain that interfered with school attendance;

(2) Any menstrual pain that lasted more than a day or two, especially if it was getting progressively stronger or longer;

(3) Any itch, rash, or unusual discharge (the white/yellow discharge, after taking antibiotics, can usually be self-treated, by over-the-counter, anti-yeast preparations).

(4) Any abnormal bleeding patterns. (See Chapter Three.)

Perhaps as a result of this "education and discovery" process, the two oldest girls, Alexandra and Amelia, seemed to become more open and comfortable about disclosing their personal health "events" and not only made a decision to get a gyn exam, but they also decided, apparently jointly, to choose courses in college that would be valuable should they later select a career in the health sciences.

Knowing the Changes Leading to the First Period

The age at which the first period occurs or fails to occur is a frequent source of concern to both mothers and daughters in our society. Both are usually reassured when they understand the basic sequence of pubertal changes. (Unfortunately, these changes become "obvious" about two years earlier than they used to. At about age 12.5 years, just when most girls are thrust into the tremendous social changes of junior high school, the physical changes that make them feel conspicuous make their debut. More about that in Chapter Twelve.)

When Catherine R. brought her fifteen-year-old daughter Cathy to my office, both shared one concern: "Was something wrong that Cathy had not yet menstruated?" My answer was that the first period "normally" occurs between the ages of 9.1 and 17.2 years, as the end result of an adolescent growth process, summarized as follows:

The **breast bud** signals the start of puberty. This small lump under the nipple in one or both breast areas is first seen at age ten or eleven. It appears under an unchanged nipple and often frightens the girl or her mother, who suspect it could be a cancer. The breast bud could occur as early as eight or as late as fourteen years of age. Once it appears, puberty should be completed within three years.

The **adolescent growth spurt** in height and weight typically, though not always, precedes the first period. When darkened, coarse, **curled pubic hair** appears, the periods should begin within months, if they have not been occurring before. Especially is this true if the pubic hair is not confined to the central area, the mons, but spreads to the medial aspect of the thighs. "Late-bloomers," defined as those who start their bodily changes later than average, usually inherit the trait from their mothers. When studies are done because periods are absent, or pubertal changes have not started by the appropriate ages, ninety percent of the time no cause is found. In the remaining ten percent, the cause is usually excessive thinness, or, very rarely, marked obesity.

Mesomorphs, or those individuals who are heavier, seem to start and finish puberty earlier than **ectomorphs**, the thinner types.

Since estrogen has the greatest tendency of all hormones to close the growing ends of the long bones, the thinner girls who have their pubertal changes later, and therefore start estrogen production later, tend also to be much taller.

"Early and Late Bloomers"

The effect in boys of an early or late onset of puberty contrasts sharply with the effect of either in girls. Early-bloomers among girls tend to have more problems psychologically and emotionally from pubescent changes than do the early-blooming boys, who often become the sports heroes or the president of the class. The opposite effects are seen if puberty is late. The girls generally do well and the boys tend to feel inferior, and are frequently stigmatized by their peers. But, as luck would have it, and since "never" and "always" are terms foreign to medicine, an exception to these "rules" occurred a few days before this writing. A thirteen-and-a-half-year-old girl was brought for an evaluation, to see if she "was normal." In the private school she was attending, she was the only one in her class who had not yet menstruated. That fact, plus her attractiveness, had resulted in her being **scapegoated**—shunned and mocked by her peers—to the extent that she had attempted suicide. She had only been released from the psychiatric hospital the day before. Her psychiatrist suggested to the parents that she see a gynecologist.

No pelvic exam was done because everything that could be seen by a simple glance confirmed that the periods would probably begin within six months. (Of course, a rectal-abdominal exam to make sure a uterus was present would have been preferable, but the "patient" wanted none of that.) The periods of her mother had begun just after her fourteenth birthday, so the physical changes already evidenced highly suggested that she would begin her periods at precisely the same age as her mother—which happens typically.

Catherine R., the mother of Cathy, our fifteen-year-old patient, and the one who asked the original question, had **her** first period at age sixteen-and-a-half. Thus, her daughter should be late, too. Besides simple reassurance, I suggested that her daughter get the same general checkup and tests, and initiate the same good health and exercise program as suggested for Betty's daughter in the previous case history. Cathy's general physical exam suggested that pubertal changes were occurring and that the first period could be expected about the same time as her mother's had occurred, or perhaps sooner. (It arrived, in fact, the night before her "sweet sixteen" birthday party).

Correcting Heavy or Irregular Bleeding

Anna R., the mother, was obviously upset. Her daughter Carmella, age thirteen, was more than upset. She was terrified. The problem was both the amount of bleeding and its sudden and unpredictable appearance. Carmella refused to go to school, having had bleeding that "everyone had noticed" on at least three occasions. Reassuring Anna and Carmella that erratic and/or excessive bleeding was common the first two years of periods, I hastened to add that I would have blood drawn right away and a few of the tests done immediately so that treatment to correct the problem could begin as soon as possible. Once a bleeding disorder and significant anemia was ruled out, coupled with normal findings on the history and regular physical exam (no vaginal exam), I prescribed treatment. (Even anemia from earlier periods could increase present bleeding—however illogical that might seem.)

Since neat, regular (though often crampy) periods require the presence of progesterone, which is produced only after ovulation, the use of **natural progesterone** was advised. Not only is it safer than a synthetic hormone, used so often in the past for this problem, but it often corrects the basic problem and helps trigger the initiation of regular ovulation.

The immediate blood tests were normal. Carmella had neither anemia nor a bleeding disorder, and the progesterone I prescribed for her brought on regular twenty-eight day cycles within three months. The regimen was continued for only six months, and the "problem" has not returned. Carmella is now in college and doing well.

Because progesterone, in the doses necessary to regulate periods, can produce drowsiness, the entire dose should be taken later in the day—part of it before dinner, and the larger part at bedtime. The same progesterone was prescribed for her mother, whose periods had also become very irregular. Anna's endometrial biopsy—tissue sampling of the lining cells of the womb (required because she was over forty years of age)—showed that Anna was missing progesterone also. Since Anna's "terrible periods" were due to the absence of progesterone, the hormone capsules produced normal bleeding patterns for her also.

Realizing When Being Thin Can Be Unhealthy

She called herself "Crazy Carol." At five feet-eight inches tall and weighing one-hundred-nineteen pounds, no one, not even Carol herself, would say she was overweight. When I first saw Carol, she confessed that she had just "dismissed her fifth and last psychiatrist, and thrown away all that damn drug stuff." **Elavil**, an antidepressant medication, had been the latest solution prescribed, although the psychiatrist herself had told Carol that psychiatric drugs were probably not what she needed most, adding the suggestion that "her hormones probably had something to do with her violent swings of mood."

(Chapters Four through Eight contained information that explained why mood-swings of marked degree are common in very thin women, but a brief review will help you understand Carol's "problem." Please note that, in every such case, hyperthyroidism should be ruled out. (A **sensitive TSH** is probably the best blood test available now to pick up thyroid problems, though not the only one.) But these changes in mood in thin women are rarely of such severity that psychiatric help for them is needed, and certainly not as the first resort. However, in some cases, the cause of the disruptive mood swings is, in fact, a major psychiatric illness called Manic-Depression. This has genetic and/or environmental origins, and has little to do with hormones. Sometimes, however, estrogen deficiency itself can be induced by a prolonged bout of depression. Moreover, the clinical, psychotic depression itself can result in a loss of appetite and marked weight loss, so that a vicious cycle is set up involving loss of appetite, depression, weight loss, and then hormonal deficiency from lack of sufficient body fat. The resultant lack of estrogen may prevent antidepressant drugs from lifting the depression enough to get the patient back to normal.)

Fortunately, most of the women who experience swings of mood have no mental illness, even if those swings in mood seem excessive. Thus, for these "normal" women, it is most essential in their management that they be convinced that they are not "crazy," and that the problem can be helped. At the very least, they need to be assured that the condition presented is not unusual, and is one that can be explained medically.

The discussion with Carol began by referring to the relationships between low body fat, hormones, and temperament. I stressed the fact that very thin women, **if** they have any serious complaints at all, tend to report alternating moods of at least three distinct types, occurring at approximately weekly intervals, with a transitional one-three days between each mood change. There are three **basic moods** in the mood-swing syndrome. The first is the time of intense mental, emotional, and physical energy, when little sleep is necessary or perhaps possible (women in this phase incur various labels—crazy, hyper, antsy, compulsive, climbing the walls, and jumping out of their skin—among others). The second is the interval of being exhausted, irritable, and anxious or even panicky, sad to the point of being mildly depressed, with an inability to sleep and sometimes a loss of appetite, (but worst of all) a lot of self-hatred that sometimes eventuates in doing "things" to bring pain or harm to herself. (Women in this phase are variously described as crazy, out of it, on the verge, blue, down, apathetic, selfish, helpless, or confused.) Fortunately, there is a third type of mood: the time of feeling nearly perfect, with joy and serenity, when all their bad feelings melt away, every problem seems solvable, and when anything is possible. (This is the phase that gives the husband hope, keeps him sane, and in some instances prevents him from giving up on his mate!)

At the time I was describing these possibilities to Carol I had no idea how right on target they were, though in Carol's case the reality was worse than the theory.

The facts were that Carol had been self-destructive often. Her two suicide attempts were more typical of psychotic depression, but several psychiatrists had concluded that in her case they were "grandiose" attempts to get "a little attention" and that she had "no intention of checking herself out at anytime in the foreseeable future." In other words, she was not psychotic. The latest doctor had therefore stopped all her antidepressants and sent her to me! Fortunately, over time, I was able to help Carol to find insight and to start the journey of self-awareness, self-acceptance, and self-respect that was to make the small little hormonal interventions I supplied work better.

While she still sees a psychiatrist regularly, Carol has not needed any drugs to treat her moods, and her relationships have improved dramatically, especially with her children. Now twelve pounds heavier, thanks in part to the side effect of the contraceptive **depo-provera** shots her family doctor has given her every three months for the past two years in order for her to avoid her fourth pregnancy, the emotional and physical highs and lows are not as noticeable, and certainly not as disrupting. Occasionally, when she starts crying "for no reason at all"—usually with her periods that now occur (as a result of her hormone injections) only every few months—she will apply the lowest dose estrogen skin patch, in order to, as she puts it, "break her fall into the blues world."

I think it is worth repeating at this point (since the problem is so common) that thin women who take oral contraceptives often have emotional, mood, or memory difficulties, during the one week in four when no hormones are taken (the so-called "off" week). Since, for all practical purposes, ovarian production of estrogen is stopped by the pill, the women who have little or no body fat to store or manufacture estrogen, often experience, because of the sudden change in hormone levels during the week without the pill, a myriad of menopausal symptoms—from "mild depression" to diarrhea, from migraine to "muddled" thinking. A tiny dose of estrogen that week—I usually suggest applying just one skin patch of estrogen during those seven days—can magically eliminate the problems.

In milder cases, the patient's use of a daily diary—by relating the mood to the precise week of the menstrual cycle—often reveals to her how problems can be tied to the twice-monthly rise and fall of estrogen and the once-monthly rise and fall of progesterone. This awareness alone—of the chemical basis for mood changes—can be curative. Often benefit is achieved when the patient plans heavy work and big projects for the days the estrogen level will be highest, and saves the smallest, easiest, most pleasant or emotionally reward-ing, or perhaps the most "self-fulfilling" activities, for the days when the level is low or falling. This benefits not only the patient but also those close to her. The relaxation exercises of Chapter Seven are especially important on the hyper days, and the journal of self-appreciation is especially important on the down days. A lot of **T.L.C. helps at any time,** but especially in the form of some **house-hold assistance on the down days.**

Dealing with Your Teenager's Request for the Pill

Questions from a mother such as, "I think my daughter is sexually active; will you give her the pill?" provoke many thoughts—medical, religious, practical, and philosophical. (Not only when the mothers, like Patricia T. in this case, ask the question, but also the many times when their young unmarried daughters still living at home have come in without their mothers' knowledge, made the same request, and asked me to lie if their mothers at their check-ups should ask me if I have ordered the pill for their daughters. The law in Pennsylvania on the treatment of minors without parental consent is complicated.[2])

Patricia's daughter, Sally, nearly eighteen, was soon to leave for college. Because Sally's periods were heavy and also painful, the mother asked, "Wouldn't the pill help those problems, too?" "Yes, probably," I replied. Thus, after a complete checkup, I ordered the pill. Since Sally had finished high school, had a stable sexual relationship with a fine boy, there were few, if any, of the common reasons to object to her use of the pill, aside from the fact that both partners were quite young and had their plans to finish college.

Unfortunately for Sally, the month arrived when for some unknown reason she did not begin her next pack of pills on time. As a result, she came home from her first, and last, year of college, two months pregnant. Happily, she had what young people refer to as a committed sexual relationship, so she proceeded to have the baby and get married.[3]

Most often the problems with sexually active children are not so safe and simple, despite the addition of a very effective new contraceptive that minimizes the need for patient compliance. The intramuscular injection of **Depo-provera**, which has been considered the most effective method of birth-control for over thirty years, is now available in the United States. (Weight gain and menstrual irregularities limit this injectable contraceptive's acceptance by most teenagers.) Admittedly, the oral contraceptive pill is a highly effective method for preventing unwanted pregnancies, but compliance or proper use is quite often a problem. Neither of these drugs, however, are of value in preventing sexually transmitted diseases.

Many people, after reading about cases like Patricia's daughter, suggest that if the pills were provided free, the problem of an unwanted pregnancy would not have arisen. This has not been the experience in any country of the world where free pills have been made available, and where abortion was also readily available. The greatest number of unwanted pregnancies, as proven by subsequent abortions, have consistently occurred in those groups receiving free pills. Teenagers especially, repeatedly prove themselves to be too irresponsible to take the oral contraceptives faithfully or correctly. At every international meeting of Planned Parenthood since 1971— when abortion became a legal option in most countries (1973 in the United States), dismay has been expressed, by governments and private health service agencies alike, at the widespread use of abortion as the "contraceptive method of choice."[4]

Being responsible and self-disciplined marks the attainment of adulthood. Teaching both is a parent's and the school's greatest challenge. Even though a parent knows that a son or daughter is beyond obeying their directives, the parent should still make it perfectly clear what he or she recommends. (In the matter of **smoking,** to which **3000 minors become addicted every day,** smoking at home should be made very, very difficult, unless the parents themselves smoke, in which case hypocrisy raises its ugly head.)

The largest car-leasing company in the world asserts that acceptance of responsibility for the use of a motor vehicle is not likely until the age of twenty-five, at which time you may lease a car from them.

Despite an obvious relationship between age and good judgment, many educators are convinced that dispelling the ignorance about sexual matters will help lessen the sexual-related problems in our society.[5] Another dubious first for the United States is our world leadership among developed countries in sexually transmitted diseases (STDs). There are four million new cases every year of potentially sterilizing "Chlamydia" infections, most of them among our young people. Twelve million new cases of STDs occur each year. The annual cost for just three of the diseases—gonorrhea, herpes, and chlamydia—is $5 billion. Without a doubt, **something** has to be done! (Even though our children would be the first to tell us that they "know all about sex" before they even start first grade.)

Certainly, gender differences have already brought many complications to the educational process, especially in urban schools, even before sex education was considered. Peggy Orenstein's *School Girls: Young Women, Self-Esteem, and the Confidence Gap*, written in association with the American Association of University Women (AAUW), was one of the first in a long series of studies graphically supporting the AAUW's repeated assertions that simply allowing boys and girls to "compete" on their own terms in our schools results in too much damage to the psyche of our daughters and places them at a marked educational disadvantage. The AAUW's claims that bias against girls is an everyday fact of life in our school systems are definitely worth our close attention and concern. Now that sex education is being added to the curriculum, the incidence of exploitation, discrimination, or abuse could be multiplied.[6]

Unfortunately, the 3000-plus teenagers who get pregnant every day, forty-five percent of whom give birth, represent only the tip of the iceberg of what's happening to our children as a consequence of our failure to involve ourselves in their lives and in their education. (In a recent study, more than 1000 sexually active girls sixteen years of age or younger were asked what topic they most wanted to have information about. **Eighty-four percent checked the answer, "how to say no without hurting the other person's feelings."**[7] Part of what is needed is a recognition that there is a clear connection between sexual exploitation or abuse of a female child or young adolescent and subsequent teenage pregnancy. Many times the "sperm donor" turns out to be a man twenty years her senior, who is taking advantage of a young girl's feelings of worthlessness that resulted from earlier abuse. Without providing remediation and personal understanding to such abused individuals, the best sex education program will be ineffective.)

Thus, while I heartily agree that ignorance in any area that is obviously relevant to our children's lives, cannot be a good and must be addressed, there are many different facets to that ignorance, most of it residing in the would-be educators, both parents and teachers alike. (Doctors can't get most of their mature patients to follow their suggestions about mammograms, hormone replacement, even regular pap tests and check-ups, so to think that primary physicians can make a significant impact on the social practices of teenagers is surely presumptuous.)

One thing is certain: girls, even many adult women (besides lacking respect and admiration for their own wonderful uniqueness, which would enable them perhaps to be more assertive and less dependent on what others think of them) cannot seem to integrate their sexuality into their thinking or behavior. One very important reason is their often total lack of understanding of their own biological cycles and inner rhythms. (**A giant step toward ending this ignorance** would be to have adolescent girls keep a daily journal correlating as many facts as possible—their feelings, thoughts, emotions, the day of the cycle, the theoretical level of the various hormones, the day of ovulation, and perhaps even the phase of the moon! If their mothers would share some of their own experiences and insights, it could, in most instances, send their daughters a very affirming message about the wonder and uniqueness of their bodies.)

However, when any sex education program is to be offered, parents must be in full control of the school environment, and the children, parents, and teachers equally involved in a precise sex education curriculum, before I would unreservedly support sex education in elementary or junior high school. In the education of our children, bad information, especially sexual information that can set a fire in their imagination—and initiate sexual desire and arousal in the classroom itself, with devastating consequences, is a worse evil than ignorance.

Having given sex education lectures and courses with my wife at various high schools over the last twenty years, I am convinced that we teach the most useful information too late—female physiology, psychology, and what I would call **human values.** These values include good health practices and appropriate understanding of what is happening or going to happen to their bodies, self-respect, self-confidence, assertiveness, insight into the male psyche and into the media message, **how to say no and make it stick,** how to protect each other, and how to use the legal system. The age of fifteen should be the latest time to begin for typical suburban schools and ten for the inner city ones. (I fully realize these ages are too late to prevent many of the tragedies due to ignorance, but there are other considerations involved, some social, and some "political" or "legal.")

Providing accurate sexual information in our elementary and secondary schools in no way ensures mature or responsible behavior in the area of sexuality. Responsible behavior for most teenagers would mean the avoidance of all early sexual relations, contracepted or not. But, **most sex education courses do not give the students what they need most—a sense of meaning regarding their sexuality, or guidelines on what makes "human" sexual relationships so special and unique**.

Girls, who are much more sensitive than boys to cultural influences, are pressured now, more than ever in our history, to conform to the **new standards** of the nineties, primarily as they are translated by their peers. The exposure to twenty-one hours per week of television sex and violence only adds to the tendency, of adolescent girls especially, to confuse love, sex, and popularity. Boys and men typically fail to appreciate or believe that most of their sexual activities signify a commitment to a future sharing of more than their bodies.

Both sexes have daily problems of anxiety, which they invariably hide lest they be ridiculed. But, for the girls, the formal and informal experiences in the school environment provide them with much more reason to be afraid. This environment does not provide sufficient supervision of student contacts. Estimates place the incidence of sexual harassment at seventy percent, and that of unwanted sexual touching at fifty percent in our school classrooms and hallways.[8] Even allowing for considerable exaggeration, no fair-minded educator can deny that a shameful situation exists in some of our public schools. The "old-fashioned" teasing of the past has now become physical and mean-spirited.

Clearly, if schools are to claim the right to teach sex, they must offer clear sexual and physical harassment policies, which protect the students' basic right to a safe environment and establish norms for conduct toward the opposite sex. Tragically, it is difficult to find a school that teaches "reverence" for anyone, much less for the fragile and confused adolescent girls, starting their own journey into a female-unfriendly society. Students have theoretically been protected since 1972, by Title IX of the Education Amendments, which banned discrimination based on sex. Ignored for twenty years, successful lawsuits, even involving incidents in elementary schools, have begun to shake more and more school administrations out of their rigorous adherence to the status quo. Those who say girls also "harass" boys ignore the reality that it is not a question of simple harassment, but an assertion of male "dominance" and female "weakness."

Despite all the "information" available to our daughters, they usually have little appreciation of their sexual, much less their reproductive potential. In their innocence, they typically remain unaware of the powerful desires they can arouse in boys (and men). This ignorance can and often does result in serious and unwanted consequences. Nearly half of our girls ages fifteen to nineteen have had sex, twice that of 1970, with twice as many also having multiple partners. Five times as many fifteen-year-olds are sexually active as a generation ago.[9] This early sexual activity extracts a high price from women—the shame, sadness, and anger after rejection, the agony experienced when one's reputation is "lost," the unwanted or un-supported pregnancies, and the sexually transmitted diseases which now include AIDS. In the movie _Kids,_ virgins were the "prize" most sought after, because they were not likely to have AIDS.

In the wake of a failed love affair, the adolescent, who feels more pain from rejection than she probably would feel at any other time in her life, is left with a callousness towards life or violence, as well as a cynicism, that places a cloud over all future love-relationships. These more-or-less permanent scars are indeed tragic, because the victims have been seduced by their own urgent need to conform and to be accepted.

Alcohol is often involved when unwise sexual choices are made, yet it is easily available to adolescents. Many parents encourage their teenagers to drink beer or wine at home so that the children will be less tempted to experiment secretly. An added "benefit" is that the child or young adolescent will also gain an awareness of alcohol's effects. Unfortunately, this represents to the emerging adult tacit "permission" to drink, and often eventually makes it necessary for the parents to keep all the alcoholic beverages in the house under lock and key as their children learn to use alcohol for the same purposes their parents often use it—to escape unpleasant everyday realities, or to loosen their inhibitions.

The same principles relating to age, knowledge, and mature judgment are involved when courses in "safe sex" are demanded for the children in the public junior and senior high schools. The intention is to protect those who choose to be sexually active from the consequences of their actions. Many school and public health officials insist that condoms should also be provided, especially to those who request them, if not to everyone in school (since, they say, some of the children will undoubtedly be afraid to admit they are sexually active, and thus will not ask for them).

The debate about how to protect children, adolescents, or young adults from the harmful results of their own sexuality is not a new one. A personal experience that occurred a generation ago provides a clear example of that fact. During a wonderful three-year tour as an army physician in Paris, France, I was singularly blessed to be "assigned" for a memorable three hours to President Kennedy and Vice-President Johnson. Having been "placed" just a few yards from them by the secret-service persons in charge, with my ambulance and crew a short distance away, I was to render any emergency care, should such care suddenly become necessary. Besides providing me with considerable personal affirmation, the assignment allowed me to experience JFK's incredible personal charm. One year later, while again exposing himself to large crowds in a wide open area, he was assassinated.

However, one of my duties during that same overseas tour included being responsible for the public health of the enlisted men, officers, and any dependents accompanying them. For the younger soldiers who were without accompanying dependents, this included not only treating their syphilis and gonorrhea, but also giving weekly lectures on "venereal" diseases, as they were then called. It also meant deciding whether the enlisted men were to be routinely issued condoms. At that time, I thought providing condoms at the off-duty times was sending the wrong signal to the young men who were thousands of miles from family or loved ones. Even though some of the higher officers disagreed, the Base Commander supported my decision, and thus they were not provided. Despite this policy, those who chose to use condoms simply bought them in the regular French stores, where they were easily and cheaply available.[10] As a result of all this, by the time I had completed my time of service, I had observed what study after study has shown throughout many societies of the world—that men irresponsible in their choices of sexual partners are too often irresponsible in practicing safe sex or in using their condoms consistently, just as girls in similar situations are lax—both in insisting that condoms be used and in taking the freely-provided oral contraceptives to prevent pregnancy. Instead, they resort to abortion when needed and skip any regular programs for diagnosis and treatment of potentially very serious sexually transmitted diseases.

One practical point: rightly or wrongly, a girl in junior or senior high school who uses the pill or a diaphragm is apt to be labeled a "slut" by her peers, if only because she has thus removed any right to claim "innocence" to whatever happens subsequently in her relationships. "Date-rape" especially elicits little peer response when the girl's "boy friend" is the rapist and the girl herself provides the contraception. The girl who takes these "precautions," frequently judges her own priorities, or "morals," harshly, and when sexual intercourse occurs against her will, she blames herself for provoking the attack!

A very recent situation in Lakewood, California shows the problem in a slightly different light. Fourteen high school athletes, who called themselves "the Spur Posse," went on trial for raping many girls, one as young as ten years of age. Some of the parents of the accused expressed pride in their sons' "virility." One parent compared the situation to that of an athletic hero, Wilt Chamberlain, who boasted of having relations with 20,000 women during his "career." The boys themselves pleaded innocent, one saying, "The schools pass out condoms and teach us about pregnancy, but they don't teach us any rules."[11] In fact, the schools are proscribed by law from teaching any "rules," whether those rules be accepted by nearly every person in the particular community or not.

(The 20,000 women who were **allegedly** involved with Mr. Chamberlain have been "explained" by claiming that such women needed to confirm their worth or at least their desirability by proving they could attract a "great man." Laura Schlessinger, one of the many wonderful health professionals whom you will meet in Section Two, counts this among the many "stupid things" a women can do to prove she hasn't learned to value herself.)

As easy as it is to prescribe condoms or hormones for contraception and disease-prevention, it is in no way easy, or often even possible, to prescribe guidelines for the relationships that are involved. In fact, the physicians' greatest challenge is to find help for those patients of whatever age whose problems derive from a failure to love, honor, and obey their own needs (in fact to even be aware of what their needs are, or the **important ways in which they need help**). Unsatisfactory or painful relationships are often the result of what I would call this **foolish selflessness. For better relationships** it is well for a woman to remember that learning what her needs and yearnings are, and then paying attention to doing something about them, sends out a **very important signal: I am worthy of attention and care. I accept who and what I am, and I shall continue to act to make myself better.**

One of the best ways for a teenager to show that she cares about herself and her future is **not to smoke. One million new teenage (or younger) smoking addicts** are created in our country every year. The terrible consequences to their future health and happiness cannot be overstated. **Adults must support the laws against minors smoking!**

The next five chapters comprise an analysis of the obstacles to **successful relationships**, including the many specific ways in which a woman's personality, temperament, and what she thinks about herself interact with the intimate others in her life to affect her struggle for **success as she defines it**.

Before proceeding, a few comments on the **body Section** of this book should prove helpful:

Reviewing the Main Suggestions of Section One

Recognize that your health is your responsibility; initiate a program of regular **safe exercises, including the relaxing bodymind exercises**; eat and drink according to simple guidelines that include **complex carbohydrates, fiber, multivitamins,** and a number of safe and possibly very worthwhile natural dietary supplements; provide **humidification** when necessary to protect your skin and respiratory tract; use the **mildest cleansers** for the skin and the **mildest detergents** without added chemicals in your wash; keep a health and feeling-awareness **diary** and get **regular gynecologic checkups;** do your **Kegel exercises** at the first sign of a bladder problem or to improve your sexual response; **inform yourself** on the causes of abdominal pain and which gyn events are normal and which require professional attention; and finally, begin a conscious effort every day to love and honor yourself by **devoting time to achieving self-awareness, self-acceptance, and self-respect**. Remember that when you lack the confidence to make your own decisions, you are much more likely to become dependent and to be controlled. Your well-being requires that you be assertive, not controlled.

Also recommended is gaining an understanding and appreciation of the ways that your hormonal changes—or the lack of them—can affect your health and happiness, and then promptly checking with a physician who is knowledgeable and interested in such matters, when such an action seems appropriate.

James House, an epidemiologist from the University of Michigan, summarized a number of scientific studies in a landmark paper relating the quality of a person's social relationships to that person's health. He found considerable evidence for claiming that **a lack of a satisfactory love-relationship was as great a risk factor for disease and death as anything else, including smoking.**[12] With that amazing discovery in mind, we proceed.

NOW TO THE WONDERFUL AND COMPLEX WORLD OF RELATIONSHIPS!

Section 2
Healing Your Relationships

THE SECOND CHALLENGE:
Accepting the Work of Love

"Men and women are no longer helpmates, companions, and
supporters to one another; instead our relationships are
characterized, at best, by confusion and frustration,
and, at worst, by hostility, violence, and hatred. . . .
(Women) tend to think of men as emotionally monolithic and
insensitive beings who will never be able to speak to, nourish,
console, or feel with them . . . (and) have virtually given up
on men . . . (instead of) perceiving them as good
human beings who have (also) loved and suffered. . . .
Only when men are embraced by perceptions
that honor them will they be able to change."
—Daphne Rose Kingma,
The Men We Never Knew:
How to Deepen Your Relationship
with the Man You Love

10

Looking at "Love"

"If you know, accept, and appreciate yourself and your uniqueness, you will permit others to do so. If you value and appreciate the discovery of yourself, you will encourage others to engage in self-discovery. If you recognize your need to be free to discover who you are, you will allow others their freedom to do so, also. When you realize you are the best you, you will accept that others are the best they. But it follows that it all starts with you. To the extent to which you know yourself, and we are all more alike than different, you can know others. When you love yourself, you will love others. And to the depth and extent to which you can love yourself, only to that depth and extent will you be able to love others."

—Leo Buscaglia, in *Love*

Mother Teresa's declaration that we seem to be the loneliest people on earth speaks precisely to the lack of "connectedness" that is epidemic in our society. The loneliness, senselessness, or emptiness in **our** lives is the very thing that could be changed if the intimacy that women need (and that men must give in order to judge themselves adequate providers), can be achieved. But the connectedness we seek definitely requires us to better communicate our different needs so that we can resolve our differences. More than anything else, **we must find better ways to handle our anger.** That search will provide the hardest challenge of this chapter.

143

Starting with a *Philosophical* Look

The first requirement in our quest for a love relationship is to recognize something **profoundly simple—we can never love anyone more than we love ourselves**. However obvious this statement may seem, it is still true. Our failure to understand and accept this truth and to act accordingly to make ourselves lovable, constitutes the quintessential reason that our relationships fail. When we deny we "need" relationships of love, we are in fact confessing that we have no intention of loving ourselves, that in fact we have "given up" on ourselves as unworthy of loving or being loved.

No normal human being can escape the fact that she/he is social. Psychotherapists, in fact, have stopped treating humans as if they were ever separate individuals, simply trying to preserve their own lives. Each person is now seen as seeking more than the "safe life," or the self-preservation demanded by the subconscious mind, that Freud emphasized. Even working and loving to the extent that one experiences the feeling of being "fully human and fully alive" does not satisfy man's deepest yearnings. Rather, a man's or woman's ultimate quest is to continually **express** his/her aliveness, to enter into relationship, to connect regularly, daily if possible, with another life outside himself/herself.[1] Of final importance is the truth that a permanent love-relationship is far and away the best way for men and woman to express their aliveness regularly, safely, and in a progressively more fulfilling fashion. (The permanence adds the safety and security required for achieving and maintaining intimacy.)

As human beings, we use our **reason** to realize the benefits of a permanent, safe, close relationship, and most of us eventually use our **free will** to pursue such a relationship. The philosophers and theologians agree that this recognition and this choice demonstrate **humanity's greatest gifts**. (The only difference between the two disciplines in this matter of relationships is whether "God" is of any importance.)[2]

Understanding the *Psychology* of Childhood Traumas

After the western tradition had reached an agreement on man's powers of reason and free will, Freud came along to emphasize that while the goal of intimacy is readily seen as desirable, it is incredibly difficult for us to achieve. By insisting on the existence and power of the unconscious mind, Freud was able to show that, while man **is** indeed logical and free, this logic and freedom exists only to the extent that his thoughts are correctly formed and his decisions are conscious, that is, not driven by forces or experiences from his past, of which he is not even aware.

Because the concept of childhood programming is a very valid one, the initial step following a decision to try to heal your present relationships is to accept and pursue the possibility that some of our major problems with our relationships are a result of problems in our childhood years. There is, in fact, a vast literature that proclaims that the causes of our adult emotional problems are to be found by searching for the early childhood traumas inflicted by our primary caretakers. As a personal example, the title of my first psychiatry text was *Juvenile Delinquency Is Parental Delinquency.*

Generally accepted theory states that as adults we keep repeating some unacceptable techniques or habits of relating to other people that we learned in infancy and childhood. These reaction patterns from our early years were of great importance to our survival in infancy and childhood, but are inappropriate now. Some of these unacceptable approaches to others are present in all of us.

Problems in our past occurred despite the fact that most of us had caring parents, who did the best they could. Regardless, the "childish" reactions remain to influence or control our present ways of dealing with people. Now, in order to be capable of maintaining a close adult relationship, we need to learn adult ways to handle the full range of problems that develop when people seek closeness.

One has no difficulty accepting the premise that, in the process of raising, teaching, or training us, our parents, by their actions or lack of action, sometimes adversely affected our ways of reacting to the demands of living. Thus, in the language used by psychology, our parents **wounded** us in some ways. Whenever, for example, our anger as infants, which gave us the strength and energy to protect ourselves by alerting our parents to our needs, was shamed, invalidated, ignored, or punished, we were hurt. Such actions on our parents' part, especially if repeated often, could have led us to hide or deny that emotion whenever it arose in ourselves. The same denial could have been repeated for any emotion that our caregivers judged unacceptable. As a result of being denied expression of our valid emotions, we now find ourselves with an impaired ability to feel, accept, admit, or consciously act on our emotions. As John Bradshaw points out, for example, many adult sexual problems are due to the fact that the sex drive is universally shamed before children are even aware of it.[3] Along the same lines, Daphne Rose Kingma, in her work as a psychotherapist, finds that many men will not commit to marriage because they never again want to experience either the overwhelming control or the stifling dependency that they once experienced in the relationship with their mother.[4]

The knowledge that the wounds we suffered in our early years of life are neither the fault of our parents or of ourselves, because everyone was presumably doing their best, yet every child was wounded, does not always prevent us from blaming our parents for our present inadequacies. In this matter, Fritz Perls was very quick to point out that as long as we hold on to resentment towards our parents, we will never grow up. Moreover, the application of modern psychological principles for nearly a century has failed to provide much evidence that simply going back to childhood, discovering the mistakes of our parents, and blaming and shaming them, provides much benefit. "Healing the wounded child" does little to help the present adult achieve love in his relationships. Rather, each person must be convinced of the need to discover, then take responsibility for, his or her **present** failings or deficiencies, and to change them.

Furthermore, we must achieve the recognition that the way **our** family related to each other is not necessarily the best way or even the normal way. Unfortunately, we tend to hold the perception that our view of the world, and our ways of doing things, are superior. This obstinate bias on our own behalf is the primary reason that the power struggle is maintained in most modern marriages. After all, what kind of love is possible when there are incessant attempts by one or both partners to change the other to their model of what the spouse should feel, want, or do, and when the main thrust is to get the other to conform, to reform, and/or to "get with it."

Using Anger as Your Guide to Marital Problems

Women, individually and collectively, are often condemned as "witches" or "bitches," when they attempt to express their anger to men. This is a prohibition that starts in infancy and continues unabated throughout their lives. In order to be a "lady" (feminine), they must deny their anger and bury their reactions to the ubiquitous male control or oppression.

Unfortunately, the process in all human beings is that buried feeling and emotions, especially anger, never remain buried but rather continuously gather strength and eventually erupt. To use the words of one of the modern experts of psychodynamics, Virginia Satir, "Repressed anger is like a hungry dog in the basement." Eventually the anger will have its day, to be manifested as pain or sadness, violence, mental or physical illness, or a limitless variety of other tactics disruptive to the relationships. (Even boredom is actually hostility buried so deeply that no emotion is allowed expression.)

Unquestionably, anger and the other emotional defenses against abuse, neglect, or violence are utterly necessary and useful in our pursuit of happiness, provided we consciously follow a few simple rules for expressing them. Each conflict that is faced, discussed, and resolved provides another stepping stone to greater connectedness.

Tragically, it is estimated that in perhaps ninety-five percent of committed male-female relationships, the individuals involved are unaware of, or are unwilling to use, the techniques available to resolve conflict. The result is that they remain locked in a struggle for power that can be waged in an endless variety of ways. This chronic battle exists in the relationship precisely because each individual has been unable to consistently confront, analyze, understand, and use his/her anger (or sadness, pain, or resentment) in a constructive or mature manner.

When considering the subject of **anger or any other emotion, it is absolutely essential to remember that such human reactions are**

never inappropriate, however misguided we are in expressing them. Anger, as a universal human emotion or power, is to be seen as a gift that alerts us or wakes us up to the fact that a human need is not being met. Looked at in this way, it is easy to see how the **energy supplied by the anger that is inevitably generated in any close relationship can motivate us to search for our own needs.**

The process of using our anger for improving our relationships requires that we first become experts on discovering our needs. There are few shortcuts in this work of love, which demands time and effort. But the goal of self-discovery, which is to learn to appreciate or care about ourselves, is surely worth the effort, because (as the golden rule so plainly states) **self-love is the essential condition for our loving anybody else.**

Marital problems are often blamed on a woman's physical ailments when, in fact, the opposite is true. The marked tendency that women show to repress all **unfeminine** emotions or behaviors, especially anger, undoubtedly causes for some of them an assortment of physical and psychological problems, including problems with weight, eating disorders, headaches, migraines, depression, crying spells, sadness, sleep disorders, palpitations, anxiety attacks, and multiple gastrointestinal disturbances. One very frequent source of a woman's anger is a husband who totally denies that he has any needs of his own. Typically, he himself is not able to discover or at least admit to any problems. Millions of women every day are adversely affected by their relationships with men who are emotionally detached, who hide all weaknesses and deny all their mistakes. Seemingly "invulnerable," because they show no problems at all, such men nevertheless subtly, and largely unconsciously, give their wives the job of acting out emotionally their suppressed feelings. Wives often allow their husbands to get away with something like this because they believe the problem is not their husband's, but theirs. When they eventually see that the husband is the source of the problem, they often **selflessly** forgive him anyway. This is precisely an area to which I was referring in the opening section, "Understanding the Message"—my exhortation to be selfish enough to become aware, accept, but also *share* the *truth* of your feelings. Your goal is not **peace** (which in burying your feelings would be a false peace anyway) but rather **intimacy,** which requires the **complete truth.**

Refusing to Allow "Him" to Dump His Anger on You

When a man in a relationship is a statue, without visible feelings or needs, the woman must emotionally express or deal with all the feelings that are experienced by either partner, in order for that relationship, that connectedness, to continue. The closer the woman is to him, the more sensitive she becomes to his unexpressed needs, and the more likely she is to "act out" **his** feelings. The metaphor that Barbara De Angelis uses, in *Making Love All the Time*, is that both spouses have their own "tank" of feelings, with an intimacy "tube" connecting the tanks. Whenever one spouse pushes the level of feelings down, the level of feelings rises in the mate, often to the point that the feelings spill out in emotional outbursts. A result often seen is an emotional, or "crazy" wife, who will be treated by her doctor, especially if that doctor happens to be a male, for the disease of expressing unacceptable emotions.[5]

When the man is the partner walled-off from any feelings, the good ones as well as the bad ones, he will frequently resort to a favorite male ploy, namely, passive aggression. These techniques are basically non-actions and include such familiar things as forgetting promises, key anniversaries or appointments, and being late or skipping agreed upon chores. The man lets his negative feelings out by essentially doing nothing, while managing to vent his hostility or frustrations with his wife by keeping her in a stew.

Barbara DeAngelis writes quite kindly about men but nevertheless strongly advises that women seek a woman's viewpoint to guide them to see the reason for their angry reactions. With help and insight she can discover the cause to be in a husband's refusal to take the lid off any of his bottled-up emotions. (DeAngelis urges a female professional as an advisor because "a woman in our culture tends to sanctify the opinions of male service-providers," who are not very likely to accept a husband-blaming scenario.)

Regardless of the primary cause of anger in either partner, it is essential that both the man and the woman be convinced that any negative feelings that exist in the relationship should be welcomed as gifts, because such feelings can supply the insight and energy necessary to alert each to his or her own most important needs. This **union of the calm, has-it-all-together male with the hysterical,**

overly-emotional female has been aptly designated as the most typical American marriage.

Working for a Goal that Provides Something Much Better

A century ago, Sigmund Freud asked his followers to find out "what women want," admitting that he did not know. Most of what has been written since, in answering that question, has portrayed women as powerless victims of man's domination and selfishness. The repeated assertion is that women will never get what they want from men, and that, in fact, men must be deaf, dumb, and blind to have failed to realize what women have been asking for throughout the 20th century.

The appraisal that women will never get what they want most from men will remain true, unless women accept the challenge now clearly presented to them. Explaining to men precisely what **"it"** is that women want to receive from them has never been enough. Rather, it is essential that women help their mates recover the ability to give them what they need. Because men are unaware that they have hidden, even to themselves, the talents required to provide to women what women desperately need, it is essential that women "educate" them.

What do women want? Most women want an adult male companion who will **care** about them, that is, who will appreciate, affirm, respect, and reverence them, who will experience the feelings of joy, sadness, fear, or anger with them, and who will use, not the male language of action, but the feminine language of words, to express this **empathy**, this ability to **feel with** them. The staggering problem in all this is that man's "feminine" talent for feeling had to be buried, repressed, or destroyed in the process of becoming a "real" man. To be "male" in our culture has been to be required not to feel, and, in that unfeeling state, it is utterly impossible to feel the loss of one's own ability to feel. Often, the only acceptable male emotions are variations of anger and pride. **The only intimacy with which many men feel at all comfortable is sexual intimacy in a committed relationship**. Any experiences or expressions of joy, sadness, fear, despair, weakness, shame, or vulnerability are limited to various forms of athletic competition. Even then, the emotions are usually vicariously experienced as a spectator, not as a participant.

Not knowing what they are missing, as Daphne Rose Kingma states, is what has always made a man a man. Therefore, when women show men the talent they have hidden or buried, they will also enable men to experience the joy and satisfaction of finally being able to give to a woman what she most wants to receive![6]

It has been the tragedy of our society, centuries after the enlightenment, that men are still "emotionally disenfranchised ... (and) experience their inaccessibility to their emotions as an unbearable void. It is the hidden pain about this void that women must finally address," not with the criticism and anger that successfully fueled the feminist movement for equal rights, nor by serving men from a "one-down" or "victim" position, but rather by loving them and guiding them in the long and difficult process of reclaiming their "feminine dimension."[7]

In order to have men reveal themselves emotionally, and to teach them the verbal language for expressing a full range of feelings, women must first develop empathy in themselves for what being a man has demanded in our culture. This means acquiring an understanding of the "down side" of the male experience, that is, the emptiness, the shallowness, the loneliness or isolation resulting from always having to be stoic, steadfast, brave, proud, and "perfect." How many comforts have been denied to men by their having been allowed to express only anger and pride, with the other emotions allowed expression only by their work, by competitive male "games," or through sex?

Thus, at the beginning of this second century after Freud's challenge to find the answer to women's needs, the overwhelming consensus is that not only the intimacy that women earnestly desire, but also the fate of this planet, depends on the resolution of the conflict, confusion, frustration, hostility, and anger between individual men and women. I completely agree with all those who insist that this resolution can come about only if men can reclaim access to those feelings and emotions, those talents and qualities, that each has had to bury in the depths of his psyche in order to be accepted as a man.

Several generations ago, Carl Jung, in *Modern Man in Search of a Soul*, stated that one-third of his patients had no definable neurosis, but were undone simply by their awareness of the senselessness and emptiness of their lives.[8] As the curtain falls on this century, the great majority of American women, and men too, would confess to wanting increased joy and happiness in their lives, and most would be willing to work for it, if someone could show them the way. Which leads us to emphasize one way, however, that is definitely wrong: the technique of **using** the children.

"Transferring" Emotions to the Children as an Escape from Each Other

The emotional dynamics in **every** family follow very closely the patterns seen between the parents. John Bradshaw, in *Creating Love: The Next Great Stage of Growth*, says that Sigmund Freud's greatest legacy was convincing parents of their children's vulnerability, and of the utter necessity of their best efforts in raising children.[9] These best efforts require that parents understand that any of their buried or unexpressed feelings are going to be transferred to the children in the same way, for example, as anger can be transferred from husband to wife.[10]

The transfers of negative reactions, whether between the parents themselves or between parents and children, have been referred to using the metaphor of the "seesaw." Whenever one parent pushes down the level of his own emotions, the level of that emotion can rise in either the children, the other parent, or both.[11] The emotional transfers, as well as other dynamics between spouses, provide the focus of this chapter and the next, Chapter Eleven. In the latter chapter, the mistakes that lead to total failures in relationships are emphasized, with a view to changing the pattern of failure.

By the same "see-saw" mechanism that we saw active in the most typical American marriage (where the husband has the anger, but the wife expresses it), the parents' personal unhappiness with each other can be transferred to their children, bringing devastation to their children's psyche and emotions. Inevitably, such children will feel responsible for the parents' misery. The children then either act out the forbidden feelings by doing angry or disruptive acts, becoming "problem" children, or they hide the transferred feelings they have picked up and thus "internalize" them. In the latter case, the buried problems can re-emerge at any time, but especially when, as adults, they attempt to enter into close relationships.

Unfortunately, the modern solution to conflict is divorce. Obviously, when divorce is the option chosen to counter a lack of caring, of attention, of acceptance, and of communication, the consequences extend well beyond the lives of the man and woman involved. Marriage failures affect, even more than the experts originally claimed, the present and future development of the children.

Continuing with the Psychology—Marrying Our Match

John Gray, in his recently revised *Men, Women and Relationship: Making Peace with the Opposite Sex*, emphasizes that women especially, from day one, have great plans for changing and improving their husbands, and that there is really nothing the husbands can do about it.[12] Nevertheless, the universality of the practice of trying to change our partners does not alter the fact that the person seeking to change a partner is **always** acting on their own behalf, not their partner's. Susan Jeffers adds the warning to women, "If you want to be alone, push for change."[13] There are, of course, an infinite number of imaginative techniques that persons in relationships develop, in order to exert their own willfulness.

In psychology, the point is made that what you can't stand in someone else is, for whatever reason, what you had to reject or eliminate in your own emotions and actions. Thus the traits that anger, disturb, frustrate (or **attract!**) you, provide the key to your **disowned-self**. Those qualities or actions of your mate that you insist he change, which may have attracted you to him initially, are invariably closely like or identical to the qualities that you buried in your earliest years. Thus, you might feel shame at his sexual openness, insecure in the face of his confidence and forthrightness, or embarrassed by his frankness and honesty. Of course, the wife often displays skills, especially in communication of feelings, that the husband repudiated before his conscious memory had developed.

Sigmund Freud called our attention to another aspect of "attraction," labeling the tendency to choose mates that have the most dominant traits of our primary caretakers, more often the negative ones, the "repetition compulsion." He claimed that the unconscious mind resists change, therefore it constantly strives to stay with the familiar, to reconstruct the past. Fritz Perls referred to this as reproducing "unfinished business." Both theorized (and this is still the majority view) that this represents an attempt to try again to correct past mistakes and bring about happy endings. As Susan Jeffers puts it, if you are wondering why you are always choosing the "wrong" man, he is probably the "right" one to teach you what you need to learn, that is, how to resolve your own unfinished problems that impaired your past relationships, and which continue to interfere with your present ones.[14]

As a practical matter, psychology insists that we choose to marry the person who is eventually going to disturb or upset us when we come back to our right minds and the unconscious interval of romantic love is over. **Romantic love** is, in fact, entirely a prelude to **conscious love**, since there exists in the former stage an utter co-dependency, such as is normally found only in infancy. As in infancy, no one has a separate identity, as mother/infant or lovers are fused in erotic, or unthinking love. Part of the unwritten or unspoken contract at this stage is an "agreement not to disagree." The time when grievances begin to be expressed marks the onset of the power struggle and the end of romantic love.

Since the mate that most of us who marry for love select is the one who, theoretically at least, is most capable of inflicting the same wounds that our parents did, is there any wonder that the infantile stage of romantic love is eventually followed by a reenactment of the **childhood situation where control was the primary issue**? The stubborn persistence of the power-struggle phase in most marriages makes our initial confidence in each other seem foolish in retrospect. But why should we be surprised at the usual result, since our initial decision to choose a particular person was made by our unconscious mind, which is concerned only with survival and with maintaining the familiar. This incredibly important decision in our life was probably not based on a conscious and rational evaluation of the facts.

Thus, we (subconsciously) select our mate because we just "know" that he or she will help us to reclaim the qualities we had to deny or disown. Without even thinking about it, we experience rapture from the prospect of once more recapturing the wholeness and the joy of infancy.

Discovering the Amazingly Effective **No Fault** Theory

Besides accepting the theory that we marry our match, who fits our real needs perfectly, another essential concept for healing family relationships is that **no one** is to be blamed for the problems in a relationship. This lack of fault includes everyone: the parent/child/man/or woman. Regardless of the way the power struggle is waged in any particular relationship—even those with the total absence of any visible anger—the peaceful resolution of conflicts or the satisfying of each others' needs remains impossible, until each partner accepts responsibility for his or her own actions and reactions.

How, in fact, can anyone be blamed for handling the differences or the conflicts that inevitably arise, which generate the anger in all human relationships, when they are simply using the techniques that each was taught (or at least that each learned) in infancy and early childhood. Crying, screaming, whining, shouting, biting, withdrawing, being sad or depressed, are not **adult** ways of expressing anger. Even though we realize this, we persist in acting in those fashions anyway. Eventually, it is hoped that someone—you, your partner, or both of you—will make the decision to "grow up."

Changing a "Living Arrangement" into a Loving Relationship

> *"No one can develop in this world and find a full life without feeling understood by at least one person. Misunderstood, he loses his self-confidence, he loses his faith in life, or even in God. He is blocked and he regresses."*
> —Paul Tournier, *To Understand Each Other*

When we fail to convince our spouse that we are right, and that he or she is wrong, the solution often chosen to resolve the impasse is to exchange our present partner for a new one. One alternative suggestion: Instead of continually seeking to find the right mate or "the first true friend," why not instead seek to **become** the right mate or the first true friend.[15]

In *The Angry Marriage*, Bonnie Maslin suggests that, in any intimate relationship, the partners abandon their childish behavior in handling conflict and use a "new language of love . . . to create an adult marriage, to express through words what has been discovered by insight—to give words to hidden needs so that they are visible, evident, conscious, and therefore lose their ability to dictate behavior."[16] The first suggestion from the new language is to start any expression of "grievance," redefined by that language as "your need," with the word "I." The "I" is an acknowledgment that **you** have a problem that is producing anger and pain. Insights about the relationship are to be shared with your mate as self-reflective statements, which means stating them as **your** feelings, fears, hopes, or reactions, and never as accusations, which will only inspire anger or retaliation in kind.[17]

On the other hand, when you express a grievance by personally attacking your spouse, you ignore any responsibility on your part for his actions. You also deprive him of the knowledge of your accompanying fears, sadness, or anxieties, while you are also failing to provide him with any evidence that you care about him. For example, a wife who has "had it" as a result of her partner's criticisms, and so tells him he is a worthless lout, doesn't accomplish much. A better way for a wife who is always being criticized to express her complaint is to tell the **complete truth**: "When you tell me what to do, I feel as if I'm being called 'stupid,' and then I just swallow all the anger that gets stirred up inside me, and I try to bury it. This burial takes so much of my energy and attention that no other emotion or feeling is left over to share with you." By including her responsibility for her own reactions, she not only keeps the door of communication open, but she also provides him with an up-to-date assessment of her feelings. What she may be saying, in effect, is that for her a pervasive sadness, a lethargy, depression, or often even a loss of any interest in sex has resulted from her suppressed anger. This information is offered as an invitation for him to respond with his own present feelings. The principle to be remembered is that **when people of good will are communicating, they can't lose**, especially since the alternatives to communicating are separation or distancing. (The key here, of course, is whether there is any good will left. When couples bury their feelings until all the good will is gone, even counseling may be futile.)

Avoiding the **Numbing** Process

Barbara DeAngelis describes the process of how simple disagreements can lead to total numbness, or loss of passion for anything, and finally, depression. She calls the sequence of events, the four R's. First you notice your husband doing something you don't like, but you **resist** saying anything. When he repeats his actions, you begin to **resent** what he does, but still you say nothing, perhaps out of fear for the consequences. Since your husband is still unaware of the problem you are having, he continues the actions you find hurtful, so you make the decision to **reject** him, to shut him out, to distance yourself, to clam up. If the emotional tension that has built up in you is not relieved, you up the ante and go to the next level of separation, that is, **repression.** "It doesn't matter anymore," "Let's forget it," "Nothing's worth fighting over," "Let's just go on and ignore that difference," are all instances of this last stage. This stage of numbness will affect everything you do subsequently. **You get rid of the pain only by burying _all_ feelings, including the "good" ones like joy, passion, or aliveness**. Keeping all feelings buried is a tremendous strain. The resultant anger must also be hidden and can be turned inward as depression.[18]

On the other hand, as Bonnie Maslin points out, if the person with the need or grievance is a ventor, a person who explodes publicly, the anger does not go away simply because she/he lets out all restraints. Such venting hurts the person who is attacked, of course, but both feel worse about themselves and their marriage. Thus, these outbursts never provide a solution to anger.[19]

It is important to see **feelings** (what you **feel in**side) and **emotions** (our outward **motions** that express those feelings) as gifts that signal or alert us to the presence of an unfulfilled need, and to see that in every complaint lies the clue, not only to one's own hidden need, but to the mate's own _complementary weakness._ By accepting such an analysis, we can recognize the _twin_ contributions required to generate any conflict. For example, a wife who fights her husband's domination in simple matters, such as control of the temperature in the car or house, with great outbursts of temper, is discovered after careful analysis to have developed, in her relationship with her parents, a hidden need to fight viciously any semblance of domination or control, while her husband brought his own need or weakness, namely, an exaggerated need to be valued, to matter to someone, and to have someone listen to what he wants. The battle is joined because each has a grievance from the past that has never been successfully exposed and resolved.[20]

(When you make progress in discovering why you react in predictable and unvarying ways to the same types of stresses, you might then be able to understand why your relationships with not only your spouse but also your business relationships or those with your friends repeatedly run into snags. For example, **I have always been like my father in never wanting to openly confront or challenge any man or woman**. Though neither my wife, Marianne, or most of our closest friends, would now describe me as a shrinking violet or martyr, I now know that "suffering offense in silence" is an approach that I often used in my life, and the approach that I still employ in many of the relationships that I presently value. However, whenever this inability to share my needs exists, the relationship never becomes close. If I had realized this fifty years ago, the history of many of my closest relationships would surely be quite different, and these experiences would have been much more rewarding. Without once consciously realizing what I was doing, I would do "anything" to please and to preserve a relationship. When the resentment had built up sufficiently to convince me that they really didn't value my friendship enough to give me what I wanted (though I would be afraid to ask them for anything), I would very quietly disappear from their lives. I am still working on this "problem.")

Marrying Your (Apparent) **Opposite**

In *The Angry Marriage,* Bonnie Maslin refers to the relationship with our parents as our **first marriage** and that a **person's experiences with the parents can provide the key to finding the source of conflict in the second marriage**. For examples, the compulsions that are brought to the second marriage, such as the need to control or be controlled, to keep spouses at bay or in their place, to find approval, to protect ourselves from abandonment, or to avoid sadness at any cost, may have been derived from the techniques we learned in infancy and childhood.[21]

Nancy Friday stresses that, unless father did a considerable amount of mothering, our first marriage was for all practical purposes to our mother.[22] In supporting that opinion, John Bradshaw adds that women who cannot escape their mother's domination "often become victims of abusive men."[23] (Judi Hollis insists that the man most women "marry" is their mother's duplicate.) Another common example of the powerful influence of that first marriage: the woman who is preoccupied with the task of improving her husband, or to totally remake him, as her first priority, may have taken from her past the thing she hated the most, namely her parents' excessive control. Now, she makes control her own basic need.

One common example of the marriage of opposites occurs when a woman who was smothered or totally controlled by her mother's love, which of course was not love at all, marries a man who was neglected, that is, who never experienced his mother's love. As a result, neither was able to learn satisfactorily how to escape the first stage of living, that stage generally coinciding with the first eighteen months of life, during which we are fused, or attached to mom. As a consequence of the hunger, pain, loneliness, fear, and insecurity that was produced by their not being cared for in the earliest and most helpless stage of relating, both begin the next stage of "psychosocial" growth—the **exploration** of the world around them—with much fear and anxiety. The psychic damage produced in the first phase of the growth process was never recognized consciously and repaired. Thus it remained to impact in a negative way all of the subsequent stages in social development and now impairs their ability to love. Their experiences of love remain enmeshed in exaggerated negative feelings of dependency, control, and need. When they marry each other, they each stand in a personal quicksand in this matter of loving, not on the solid ground of successful loving experiences. For such individuals, expressing their love freely and easily as mature adults constitutes a very difficult challenge indeed, though not an unsolvable one.

Thus, all the various "relationships of opposites"—which includes the emotional/stoic, angry/calm, nurse/patient, sociable/recluse, dependent/independent, controller/compliant, or pursuer/distancer "love-matches"—most likely occur because the individuals handled identical, or nearly identical, problems of relating to their primary caregivers, in exactly opposite ways. (Ideally, this fact should make it possible for each to provide the other with the "qualities" he/she is lacking.)

Sadly, what happens is that a complementary weakness or need produces conflict, for which the man and the woman are **equally** responsible. But, the truth that both bring their immaturities with them is a fact that few spouses want to hear or will accept. This is especially true, for example, when a woman has a husband who is abusive, distant, an addict, a workaholic, lazy, oversexed, inept, an adulterer, or a deserter. Should a doctor foolishly suggest that the wife might contribute something to the troubled relationship, the likelihood is that the patient will start a search for a more perceptive doctor, one who would be smart enough to see that her husband is the one with all the problems.

Some spouses, in fact, even steadfastly deny any responsibility for choosing their mate in the first place, even though an investigation often reveals that it was not only totally their free choice but also one made totally against advice.

It is definitely true that the chances for saving or improving any marriage are eliminated when either partner denies having some responsibility for the problems that exist or refuses to do anything about them. The acceptance of some responsibility is absolutely necessary, even when, to any outside observer, the one mate is obviously the "sinner" who needs to be converted, and the other the "saint" who is virtually perfect.

Seeking *Counseling* for Your Marriage Problems

It is quite important for couples seeking deeper intimacy in marriage to recognize when counseling is necessary. Counseling will help in almost every case, even when it is not absolutely necessary. Over four-and-a half million couples now visit 50,000 licensed family therapists each year. The "stigma" of such resort to outside help for one's marriage has virtually disappeared. As an example, when Vice-President Al Gore stated in 1992 that his family had been in family therapy, no one batted an eye.

The ready availability of counseling does not mean that the books specifically dealing with healing relationships should be ignored. They can often also be of crucial benefit. In addition, it is important to realize that outside help or marriage therapy that tries to cure troubled marriages by simply attempting to help settle the disputes, arranging deals, or brokering treaties between warring parties, is futile. Having someone else resolve their problems simply saves the couple from the necessity of facing each other honestly and communicating, thus blocking any improvements in their own ability to handle conflict.

That half of "angry marriages" do not end in divorce demonstrates the truth that anger, rage, or resentment do not signify the absence of love. Rather, the lack of any connectedness, even the connectedness that anger maintains, reflects the absence of caring. Couples prove this fact every day when one or the other tolerates a sometimes-hostile spouse long after an indifferent one would have been dumped. It is the appearance of indifference that signals a distancing, a severing of connectedness, and an absence of love.

Tensions or conflicts that produce fighting in one form or another are inevitable in any close relationship. This fighting can take place under an endless variety of forms. I've seen many couples that for all intents and purposes "never" fought, but their eventual divorce came as no surprise to anyone, perhaps because they were never "loving" either. Children, the media, society, neighbors, parents, boss, workmates, weather, and circumstances all provide excuses for avoiding the "real" problem, namely, **our reactions** of anger to our partner.

Couples fight because there is always something that each wants, or needs, that they believe only their partner can provide. Often this need involves your partner not doing something that hurts you. Since communicating skills are either primitive or seldom employed, the partners rarely realize the real reason they are fighting. In fact, anger is frequently the only way some couples have left to communicate or connect with each other. Their fights, in effect, represent desperate cries for love, affirmation, support, respect, appreciation, or understanding, as each is searching for someone to care.

Acknowledging Our *Anger*

The truth that our anger is sometimes displaced, or buried, is indisputable. Why should a simple disagreement with something your husband says or does turn so quickly to an "explosion" of disapproval of your husband himself? The answer to why a little thing sets you off is that you have been hiding your anger, frustration, pain, or sadness. Men are tremendously more inclined to ignore their negative emotions, which then become even more powerful motivators of their subsequent actions. When this is the case, the wife's smallest failings can flip a man into a rage. In addition, men may dread emotional exchanges because they sense that all the destructive emotions arising from their huge buried burden of unresolved feelings might spill out if they try to express one of them. This dread makes it virtually impossible for such men to share, express, or, using the language of love, "make a gift of" some past grievance or pain to the ones they love. It is essential to maintaining intimacy that such gifts be exchanged, regularly, and that we begin to seek more awareness of, acknowledge, then share the truth of our feelings as completely as we can. Otherwise, they become so important that they begin to influence in a negative way our thoughts and actions toward our spouse in the present moment.

Since there is no love after communication stops, and since intimacy depends on the frequent exchange of our desires, needs, and emotions, especially the ones that are most important to us, we must develop ways to get rid of our acquired barriers to connectedness. The hidden causes of our fears, anger, or sadness must be sought for and discovered, if we are to prevent them from directing our lives.

When we accept a need or a weakness in ourselves, we simultaneously hope that our lover can also accept it. Thus, when we present such a need as a gift to the one we love, we demonstrate our trust that he will accept it, too. Once our fault is accepted, it will cease to hurt us so much, or we might even be enabled to let it go.

Why should our mate accept our personal blemishes? For the very reason that each blemish is authentically us, and this exchange represents a true giving of ourselves, a sharing of the complete truth of where we are at that moment. If you want intimacy with someone, you must first be able to be vulnerable. No student of love disputes this fact. But being vulnerable means exposing ourselves and opening ourselves up to something that may produce pain or unpleasantness for us, something stronger or more powerful than we are, which has the potential to cause shame and blame. We choose to take that risk because if it happens that we are not shamed and blamed, and our mate accepts more of what we are, the bond of safety required for intimacy and the bond of intimacy, itself, are forged ever stronger.

The tragedy of our present society is not just that men and women do not communicate to each other clearly in the ways that matter most, that is, on the emotional or feeling level. Rather, the greater tragedy is that they choose to do little or nothing to remove their ignorance of the techniques that would transform their relationship—the techniques of communication.

Working Hardest on *Communication*

When women shout that men are remote, don't express themselves, are like statues or barbarians, are wise guys, condescending jerks (or in some cases, nonstop performing comedians), they show that they are missing a **vital truth that applies to virtually all men. This truth is that men are so sensitive, yet so unskilled in resolving their emotional problems, that they will flee any attempts to make them react emotionally.**

I heartily agree with Daphne Rose Kingma's hypothesis that in every troubled relationship between a man and a woman it is the woman who must be the mediator and initiator in the healing process, since this is every woman's special talent. One caution that must be unfailingly observed in this work: **safety must be absolutely guaranteed and maintained, otherwise the man's flight from vulnerability will not be reversed but rather made permanent**. (I'm referring to every negative attack on the person himself: criticism of his personality or temperament over which he has little control, mockery, sarcasm, skepticism, or cynicism. In no other situation in our lives is Edna St. Vincent Millay's poetic statement more applicable: ". . . love is the inexpressible comfort of safety.")

Learning How to Write Love Letters
(Among Other Great Ideas)

The entire "Marriage Encounter Movement," as first popular-ized in the sixties, was predicated on the belief that open and honest communication was the fundamental secret to staying in love. And, of course, it is. The daily **ten and ten**, that is, the ten minute love letter followed by a ten minute discussion did, in fact, help many married couples to better relationships. In practice, however, too many spouses (women much more often than men) thought honesty in relationships meant telling your mate what you hate about them and then expecting miracles to happen as a result. Sadly, these supposed love letters often lacked any expression of love. Such unstructured, unguided statements of pain or grievances rarely led to intimacy. Most often, especially when the participants were really at war, they produced casualties. Such casualties included many unbelievably bitter divorces, precisely because **the expressions of grievance were not always accompanied by expressions of love, and so they pro-vided plenty of reasons for the individuals involved to hate each other intensely.**

One other serious omission of the "ten and ten" technique was that not enough stress was given to the vast difference between men and women in their ability to express their feelings in words. This lack of an appreciation of the fact that **many men are indeed as loving as their mates, but that they never share their appreciation, concern, or devotion in words**, resulted in men being placed in an unacceptable "one-down" position. Unfortunately, men have been culturally indoctrinated to express their love exclusively by their actions, including their sexual actions. In addition, most men think that being a good protector and provider for their family proves quite convincingly their love for their family, since success usually requires hard work, courage, risk-taking, tenacity, and even suffer-ing.

To accomplish its purpose, a love letter obviously must express love. In fact, it must be intimate. This means that two independent and equal human beings become vulnerable to each other by sharing in writing something of themselves. As their feelings are disclosed and accepted, the bond of love and security between them is strengthened. Barbara De Angelis presents an **emotional map** of the **five levels of feelings** that must be expressed to make a love letter complete: 1) the anger or **grievance** must be expressed, to be followed by 2) any of your **other reactions** and 3) **feelings** that now accompanying your anger, such as sadness or disappointment and feelings of anxiety, insecurity, or fear for the future of the relationship. Then 4) some **personal responsibility** for possibly provoking his actions must be offered along with **your hopes** that things will improve. Finally 5) you must **reassert your love**, understanding, or appreciation for him.[24]

In seeking intimacy, a couple must always communicate with **complete truthfulness**. This means never burying or hiding or denying the negative emotions that they might be experiencing at the moment communication is attempted. Anything short of the whole truth can be deceptive, and such "dishonesty" will eventually destroy the love. For this reason, the love letter, or the "ten and ten," is not complete unless the writer includes all "the necessary parts." Besides the grievance and the accompanying reactions and feelings, there must definitely be an admission of some personal responsibility for the writer's reaction. For example, in writing, "**I have a problem** with handling put-downs," I must then **add the feelings** that now go with that reaction. For example, "They fill me with uncontrollable rage, so that I wish I could cut out your tongue or strangle you." (Obviously, ending the letter here would be disastrous.) The writer then expresses **the fears or anxieties that accompany the reaction** to the grievance, again **stressing that this part is one of the *writer's* problems**. After some hopeful **wish for better things** together, the love letter must be finished with an **expression of "love."** As one example, finish with "I love you, and I [affirm, support, respect, appreciate, or understand] that you do love me. I welcome and reciprocate that love, and I would like it to continue, despite these setbacks." If you cannot reach the loving part, do not send the letter.

Writing Love Letters to Help Yourself

The love letter is especially effective in resolving deep emotional conflicts that are too loaded to initiate face-to-face. Keep in mind that the purpose of love letters is not to change your partner or to make a point or to win an argument. In fact, it is best if you keep the head games out of it. The purpose is to get in touch with and to expose your own negative feelings, to clarify your own wishes and what you intend to do, and to experience and share the love that you feel within you. This sharing, this exercise in connectedness, or really doing something loving, guarantees to make **you** feel better.

In fact, remember to follow the rules of the love letter and you can't lose: first the grievance and accompanying feeling, such as "I hate it when you . . .;" then the hurt, the pain, the disappointment, as in, "It hurts me when . . .;" followed by any fears or anxieties the mate's actions produce in you, for example, "I am afraid that some-day we will not be together. . . ." At this point in the letter, it is time to share how what you say or do might be contributing to the problem: "I'm sorry when **I say mean things to you**. . . ." The final sections begin with your ideas, wishes, or suggestions for the future, such as, "I want us to plan time for each other . . .," followed by your expression of caring for your mate as a wonderful person, as in "I appreciate (love, care, support) what you have already done for me, such as. . . ."

It is suggested that you first practice the love letter technique by writing a few love letters to your friends. Don't mail them, but instead exchange these letters with your mate, and have him read your letters back to you. Once you master and appreciate the value of the technique, you can commence writing to your husband, and he to you.

Writing love letters to yourself is also highly recommended, especially when you are down on yourself, confused, or depressed. In fact, **the writing exercise as a way to express strong or difficult emotions can be used throughout life, whether one is in a close relationship or not**. Going back daily to an unresolved problem, whether new or old, until we have full awareness of what is causing us pain, anger, anxiety, sadness, or depression enables us to sort out the problems and deal with them. (This technique of expressing emotions in writing is yet another example of "journaling," which has already been recommended for gaining awareness of our needs, our health habits, our goals, our symptoms, our "talents," and the things that disturb, frighten, or move us. Writing such information daily can be an invaluable resource in adjusting to any difficult life passage, be it physical pain, mental or physical cruelty or abuse, menopause, an unfavorable diagnosis, infertility or miscarriage, infidelity, separation or divorce, or death of a loved one.

Some other techniques of communication between persons seeking intimacy, including verbal ones, which are safe when the emotional conflicts are not so overwhelming, are included later in this chapter and in Chapter Eleven.

Getting Your Needs *Across and Understood*

When someone loves another person, he or she naturally presumes that the beloved likes what the lover prefers. Yet, why is it that "doing unto others as you would have them do unto you" often moves couples away from intimacy, not toward it? Though George Bernard Shaw scornfully answered that question by claiming that no other person could imagine or match his good taste in things, the simple fact of the matter is that the basic principle of a love relationship is to **do unto others what they would have you do unto them.** Unfortunately, the obstacle to providing what the other wants is generally our mutual failure to explain clearly and understandably to our mates what we want them to do for us. Whining and complaining are generally very ineffective ways to communicate to a man, being poor substitutes for stating a specific need or grievance. (Women readily admit that they complain to each other all the time. Happily, this provides them not only emotional release and resolution but also an intimacy rarely ever achieved between men.)

The obstacle to your being closer to your husband is rarely that either of you lack for a caring mate. In fact, in most cases either of you would probably accept an expression or confession of need by the other, if it were made. Unfortunately, such "true confessions" are rare, and our confusion, misunderstanding, frustration, sadness, or anger is the result of our **mutual failure to clearly inform the other of even our most basic needs.**

Why don't men and women declare their needs to each other? The answer for most of us is that we really do not know what our needs are, because **we have never taken the time to discover them.**

The statement commonly made that "if my mate really cared about me, I wouldn't have to tell him/her what I want," ignores the reality that the sexes are so different that any consistency in knowing what our mates want is virtually impossible. Even with verbal communication, the messages can be distorted. In Chapter Thirteen, on "Sexuality," failure of communication is presented as a frequent cause of sexual problems. This fact is illustrated by the two very common "scripts" that can do harm to a sexual relationship: 1) "My husband, if he is a real and normal man, should know how to provide me with great sexual pleasure," or 2) "How can I, with all the negative sexual training I have received since infancy, ever be expected to know, or to explain to my husband, even if I did know, the specific sexual techniques that would be best for me? Certainly most men would be offended, or shocked, or worse." In truth, it would be a rare man who would be any of those things. Neither script is true.

Selecting Among **Non-Written** Ways to Communicate

That one partner does not typically hear what the other partner is saying is the reason that marriage therapists insist, from the beginning, that the **mirroring** technique, or exercise, be practiced and mastered. Simply put, in this technique, one person states very briefly a desire, feeling, or need, and the other then says what he/she has just been told. The same thought is repeated until what has been said is acknowledged by the sender as correctly heard. This process continues for a specified length of time, usually agreed upon in advance. Satisfying results are often immediately felt. Just knowing that the spouse has heard what you said, that he/she has listened, perhaps for the first time, can reverse a trend toward decreasing connectedness. With an even simpler variation, referred to as the **duplicating** technique, the original speaker's words are repeated exactly. One caution: for deep emotional conflicts that seem overwhelming, the face-to-face methods should be postponed until the love letter approach has defused all the explosive issues. Some marriage counselors suggest an even simpler technique of oral communication, called **paired listening**, in which the ground rules are that each partner alternates speaking for five minutes at a time, while the other can do **nothing** except listen. Again, the purpose is to accustom yourself to speaking freely without fear of interruption or argument, and to learn to listen without interrupting, interpreting, or arguing. The sense of being heard and understood might well be achieved this simple way. (**A neat use of this technique**, suggested by Alice Domar and Henry Dreher, one that will quickly demonstrate that **communication can be about positive and joyous things**, is to have each partner alternately have a few minutes to exchange their thoughts on three different topics: something each likes about her/himself that was never told to the other; something each likes about the partner that also was never shared; and, something each person likes about their relationship that was never mentioned before.)[25]

Two other exercises in communication generally suggested for couples, even those who have had no formal marriage therapy are:

1) **setting aside a specific time when the expression of anger is allowed** by partner "A." The roles are, of course, subsequently reversed at some later time, but partner "B," when it is his turn, may not say anything that refers directly to, or rebuts, partner "A's" original remarks. This prohibition should preferably last forever, but must be observed for at least several days.

2) **compiling a list of as many wishes or needs as you can** think of—a "wish list," not a litany of "gripes"—then exchanging them with your spouse. (With a few seconds' thought, any wife could quickly come up with at least forty examples. The husband might have as many, but it would probably take him days to discover them.) Some common examples: a weekly **date,** an occasional thoughtfulness or present, more hugs, spending more time listening, helping with the chores, initiating sex once in a while or being a little more active, fixing the broken . . ., or putting the clean or soiled laundry away.

In making wish lists, as in the sessions where anger is expressed, any comments about the partner's character or past behavior must be avoided. What is to be communicated are one's own feelings and needs. In every case, however, they are to be considered requests only, as nothing must ever be demanded or required. It is most important that any wish granted be seen as a pure gift, and not a form of barter or exchange. One common example of barter in a relationship would be offering "this" in exchange for "that," with the first being "flowers" and the latter "sex." Motive is critical here, since many giving activities are really about getting something back, and our spouses know it. Something offered with the idea that a debt has been created is not a gift, but rather a purchase. It is human to run away from such gifts. Too, in many relationships, one person will knock himself/herself out doing things for the other in a desperate search for approval. Again, this is "barter," not love, as should be recognized by the lack of a loving response on the part of the receiver.

When favors are exchanged with a loving motive, eventually, if not soon, surprise or unasked-for-gifts are being exchanged, generally bringing back many of the emotions from the honeymoon phase in the distant past. One special bonus from exchanging such a list is that the wishes expressed can be very useful in rejuvenating a tepid sex life.[26]

If your mate will not write wish lists, or love letters, do them anyway, since they are not primarily intended to change him but to get you in touch with your own needs and to provide an exercise in expressing and sharing love. Why is it that we so seldom act on the truth we know: that the **greatest joys of life are in the living and the giving, not the promise of rewards?**

Mind-Reading Without a License

In the absence of explicit communication between mates, guessing, or even mind-reading, appears. But, while men can sometimes read each others' minds, and women often can read other women's minds, neither can read the minds of the opposite sex. When they attempt to do so, trouble is inevitable. In *Men, Women, and Relationships: Making Peace with the Opposite Sex*, John Gray states that a woman tends to read even a man's *behavior* negatively. She interprets his silence as lack of caring, his lateness as a sign of her unimportance to him, or his forgetting as an act of revenge.[27] (Unfortunately, sometimes the woman's judgment is correct. This negative reading of a man's behavior, which may or may not be justified, suggests that it might be better for the relationship if a man would more often admit when his behavior reflects anger and when he has made a simple mistake or was simply not thinking. **The lady in question can then eventually decide how much simple forgetting is too much**.)

Putting Your Plans Into Practice

In summary, a committed relationship in which two people share a common vision can provide the perfect vehicle for the expression of their aliveness to each other. Permanent relationships can provide all the psychotherapy each needs to heal her/his childhood wounds. The process begins as each accepts in the partner the expression of those emotions or attributes that have been denied in her/himself. The process continues as each takes responsibility for or re-owns those emotions (anger, for example) that have been projected onto the partner. (This transfer of anger, whereby the woman is always angry while the man is never angry, yet it is the man's buried pain that instigates the whole scenario, was cited as one of the most common dynamics in American marriages.) Intimacy in such a situation becomes possible only when the man can accept some responsibility for the anger in the relationship, at least by accepting the possibility that the anger present may be the result of his repressed feelings.

One fact is certain: desired changes in a spouse are never accomplished by asking for reformation or conformity. Rather, such changes often happen when one or the other begins to try to change him/herself. Intimacy can exist only between equals, and persons who have a clear appreciation of their separateness. It is helpful to remember: nothing—"not psychotherapy, religious discipline, or social revolutions"—promotes personal growth and healing of the childhood wounds, which ruin our adult relationships, better than the spousal commitment to the work of love.[28]

In this chapter we have presented five of the "seven techniques" that Judith Wallerstein, in *The Good Marriage: How and Why Love Lasts*, suggests as the keys to a successful marriage. Sexuality and Intimacy/Autonomy will be discussed in Chapters Thirteen and Fourteen. Ruth Westheimer adds the necessity of maintaining some separate interests, which assures that each mate will always have a plentiful supply of new things to say.[29]

However, the most insightful ideas for bringing harmony and peace to a marriage have been presented by Daphne Rose Kingma, who ends *The Men We Never Knew* with twenty-five specific suggestions for women to help guide their mate with safety and patience to expressions of his feelings. By showing him how to express his feelings verbally, and thus not continue to be limited to using actions, non-actions, or body language to show his joy, sadness, anger, or fear, they can open up the possibilities for an unprecedented dialogue of love.[30] (You are invited to check the list—references 46, 51, 52, 76, 88, 96, 97—of the most recent and most successful guides for working with your mate. If you are both willing to work, expect to discover that the best part of your marriage is yet to come!)[31]

The next chapter takes up the unique problems for the woman who is presently without a committed relationship.

11

Learning from Past Mistakes

Four of every ten first marriages will end in divorce (down from five of every ten). However, in some areas the divorce rate is still rising, now reaching seventy-five percent, for example, in Southern California. Nationally, the failure rate for second marriages is six of every ten. **It is easier to get a divorce in the United States than any other Western country except Sweden.** Compared to an average wait of one year in this country, the wait is five years in England and six years in France. That Americans remain committed to the institution of family is shown by the fact that **our remarriage rate is the world's highest**, with seventy-five percent of the men trying again and sixty percent of the women.

If you are divorced, you are destined to repeat your past mistakes if you carry feelings of blame, revenge, or anger against your former partner into the next relationship. Barbara DeAngelis points out in *Making Love All the Time* that if you continue to criticize him, to feel like you were victimized and "got nothing" out of the time you shared with him, then you are not healed enough to be loving to another mate. It is true you must forgive yourself, but first you must forgive him. This is not to say that you approve of him, or that you should feel in any way guilty about what he was or did. Obviously, that would be a mistake.[1]

However, as Geneen Roth describes in *When Food Is Love,* before you can forgive, you must "grieve." You need to grieve for yourself and for the suffering, anger, loss, or desolation that he caused. The grieving takes both courage and time and includes sorrowing for the lost years. The process is the same as grieving after the death of a friend, or during one's own terminal illness. Denial, confusion or bargaining, rage, grief, and acceptance, must be experienced. Then, and only then, is any forgiveness possible.[2]

After the forgiveness and letting go of the feelings, the work of learning from the experience begins. To avoid the same mistake and marrying "him" all over again, or repeating the same mistakes that were unsuccessful in creating or sustaining that relationship, I suggest that you compile as complete a list as you can of your previous mistakes, starting with all the incompatibilities that existed between you. In this work, you should devote most of your search to the beginning of the relationship, rather than spend time examining all the reasons that you battled or all the techniques you both used to win. (The apparent reasons for your battles were probably not the real issues anyway.)

Harville Hendrix, in *Keeping the Love You Find,* exhorts men and women, of whatever age, to use the **single** stage of their life, including before, between, or after marriages, as a temporary opportunity, or window, to learn how to improve their communication skills, with a view toward bettering their subsequent relationships. Hendrix' book provides psychological exercises for singles so that they can devote that phase of their life to self-discovery, especially trying to find their deepest needs and deepest wounds. Perhaps love was always conditional in their life or they never achieved any confidence in their own worth. There are for all of us many possible scars from the past that still hurt. By first working alone, and then, later perhaps, working with a partner, each can undertake the very demanding task of finding and reclaiming those qualities which each has lost or buried. The more unconscious needs one can bring into consciousness, or recognize, the more control one will gain over his or her present choices and reactions.

> "If one is serious about having a full and lasting love relationship, you have to get serious about being single . . . forget the mating game [until you] educate yourself about relationships; educate yourself about yourself; train yourself in the skills of relationships; [and] do what you can to change the behaviors and character defenses that are preventing you from keeping the love you find."[3]

Remember that the person you win in a committed relationship, whether it is the first relationship or not, is typically your camouflaged **match**. Thus, if you want a relationship with someone special, someone who will impress you and whom you can respect, it is obviously essential that you work to **become special**. Recognize and do something about your most glaring deficiencies, and affirm and strengthen those qualities that make you more lovable and unique. The key is to show that you love and care about yourself. Thus, **as** you will find yourself doing things to impress yourself, you will, in fact, be demonstrating to those around you that you love and care about yourself.

Accepting Your Essential **Connectedness**

Despite your personal responsibility to undertake self-improvement, it is nevertheless true that no matter how much you esteem your own efforts, the first step toward human relatedness, the first step on the path to intimacy, still remains the "acceptance of another's acceptance."[4] One must believe, very early on in the self-improvement process, that another person accepts them. Unfortunately, for someone looking for that initial affirmation, it matters little who that other person is. This statement means that, because **self-love cannot simply be manufactured without at least some outside input, it is necessary in the very beginning of the intimacy process for us to discover it in the eyes or words of another.** Obviously, who that affirming or accepting other person is might possibly have much to do with our future happiness. Therefore, in our search for intimacy, we need to maintain a certain vigilance, values, and standards regarding the person whose acceptance we earnestly seek.

The overwhelming consensus in psychiatry now is that even before we are born, we exist in relationships, and that it is in and through our relationships that solutions to our needs are to be found and human growth is to be achieved. In this regard, John Bradshaw adds that you can read all the self-help books on self-esteem until hell freezes over, and nothing will change until you restore the "interpersonal bridge" that allows you to become connected to others.[5] It is for this reason that no addict, whether addicted to food, sex, drugs, violence, or abuse, can cure himself. The admission of personal powerlessness and the willingness to reach out for help restores the interpersonal bridge. Even encounter groups of the most informal kinds can often provide us with a crucial sense of security and belonging and constitute reality checks for what it is essential for us to know about ourselves, and for what we can't discover alone.

In or out of a committed relationship, we are all lovers-in-training, and no relationship is ever truly wasted.[6]

Facing the Challenges Unique to a *Single Woman*

Being single in America obviously presents challenges that the woman in a permanent relationship does not have to face. In addition to the lack of support and companionship provided by a live-in mate, there is also generally the perception that the woman in such a situation would be married or remarried, if she could get a husband. This is especially believed if the woman in question has not achieved a comfortable standard of living. Of course, poverty is most devastating to the single woman when young children are included. There are now, in fact, twice as many single mother families as there are "homemaker-mom" families.

There are now also record numbers of single American women, both those with dependent children and those without any. Besides the nearly twenty million single women over fifty-five years of age, there are an even greater number of younger women who are single, at least temporarily. Two-and-a-half times as many women between the ages of twenty and twenty-nine are single now, than one generation ago.[7] Included in the single group are a significant number of women who express the desire to marry for the first time, but who will never achieve their wish. After age twenty-nine, the number of involuntarily-single women increases dramatically. The most optimistic statistics for never-married women reports that college grads at age thirty have a fifty-eight to sixty-six percent chance of finding a spouse; at thirty-five, the chance slips to thirty-two to forty-one percent, and at age forty, the percentages drop to seventeen to twenty-three.[8]

Despite the record number of single women, the percentage of women in this country who do marry, at least for a time, or have children, either in or out of a permanent relationship, is also the highest in our country's history. Still, nearly one-third of all families now have only a single parent, with ninety percent of these single parents being women. **More than half the single parent families live below the poverty line.** Since the average income of mothers in this group is $16,000, it is easy to see why the number one priority of single women in recent polls is more money.[9] Also true is that seventy to ninety percent of children born out of wedlock end up on welfare and stay there much longer than children of divorced parents.[10]

In order to highlight some of the more common difficulties faced by single women in American society, I have chosen to briefly describe one of many such patients from my practice, whom I will refer to as Margaret (though that was not her name). Of the ten stupid things that Laura Schlessinger says women commonly do to mess up their lives, Margaret had done all of them before she was thirty.[11]

Margaret's husband abused, then abandoned, both her and their one-year-old son when Margaret was only twenty-one.[12] I still see her regularly for checkups because she has chosen oral contraceptives to protect herself from any further pregnancies.

At the time of her graduation from high school, Margaret had great prospects for the future, because of our cultural bias toward beauty, and sometimes toward intelligence. Despite these gifts, she had fled to an early marriage primarily to escape from home and from an abusive father. He never overtly sexually abused her, as far as I know, but neither did he once, according to her account, ever show respect for her as a woman. Her mother could barely survive her own fears and anxieties, much less protect or affirm her daughter.

The phase of romantic love in Margaret's marriage lasted nearly two years.[13] When her husband slowly but unmistakably began to distance himself, by his work and his attitude, Margaret decided that her fulfillment would lie in being a mother and then in giving her offspring all the safety, love, and affirmation she had never received. This love for her child, she stoutly believed, would be reciprocated, and thus she would finally have, for the first time in her life, someone who would eventually love and care about her.

Margaret never discussed with her husband the incredibly important decision she had made to get pregnant. She simply stopped her birth control pills. Unfortunately, when Margaret announced her pregnancy, her husband became furious and, as was typical of the way he acted out his disapproval, he slugged her.[14] This event, however, initiated his emotional and sexual abandonment, though he still resorted to physical abuse periodically. His total physical desertion, which led to an eventual divorce, occurred soon after their baby's birth.

(Obviously, not all men who abuse their wives seek divorce. In the greater number of cases, two-thirds in fact, it is the wife who decides the husband's liabilities outweigh the benefits of the marriage relationship. In the matter of the wife abused physically by her husband, certain important principles need to be emphasized. A woman must never tolerate **any** physical abuse. This statement applies, even if the perpetrator is wonderful 99.9% of the time. No religious belief in man as the head of the family should prevent a woman from taking immediate action to ensure that one episode of violence can never be repeated. No counselor could ever rightly advise differently. Moreover, it would be absurd to say that the physical abuse of women by their mates could ever, in any way, be the victims' own fault! Though both partners share the responsibility for the anger and resentment that arises periodically in any committed relationship, the one who resorts to violence as a way to handle conflict or disagreements, is totally and solely responsible for his actions.

Physical abuse must never be minimized—it is always serious! When the physician becomes aware of the problem, he is obligated to see that it is reported. If separate accommodations are not available immediately, the victim, or potential victim, must at least have instant access to help if needed, and a precise escape plan.)

Discovering that Your Husband **Hates Women!**

As women come to realize that a man's physical intimidation is perverse, and therefore totally unacceptable, a special type of wife-abuser, namely the **misogynist**, defined as the man who hates women, is now being much more frequently recognized.

Incredible as it may seem, men who harbor a lifetime hatred for women typically are not at all aware of their hatred. Equally startling is the fact that their wives do not recognize that their husbands hate women either. In fact, both the men themselves and their wives typically rate the misogynists as basically "good" husbands. They are more than adequate as sexual partners. A woman-hater is definitely **not** a Don Juan, that is, he is not a womanizer, defined as a man who is awed by his own sexual abilities. He is, in fact, a faithful spouse.

(Misogynists, surprisingly, are not sadistic lovers either. Portrayals of such sadism abound, by definition, in "pornographic" literature. Examples are quoted in every offensive detail by Kate Millett, in *Sexual Politics*, in order for her to make her point that men's sexual domination of women is nothing more or less than a demonstration of their total domination in everything else.)[15]

However, misogynists are very much into **control**, and that control typically applies to only one woman! Tragically, their need to emotionally dominate their mate is so overwhelming that they are very difficult to get away from, as the wife who seeks divorce often discovers.

Despite the fact that a neutral observer would quickly see that the misogynist despises his mate, the abuser himself does not realize his hate and continues to act committed to the marriage. Apparently, he retains the hope that someday the woman involved will learn how to do everything the way he demands. By blaming all the unhappiness in the relationship on the woman's failure to correct her own faults, the misogynist finds ample justification for his cruelty. Although his abuse is typically mental and verbal, his controlling attitude nevertheless always carries with it the threat, at least, of physical violence. Unfortunately for the victim, the behavior that the man expects from her is always in a state of flux. As a consequence, her life is generally one of continual confusion, frustration, and abject misery.

The tragedy represented in a misogynous relationship is that the woman involved thinks that everything negative that she experiences in the relationship is her fault. After all, the misogynist, characteristically, is not only good with sexual expression, but also quite charming, thoughtful, romantic, attentive, and otherwise endearing. Except, of course, for the occasions when he is enraged, overly critical about trivia, belittling, sarcastic, or demanding. Because the wife accepts self-blame, she perseveres in the relationship, and thus perpetuates the union. There is one additional tragic aspect: the anger that is present in the woman who is being controlled is typically repressed; or, the anger is turned against herself as depression. In either case, self-destructive behaviors can result, for example, substance abuse or even suicide. In the case where the anger is simply repressed, what is seen by the people who know her is a woman devoid of any emotions, a woman who would be best described as "dull" or "numb."

When a woman realizes that her mate may be a misogynist, she is neither thereby justified in condemning him, nor is she absolved from any responsibility for the troubled relationship. That would be denying the basic principle of all relationships: we select someone we deserve, or someone whom we believe will fill our needs. A man who hates women has been abused in some way by women, and is, in fact, using control as a way to handle all his insecurities toward women. The woman selected him because she was also, in some significant way, insecure, and sensed his "control" would eliminate her insecurities.

Nevertheless, when anyone realizes they may possibly be a cooperator in such a relationship, that person must seek help. I recommend reading Susan Forward's _Men Who Hate Women & The Women Who Love Them_ as one step toward understanding the situation, but seeking individual professional help is definitely advised. The shame and guilt that the person "sleeping with the enemy" inevitably feels, is best resolved in a therapeutic setting, lest the tragic choice be repeated.[16]

Despite her obvious gifts of beauty and intelligence, Margaret's subsequent choices for committed relationships, not to mention the occasional one-night or three-night stands, continued to provide graphic proof of how little she reverenced herself and how little self-esteem her family had provided.[17]

Undoubtedly, many women use sex addictively, that is, using sex with people they care little about as a way to avoid facing their pain, sadness, anger, or feelings of worthlessness. The tragedy for large numbers of single women like Margaret does not consist in their simply being temporarily without a committed relationship. Singleness can occur at any age, even though **there is no shortage of single men, especially in the "prime" marrying years, ages twenty-four to fifty-five**.[18] The tragedy for these single women, whether mothers or not, is that no one has been able to convince them that their subsequent relationships might turn out better, if they would invest some time and effort in finding out why their relationship failed, or why they are still single. (Unless, of course, it is their deliberate choice). In practice, it appears that few ever bother to determine what they might have contributed to a previous failed relationship. Rather, the judgment is that life was unkind to them or that they were simply unlucky.

When single women believe that their situation is solely due to a failure to find the right man, the perfect partner, then those who previously mated unsuccessfully are surely destined to repeat their mistake. Why will they fail again? The answer is: because no such perfect partner exists.

Starting with Sincere *Self-Examination*

As a first requirement, those whose relationships have failed need to recognize that there is something missing from their mate selection process. In addition, they need to be convinced that they can change it. How can they change the process? The answer to that question is basically that they begin the journey of self-discovery that we have described in "Understanding the Message" on page xvii at the beginning of the book and again in Chapter Ten, to which I will now add.

Laura Schlessinger pleads that women must decide that an "I love you" will not be the great excuse for not working at personal growth, or for not maintaining personal responsibility for the risks and hard decisions that maturity demands.

The journey of self-discovery can never begin too soon. Don't postpone being a loving person until you fall in love. Become the kind of person you want to meet. Become a more caring person, one who appreciates, supports, affirms, respects, and tries to better understand others.

Your first assignment in the work of making better choices is to complete your own personal "compatibility list." After all, the **chief message of this book is the need to make your own decisions**, *based on adequate knowledge of the facts*. Making sure you know exactly what you want and what you need in a mate requires that you know yourself completely: what your personal interests are, your short term and long term goals, your hobbies, your ideas of having fun, your education, your religious and moral choices, and, finally, how you have been spending your time.

If your relationship survives to the third date, don't be afraid to suggest to your date that he make his own compatibility list. In fact, you should insist on it. Share your list with friends, in order to get their suggestions, comments, or criticisms. Keep it up-to-date as you change and grow. Resist the temptation to put anything on your list that isn't totally true, in the hope perhaps of impressing or pleasing anyone. You do, after all, want them to like the real you. If you meet a person who is not like the one you are looking for, remember that you are not the person he is looking for either—regardless of how attracted to each other you may be in the beginning.[19]

In courtship, it is imperative that your decisions be guided by the head and not the heart. Dr. Schlessinger labels it "stupid passion" to allow sex before every part of you is ready, including your mind and reason. When a woman lets a man have sex with her, she usually thinks he feels the same way about her that she feels about him. Why not at least ask him first what having sex with you is going to mean to him? Please don't answer that you can have sex with a man but cannot discuss its significance to your relationship. Sex never validates you or the relationship.

Dr. Schlessinger also suggests eighteen months as a minimum before engagement to allow time to discover if he is dishonest, controlling, dependable, dependent, abusive, mean, cold, addictive, violent, negative, jealous, or a workaholic. She suggests this rather long interval because so many women find it impossible "to be cruel enough" to drop someone when they eventually discover he is unworthy of them, once the engagement has been announced. It is **very important, also, to keep asking yourself if you are looking for the best person, or the one easiest to hold on to.**

In the same vein, consider that women seem to find it almost impossible to accept the truth that they cannot change a man. Whether attempts are made before or after marriage, any woman's actions of trying to change her mate (and change is always sought for one's own good, not the spouse's) provides proof that the woman believes that her worth depends on his performance or qualities and not hers. By attaching or clinging to him in dependency, she is in no way being loving. This matter of making your own decisions and letting your mate make his own decisions is a crucial component of an intimate relationship.

Therefore, having considered many suggestions on how to establish or improve your close relationships with another adult who is your equal, you can, in the next chapter, consider your crucial but very unequal parent/child relationships.

There will always be a few who care little about what we have been describing in these last two chapters as the work of love, but most, I sincerely believe, welcome such information, which could help heal their relationships, and in the process provide their children with a working model of love.

12

Keeping Love in the Family

*"... [the] good people ... are always 'there,' who can be relied upon
in small, important ways. People who teach us, encourage us,
support us, uplift us in the dailiness of life. We never tell them. ...
And, of course, we play that role ourselves. There are those
who depend on us, watch us, learn from us, take from us.
And we never know. Don't sell yourself short. You may never
have proof, but you are more important than you think."*
—Robert Fulghum, *All I Ever Really Wanted to Know
I Learned in Kindergarten*

*"Procreation has little to do with your needs;
it has everything to do with a child's needs."*
—Laura Schlessinger, *Ten Stupid Things
Women Do to Mess Up Their Life*

If I could live my life over again, the choices I would most like to
change would be the ways I related to my children, especially my
sons. I doubt whether I would ever use physical punishment again.
My oldest son, James L., dedicated his book, *In Search of Lost Fathering*, to me, supporting his assurances that he has forgiven me for the
stern discipline I imposed on him almost from the day of his birth.
He has tried often to convince me that the guilt that I feel now is not
justified. Perhaps someday I will be able to take him at his word, but
for now I see my son's drive to become "one of the world's top

Christian childhood-and-adolescent psychiatrists" as an example of the age old tradition of sons who need to best their fathers, but who sometimes, in the process, forego things that might be a lot more fun.[1]

Without question, the most important gift a mother and father can give to their child, regardless of their moral convictions or technique of discipline, is a happy attitude toward living. This gift is given or withheld long before there is any other influence from any other person or thing, and certainly before the question of upbringing is involved. We all accept the truth that an **infant** (by definition, **a child up to the age of two years**) cannot be spoiled or receive too much love. Despite this certain knowledge, many of us still ration our attention and responsiveness during these first two years because we do, in fact, feel somehow we **are** spoiling our babies by our constant attention.

Nancy Friday theorizes, in *My Mother/My Self*, "that we get our courage, our sense of self, the ability to believe we have value even when alone, to do our work, to love others, and to feel ourselves lovable, from the strength of our mother's love for us when we were infants."[2] Surely, this seems to be logical and true. Unfortunately, as Friday herself describes the mass of mother-daughter relationships, something invariably happens, as childhood and adolescence unfolds, to wreck the mother-daughter relationship. In this chapter, I will try to dissect the various realities that prevent the ideal of a loving family from being realized.

Uncovering the Realities of the *Typical* American Family

It is a tragic fact that on any given day, four women and three children will be killed by a family member. Thus, no one can claim that the topic of getting more love in the family is not of momentous importance.

Defining a **family** as two or more persons living together in one household related by marriage, birth, adoption, or a cohabitation agreement (the last includes the 1,600,000 gay and lesbian "couples" and the roughly 2,000,000 two-parent families in which one member is explicitly same-sex oriented), there are about seventy-five million American families, with half of them having children under eighteen years of age. The number of births to unmarried mothers is now 1,200,000 per year, a figure that keeps increasing, but the **fastest growing segment of the population is the number of men or women who live alone—now numbering one of every four households.** The average age of the man alone is forty-one, and the average age of the woman alone is sixty-one.

The fact that nearly thirty percent of American families are headed by a single mother, and that half of our teenage mothers are unmarried, should provide graphic evidence that up to now, little time or education has been provided in either our families or in our schools in either self-knowledge or relational skills that would prevent such overwhelming numbers of our young women from apparently messing up their lives (and, of course, the lives of their children).

How can advice and insight on what is for most women the two most important decisions in life—choosing a spouse and having a child—be imparted to children, when one or the other parent is absent, an uncaring stranger, always at work, or when both are primarily engaged in their own power struggle. (A recent survey reported that forty-two percent of children ages nine and under are left alone at least part of the time.)[3]

The environment at school in many cases is even unsafe, especially for teenage girls. The chief concern for many teachers is control, not teaching, because of the attitude the students bring from their homes and their neighborhoods.

Parents have to provide models of love, morality, attention, character, caring, comfort, support, service, and guidance to their children. Many of us fail in teaching our children how to choose a partner because we do not have that information ourselves, or we are still locked in the power-struggle phase of our own relationships.

*Seeking a **Better Approach** to Parenting*

The old school of child raising is now criticized for all its punishing of children, that is, for using the stick approach. The new school claims to be much more enlightened and asserts that rewards, especially praise, provide the key to raising children successfully. This is the carrot approach.

While the stick and the carrot work fairly well when you are trying to control a jackass, there are at least thirty years of scientific studies that show they don't work too well with kids. There are many very clear reasons why **it is a fact**, as Alfie Kohn writes, that **children are "punished by rewards,"**[4] Unfortunately, both parents and our educators have chosen to ignore the disastrous side effects of basing training and education primarily on a system of punishments or rewards. The present result is that our children are marinated, or, in fact, drowning, in a sea of rewards or punishments all the time. However, this is but one reason that few of our offspring are learning the "5 R's," (the last two R's being "respect" and "responsibility.") The other fundamental reason our children are not learning is that the two-and-a-half million public school teachers, their students, and the students' parents do not know the core material that must be covered and mastered by every student in each specific grade. The idea that there exists a coherent plan for teaching content within the local school district or even the individual school is a gravely misleading myth.[5]

Moreover, there are now many studies showing that resorting consistently to the imposition of external forces, whether in the form of rewards, even praise, or punishments, generally produces inferior and less desirable results than those obtained by "hooking" the student's desire to learn with a clear, accomplishable goal.[6]

Sticking to the Basics—*Acceptance, Attention, and Support*

In contrast to the elementary school systems so successful in Europe and Asia, in which praise is rarely seen, in which no errors are ignored and immediate clarification and correction of such errors is demanded, the most frequent form of evaluation used by American teachers is praise, a technique that is intended to bolster self-esteem regardless of academic achievement. The result is complacency or skepticism or both, and ultimately a **decline** in self-esteem.

The same principles apply in parent/child relationships. A child who trusts his parents, who has had ample proof of their support, affection, and acceptance, will be much more likely to share, to risk, to admit ignorance, or to ask for help. **"You are wonderful" statements put children on a shaky pedestal and require little effort or**

attention on the part of the one giving such praise. Much preferable is to pay close attention to what our children do or do not do, giving specific appraisals or progress reports (and praise when it is deserved), which truly educate, because such thoughtful evaluations recognize and separate successful effort, unsuccessful effort, or lack of effort, as well as mistakes, and provide specific ongoing corrections.

Of course, it is important to believe and accept that, while children often do as we do and sometimes do as we say, they are highly likely to model their life on the ideals or priorities that we carry in our deepest, most secret heart!

Lessening the **Intimidation** and Increasing the **Communication**

In discharging their responsibilities to their children on a day-to-day basis, parents can easily forget how weak and vulnerable their children are. To lessen the intimidating force of just our immense size compared to that of our young children, John Bradshaw suggests we sit on the floor whenever possible when we communicate with them, especially when we are instructing them, so as to be nearly at their eye level. The popularity of Steven Spielberg's movies with children has been credited, partly at least, to his extensive use of child-level camera angles.

In my son's book, *The Search for Lost Fathering,* the point is repeatedly made that because fathers can be so dominating or so intimidating, the predominant features of their personalities can be crucial to their children's development.[7] But, this does not imply that mothers are not equally crucial. Camille Paglia, in *Sexual Personae,* provides concrete illustrations from the art of Western civilization to show that the way the mother is perceived by the artist in his earliest years influences to an almost unbelievable degree all of his/her works.[8]

Examining the **Mother's Role**

Nancy Friday places the blame for a woman's low self-esteem, passivity, lack of competitiveness or courage, and even her failure to achieve full adult sexuality or marital adjustment squarely on the presence of **unresolved problems** with her mother.[9] Judy Hollis also blames all eating disorders on this mother/daughter conflict or wound.[10] The fact that these problems often begin, in most cases, before the development of memory, doesn't prevent the unconscious mind from remembering them in a way that influences one's adult choices. Therefore, unless Dad did the bulk of the mothering, it is difficult to deny that some benefit will be derived from an evaluation of the mother/daughter relationship, with the intent of increasing openness, honesty, and tolerance, and decreasing competition and criticism. Whatever insights are achieved through an interaction with mother can then be used to improve the communication with one's own daughter.

The mother and daughter seeking to communicate better need to drop the masks and avoid lies and half-truths, while retaining a confidence that any attempt at greater friendship between persons of good will can survive some truthful exchange of grievances. Mothers and daughters might then understand at least a few of their recurring problems well enough to let them go.[11]

It is essential, however, when discussing the very rewarding goal of rapprochement between mothers and their adult daughters, to remember that intimacy is possible only between equals. For the reason that you will always be "her daughter" and she will always be "your mother," don't expect too much, at least in the beginning. Even a little progress in sharing thoughts more honestly with each other should be a cause for great hope.[12] (See the Appendix, pages 248–49, for a "Meditation on Mothering"—one mother's very practical appraisal of the process.)

It is important to remember that your parents' attempts to shield you from the evils of the world may have thwarted your efforts, at four or five and in early adolescence, to separate yourself from them as you tried to find your own independent identity. By their resistance to your natural drive toward more independence, or to your acquisition of more control over your own decisions, resentment and anger could have been generated, which you still carry along with you when you relate to them. If you now have children, the same dynamics are at work in them. Again, as in all close relationships, the talent that we should try to develop is the ability to handle any resentment and anger, as it arises, and as we recognize it. For pleasant and peaceful coexistence, and for more intimacy, we need to know how to manage or resolve conflict.

In each generation, too much control by the parent can produce the successive steps to "enmity," which means that all the interpersonal bridges are removed, as the child uses the four "R's," referred to in Chapter 10: first the child feels the need for **resistance**, which is soon followed by his or her **resentment**. If neither the parent or child accepts the other's wishes or needs, the next step toward separation, or alienation, is **rejection** by the child of that particular parental connection. Then, because this is so painful, or guilt-producing, this can often lead to **repression** or depression.[13] As a consequence, the controlled individual, most often a daughter in our culture, may, at some point in the relationship with her parents, in an unconscious attempt to reverse the process and reconnect to the parents, try to vent her anger, frustration, or rage, in a variety of **self**-destructive ways, which means ways that do not directly harm her parents. Any direct attack on the parent would be seen by the controller of the whole process, namely the unconscious mind of the daughter, as a sure way to "lose the parent forever."

Unfortunately, food disorders or addictions constitute one of the adolescent girl's favorite ways to bond, whether the connection is one of dependency or control. Either technique enables the daughter to preserve the parent/daughter relationship by involving them in bonds of dependency and concern.

Another technique used by adolescent girls to thwart parental influence without directly confronting or endangering the parents, or without being forced to resolve the real conflicts between parents/child, is for the daughter to transfer all dependency needs from her parents to her peers. The attempt to successfully forge an identity separate from their parents can often spur these teenagers into an early marriage. This last choice resolves nothing of importance, but, obviously does provide the formula for transferring all the adolescent's problems with mom or dad onto her new husband. Chances are, unfortunately, that the new husband has his own problems with growing up. Once the mistake is recognized, the tragedy is often compounded by a rush to motherhood!

In her book, *My Mother, My Self*—a chronicle of mother/daughter bonds and how they might be broken—Nancy Friday repeatedly stresses that motherhood is not a solution to loneliness, immaturity, or an unfortunate marriage choice. Motherhood is an incredibly difficult challenge that multiplies the effects of one's immaturity:

"Whether you call it instinct or not, most women enjoy having children, want to, and do. (Yet) For this majority, the trouble begins . . . with the emotional propositions contained in the notion of maternal instinct. . . . (M)other love (does not) well up spontaneously the moment a child is born. . . . (It is) the great American myth that all mothers love their babies. . . . (T)he tyrann(ical) notion of maternal instinct idealizes motherhood beyond human capacity."[14]

Many mothers confess that it took weeks until they "cared" for their baby, or that moment to moment they did not "instinctively know how to be a good mother. It is not easy; it is not automatic. . . . (That) myth (has been promulgated) by men."[15] Parental crisis centers can be filled with women who fear that they will harm their babies, and, as we hear or read daily, many do.

Unfortunately, it is the women who have traditionally been assigned in our culture the task of maintaining relationships. Thus, an escape to marriage is one step that is quite likely to be calamitous for the girl who has not acquired any skill in expressing and resolving her grievances and needs. The relationships that are forged in these early marriages tend to be ones of mutual and chronic dependency, the situation psychologists call co-dependency, whereby the people involved lack any of the skills and insights needed to develop a satisfactory or responsible adult relationship. In co-dependent relationships, each becomes the sole source of satisfaction and affirmation for the other, much like a mother and her newborn infant. Eventually, as in the case of the child, the stage of rebellion arrives, when one seeks to escape the unnatural fusion, the lack of personal space, or the feelings of being used or controlled by the other, and so begins to explore elsewhere.

Happily, having had very controlling parents does not inevitably condemn a child to a lifetime of allowing himself or herself to be controlled, nor does it mean he will be controlling of his children. In fact, if any child can retain a sense of his/her own worth, or the will to understand why his parents might be controlling him, or get persistent affirmation from another source (all very likely possibilities), he can readily repair the damage. For example, Karen Horney, one of the most influential psychoanalysts of the twentieth century, escaped her bad fathering. Horney's father was a domineering German sea-captain who had terrorized her and eventually tried to block her entry into medical school. The strength she acquired in that struggle started her on a path of undaunted independence.[16]

When someone accepts us as an authentic and worthwhile individual, and thus affirms us, or when we can get insight from books or counseling, we can then derive and begin to develop adult behavioral skills from any of our subsequent male-female relationships. But, without ongoing acceptance or affirmation from some source, intimacy remains an elusive or unattainable goal, even within marriage.

"Educating" Father

If it was true that a generation ago, dad's role in child-raising was frequently dismissed as secondary to mom's, or even of virtually no importance, the belief now is that the role of the male in the house can be pivotal. My experience would support the present opinion. In the beginning of my career, I often asked the navy fliers, who came to my dispensary for medical problems, and whose careers demanded the ultimate in courage, "What was your father like?" As I remember now, the invariable answer could be capsulated by the expressions, "He was fearless and adventurous," or "He was very confident in everything he did." Undoubtedly, in the case of these men, their fathers had played a large role in determining the fliers' own adult choices.

Robert Bly says, in *Iron John*, "There is not enough 'father' in our culture, and in our families." Not only do sons suffer "father hunger," but their daughters suffer also.[17] Some seventy percent of men living in U.S. penal institutions are men who grew up without fathers. Girls from fatherless homes have 111% more teenage births, 164% more premarital births, and 92% more marital breakups.[18] But, many fathers find it difficult to truly affirm their daughters appropriately, especially in early adolescence. We know, with certainty, that "sexist" fathers can do great harm. On the other hand, all agree that emotional availability can be a father's greatest asset, especially when he is supportive but not controlling, when he is available at a moment's notice, and if he strives purposefully never to be abusive, cynical, or belittling.

From her practice, Mary Pipher also found the father to play a very prominent role in the struggle of his adolescent daughter toward maturity. She too has often observed permanent damage resulting in families where a father has been too strict, distant, or abusive.[19] Mary Valentis and Anne Devane, in *Female Rage*, write of other paternal errors, seeing "good fathering" not only as a "political act, but also as a sexual one," meaning that their fathers' sexual attitude toward women in general and their daughters in particular mold their daughters' attitude or approach to men. They fault fathers who address their daughters as "Princess," or who encourage them to flirt or be "sexy." When fathers send this message, they "set (their daughters) up for later bitterness and rage, (when their daughters subsequently) discover that disappointment, abuse, or exploitation are the typical result" of this approach to men. Women praised only for their beauty, when the eventual and inevitable physical imperfections come, then perceive the changes as losses of their **only real assets**.[20]

On the other hand, some fathers, to avoid the trap of encouraging their daughters to be sex objects, encourage them to strive for traditional male skills—sports, fishing, mechanics, or computers. As I see it, there is much to commend in that attitude. The American Association of University Women would certainly agree, as their 1992 report, *How Schools Shortchange Girls* calls for the elimination of all gender bias in education. The campaign to get our daughters into math and science is now a very high priority of most feminists active in education.[21]

Countering the **Emotional Abuse,** Too

Perhaps out of fear of sending "innocent" daughters any unacceptable sexual signals, a father may avoid his daughters entirely. The "unacceptable" signals do not necessarily have to be "sexual," however. The instances of "emotional incest" described by Patricia Love in *The Emotional Incest Syndrome: What to Do When a Parent's Love Rules Your Life,* are quite convincing in showing how emotional control, in the unequal relationship between parent and child, can be overwhelming at the same time it is subtle. What loving father, at one time or another, does not say to his daughter, in attempting to show his love and affirmation, "You have never done anything wrong; you have never given me any problems or anxieties; you would never do anything to hurt me." Such praise, especially when heard often, definitely inhibits the typical adolescent from being honest about her weaknesses, mistakes, problems, fears, or anything else that might hurt the parents or spoil her perfect image. How can any child or young adult feel secure or mature normally if they are valued for being perfect when they know they are not?[22]

Besides the harm that results when children are valued because they are "always perfect," there are also many children hurt by being made to conform to the parents' needs or fantasies. In either case, the child is adversely affected. John Bradshaw claims that a child who is taught that he (or she) is not "O.K." the way he is, represents a very typical example of emotional abuse as well as of domestic violence, since violence is defined as the use of power (in this case parental power) to control the child.

> "Enmeshment, (the opposite of detachment, occurs when) parents live vicariously through their children's successes and talents. (Such an approach) is really exploitation, (and) can block psychological growth, especially if it is covert, (that is,) not consciously admitted or recognized. . . . (Such) children are often totally confused by being special to mom and dad. . . . They do not know they are being used, yet, as in all cases of violence, something deep inside cries out in the child."[23]

Children are often used as pawns in the parents' power struggle.

"Loving" a Child to Show Hate to Your Mate

Too often, I have been presented with instances in which a son or daughter has been made more important to one of the parents than anyone else in the family, including the spouse. The facts of one case were recited to me by a mother just a few days from this writing, so the details are still quite fresh in my memory. I will present this fifty-eight year-old woman's account, without comment. **Martha** lived with her husband of forty years. For as long as she can remember, every time she asked her husband to help with any project involving the house, it was as if he were deaf, dumb, and blind. Several months previously, they learned that they had to vacate their house and move to another house around the corner. Not once since has the husband discussed the move, nor has he lifted one finger to help. As far as he is concerned, it is a nonevent. Yet for also as long as Martha can remember, whenever their daughter asks dad to do anything, he responds immediately. In fact, on the day she was in my office, her husband was painting the third floor of their daughter's house!

Seeing Dad's Problems Too

Family therapists keep coming back to the theme of preserving generational boundaries as essential for family health. This requires that the children, at all times, see that mom is the most important person to dad, and that dad is mom's "numero uno." (Even the single mother in my practice, who was recently told by her teenager's school counselor that she should be her son's "best friend," expressed to me that she knew instinctively that such advice was foolish and dangerous.)

Valentis and Devane, in *Female Rage*, suggest that "much of women's rage against our patriarchal society is displaced anger against inept fathers."[24] Unfortunately, the radical feminists, like Mary Daly, Kate Millett, Marilyn French, and Adrienne Rich in her earlier writings, omit the critical truth that many men are victims too of our male-dominated culture. Paul Kivil, in *Men's Work: How to Stop the Violence That Tears Our Lives Apart*, reports that one of every six men is sexually assaulted in his lifetime, and one of every two physically beaten up at some time in their life, by a parent or other adult; and that virtually every man, by the time he is an adult, has been either beaten, severely intimidated, or humiliated through violence. Kivil's life-work has become uniting men to oppose and confront violence, in all its forms, instead of supporting violence by their silence.[25]

The vast majority of fathers, because of the constant encouragement from earliest childhood, even infancy, to act like "real men," which is usually defined as unemotional or non-communicative or non-complaining, are totally unskilled in relating intimately, openly, or authentically to anyone, much less their own daughters. Yet, we cannot deny that the young daughter, both in early childhood and adolescence, garners guidance and motivation from a father who encourages her to be all that she wants to be, without any bias or exceptions because she is a daughter and not a son. Without a father to value her as she attempts to give up the strong bonds of dependence on mother, and to assuage the guilt, anxiety, and fear that results from this process, the adolescent will often falter. Having a model of the nurturing, loving male who respects her personhood can launch her on the road to fulfillment as a person. His strength, or perhaps that of another affirming adult male, can be the difference between growth and independence, or a flight from autonomy back to dependence.

Taking a Look at the "Worst" Fathers

A final type of harmful fathering must be noted. One circumstance that is extremely likely to thwart the process called "individuation" (which simply means cutting the apron strings from mother, whether at four or five, or at adolescence) is sexual abuse. Besides the victims' withdrawal to complete dependency, lifelong feelings of unworthiness are the usual result, especially if the violation comes from within the family. Freud steadfastly denied incestuous accounts from his patients, labeling them all as fantasies, but thousands of women, whose credibility was established, have come forth in Freud's time and since to reveal sexual abuse at the hands of their fathers or other male members of the household. The newspapers, magazines, and talk shows abound with examples. While certainly not new (Rita Hayworth and Anais Nin were just two of thousands of famous female celebrities born early in the twentieth century who have reported abuse by their fathers), the crime of incest is accounted to be increasing in frequency, along with everything else involving violence against American women.[26]

All sexual abuse victims should be offered therapeutic help. For victims of **incest**—which is generally the most shaming type of abuse, because a trust has been violated—long-term therapy is almost always required. With any sexual abuse, the message that the victim takes from the unwanted invasion of her privacy and space is that she is not valuable in her own right.

Incest, usually, though not always, produces permanent self-hate, which can be expressed by depression or by a self-destructive approach to sex. Incest can also infuse the victim with a deep and enduring free-floating rage against all men.

While every act of rape inflicts a wound on all the victims, it is the *young* woman who is hurt the most, often subsequently experiencing the same complex of signs and symptoms referred to as the "post-traumatic stress syndrome," manifested by victims of war or natural disaster. In fact, eighty-two percent report permanent problems with fear, depression, and horrible dreams or flashbacks.[27] John Bradshaw quotes evidence to show that one episode of violence, especially a sexual one, can permanently alter the chemicals involved in the body's "fight-flight" reactions to acute stress. The individual can become forever hypervigilant, over-reactive, easily startled, and start worrying excessively or experiencing panic attacks. In many cases, a scene, or sense impression, can trigger the victim's initial response to the attack all over again. Many victims retain a distrustful attitude, or paranoid view of the world, are hypercritical and obsessive-compulsive, or live with constant watchful and fearful tension.[28]

I am no longer mystified by the anger of the gender-feminists, since it is apparent that a large part of their anger represents a defense against their perception of helplessness, especially in matters pertaining to **domestic** violence.[29]

Differing Views on the Challenge to Create Family Love

Unfortunately, as Maria Montessori said almost seventy-five years ago, "No social problem is as universal as oppression of the child."

Those charged with dealing with cases of child abuse invariably report that children who are seriously injured by their parents, then placed with loving foster parents, prefer to go back to the original cruel family. Apparently stronger than anything else is the child's illusion or need to believe that his/her mother or father loves him. Certainly, in the mind of a child, the parents are "God-like" and "I am bad." The child's whole sense of survival depends on the belief that the parent could never do anything wrong or evil.

The abused child can react in any or all of several basic ways: the child grows up to be an abuser also; the child abuses himself or herself in various self-destructive ways, such as promiscuity and addiction; or, the child's reaction patterns cluster around techniques of isolation, or of permanent victimhood.

Finally, Giving **Mom** the Credit She Deserves

Unfortunately, as is true for many things, our civilization has a double standard in its comparison of mothers' and fathers' role in raising children. As Mary Pipher points out in *Reviving Ophelia: Saving the Selves of Adolescent Daughters*, fathers are lauded for the slightest efforts in engaging their children in a relationship, while mothers are criticized if their involvement with their children is too distant or too close, especially when adolescent daughters are involved. Mothers are seen as having the potential to do great harm with their mistakes, while fathers are given praise for the most tentative of good attentions, and are often given most of the credit when their daughters are ambitious, independent, and assertive. Mothers often get too little credit for parenting success. In actual fact, strong mothers are more likely to have strong daughters. As an added unfairness, what daughters do, vis-a-vis their mothers, never seems to be seen as proper either. If they stay close, daughters are judged as still being passive, dependent, and childish. If they reject their mothers, they are praised for their maturity, even though they may have forsaken the most caring person in their lives.[30]

Friday suggests that mothers are not usually as rigid, controlling, unyielding, vulnerable, or asexual as they seem to be to their daughters, and that mothers will not be crushed, humiliated, or feel rejected if their daughters, especially their adolescent ones, communicate authentically and with less bitterness or anger.[31] Mothers, for their part, must accept their daughters' emerging sexuality and their desire for more independence, and actively assist in the process of educating them for their independent existence. This includes seeing that they are sexually educated, even if the mothers cannot undertake that task themselves.[32]

Recognizing That Most Children "Make It"

Despite all the possible dangers that adolescence brings, happily, most clinicians and researchers working in adolescent psychology share the viewpoint of Anne Petersen and Roberta Simmins, expressed in Sommers' *Who Stole Feminism*, that the time between ten and twenty years of age is passed by most boys and girls without major problems or alienation from the family, or permanent ego-damage.[33]

One very important truth must be noted before leaving the topic of adolescence. In Hope Edelman's *Motherless Daughters*, loss of a mother is shown to be, for most women, the most defining event in their lives. When it occurs in adolescence, it can be (and usually is) the most devastating life-experience.[34]

Reviewing **the main things to remember,** if you are or have been a "normal parent:" children typically will copy much of what we "model" for them, but not all of it or in every case; they can be devastated by the parents' unresolved conflicts; even if your children have reached a point where they no longer obey your directives, provide guidelines for them anyway, so they know what you approve of and what you believe is wrong; punishments or rewards are not nearly as effective as attention, appreciation, and support; and it is now society, the culture, or their peers that largely determine the final outcome, at least in the short term.

Summarizing . . .

The **dominant challenge** of these last three chapters has been to use the work of love to eliminate all forms of violence in our marriages, in our families, and in society. **Repairing our closest relationships should remain everyone's first priority.**

If America is ever going to erase the shame of being the **most violent nation on earth**, we will first have to change the fact that we are the **loneliest people on earth**. The ultimate violence is our **failure to connect!**

If we continue to handle the inevitable conflicts and tensions that increase in proportion to our closeness to another human being, in the same ways a child handles them, our personal and societal problems will only get worse. On the other hand, many **wonderful possibilities could become realities, if we first learn to communicate with each other** (man/woman/child) using a common language (an adult **language of love)** for the purpose of resolving conflict.[35]

13

Eliminating Sexual Ignorance and Repression

> "'Is it a boy or a girl?' is the first question asked of (and by)
> the parents of a newborn, setting the stage for role assignments,
> orientation of life, and exposure to controls that will order
> the child's activities. Preference is still confused with inevitability."
> —Cynthia Fuchs Epstein

Certainly it is no secret that "life can be one damn thing after another," or even sometimes, as Edna St. Vincent Millay has written, "one damn thing over and over." In this matter of male-female differences—whether sexual or nonsexual—both these observations are appropriate.[1]

As medical students, few of us realized, in our frenzied quest for technical knowledge, that part of our vocation was to be a type of father-confessor. We were trained to listen and to see only the medical symptoms and signs. We were to employ patience and attention, but were never to allow ourselves to be distracted, influenced, or biased by personal feelings or opinions about the person speaking. Fortunately, in subsequent years, most of us eventually came to realize that simply listening with compassion when a patient shares her feelings cures more often than pills from a bottle, and, **while a physician cannot always cure, he can always offer help,**

hope, and comfort. In the event of a marital, psychiatric, or sexual problem, a gynecologist can always do **something** toward correcting what's broken.

In fact, while gynecologists refer many women for depression or serious marital conflict, they refer fewer patients for sexual counseling. A **lack of desire for sex rarely reflects a _sexual_ problem.** Such "disinterest" nearly always reflects a marital, or very rarely a psychiatric, problem. Even some supposedly serious sexual problems like premature ejaculation or lack of orgasm can be corrected without much effort.

Perhaps it is ironic, but the most common "contentions" in serious relationships, and which are most likely to lead to sexual aversion, have been the failure of the men to do their share of the household chores. "Cleaning up after a parasite" is proclaimed a total turn-off. The man who knows the importance of helping out generally "cleans up" sexually as a result.

Some of the sexual problems that women experience are the result of their ignorance of their own sexuality, often including lack of basic knowledge of their own anatomy. Another cause is the lifelong prohibition placed by parents and society on any expressions by women of their sexual nature. The most common problem is that wives are "turned off" by the husband's concern for his own performance rather than concern for pleasing her.

Nancy Friday states that "whether we get our sexual information in school or from our friends, we are stuck with the sexual attitudes that we got from the woman who raised us." The "hardest thing to face is your mother's sexuality, and her, yours."[2] She insists throughout her book that achieving honest recognition and acceptance of your mother's sexual identity, and her acceptance of yours, is one prerequisite for achieving mature adult relationships, especially with men. You need not only your mother's approval, permission, encouragement, and affirmation, but also her acknowledgment that she herself was "sexual," that sex was wonderful, or that at least she wished it was, or should have been.[3]

Though a woman's fears, guilt, distrust, ignorance, anxieties, or poor functioning in the sexual arena are so much a function of her upbringing (which unfortunately often requires an incredible amount of effort to overcome), her innate sexuality and its power to produce pleasure and to motivate her actions is every bit as real as a man's.[4] One obvious example of cultural bias in sexuality is manifested by the prohibitions we place from birth on any expression of sexuality by our daughters, contrasted with the freedom we allow our sons. "Nice girls keep any sexual feelings hidden, if indeed they have any." Our adolescent daughters must put their primary emphasis on being desirable, but they must suppress all their desire. Only good can result from the parents' recognition of the fact that their adolescent daughters are struggling with sexual desires and conflicts.

Sex is obviously powerful. We marry for it, divorce for it, and often risk our reputations, careers, and our health for it. Thanks to AIDS, we risk even our lives for it. Besides the physical dangers for persons engaged sexually with many partners, there are the endless possibilities for psychological disaster. The reality that simply satisfying your own or another's sexual needs often unleashes unwanted unconscious forces beyond either person's control, has been a favorite Hollywood theme, as in *Fatal Attraction, The Last Seduction,* and *Looking For Mister Goodbar.* Sonya Friedman states that "a lot of women are objective about a man until they go to bed with him. Then they literally get all screwed up." Obviously it constitutes a contradiction in terms to speak of "casual" sex.

Reviewing Some Sexual Specifics

As a practical matter, there are definitely some biological explanations for men's and women's obviously different attitudes or approach to sex. Men sometimes want orgasm without foreplay, especially when they have already expended all their available energy on their job. Orgasm is seen as a way to release their frustration or tension. This two-minute quickie can be a woman's "gift," which will, almost without exception, be very appreciated by her spouse. Women have written and stated that sometimes they like a quickie too. As a bonus in such instances, her mate is seen as freed from the responsibility of bringing her to climax, and she is relieved of her "obligation" to achieve orgasm.

While an occasional quickie has its usefulness, the opposite end
of the sexual spectrum is, for the woman, in most cases, preferable.
The wife welcomes the hugs, the touch, the body massage, the
foreplay, when offered without any thought about the goal of orgasm. This prolongation of what, for men, are only the preliminaries,
she sees as a wonderfully satisfying way to relieve her own tensions
and anxieties. Without the goal of orgasm, which *supposedly* proves
something about her sexual worth (while providing clear evidence
to her consort that he is a satisfactory lover), the woman can often
relax better and enjoy making love without any performance anxiety.

The common sexual mistakes of equating making love with
intercourse, or considering lovemaking successful only if release is
achieved, are not the only ideas that are off the mark. "Gimmicks"
like using pornography, erotic novels, and fantasizing as a sexual
starter might help some people realize they still have some sexual
feeling, but over time there are diminishing returns. "Sex toys" are in
the same category. As Barbara DeAngelis asserts in *Making Love All
the Time,* all of these can help us have sex with someone, but none
actually help us make love **to** someone. **For what can any of these
"things" contribute to personal worth and dignity?**[5]

Another erroneous idea is that sexual encounters must be spon-
taneous and not planned. This unfortunate belief means that for
many couples, lovemaking rarely "happens" anymore. While faking
or forcing love, because a time has been set aside for it, is definitely
counterproductive, planning means creating the opportunity for
affection to happen, and certainly provides clear evidence of your
attention and commitment to each other.

The **all-or-nothing** approach so popular with men (defined as,
"if you want me to spend time being **loving,** then let's "do it all," that
is, have intercourse) causes many women to choose "nothing" instead. In addition, virtually every women knows that "long and
soulful kisses," as Barbara DeAngelis describes them, lasting at least
twenty seconds, can be a separate item entirely from having sex. At
least three times a day is her suggested minimum. One bonus from
exchanging kisses: if either you or your husband refuses the offer of
such a kiss, that refusal could signal the presence of a buried or of a

hidden grievance that should be dealt with before it builds up to a real problem.[6]

Making Love and Not Just Having Sex

If a man wishes to retain or increase his wife's affection for him, women suggest as a first step that he give her time and attention. They add that some of that time and attention be used to express his appreciation for her. He should also share his feelings, even (or especially) before, during, or immediately after having sex. Saying this another way: making love in bed works best when you make love out of bed also, and share good feelings and positive emotions throughout the day. A man should also be reminded that the safer his mate feels in his presence, and the more desired, the more responsive she will be. Seducing your wife, especially if done in a creative way, is an excellent way for you to express your desire.

Barbara DeAngelis offers men a very practical and beautiful suggestion for making love: "to respect a woman's body and honor her for her willingness to allow you to enter it, is truly to make love to a woman." Don't enter until invited, go slowly, let her get used to your being there. When you leave, fill in the emptiness with hugs, loving words, and assurances that she is important to you.[7]

In *Men Like Women Who Like Themselves (and Other Secrets that the Smartest Women Know),* Steven Carter and Julia Sokol provide an "A to Z" summary of practical advice, from which any woman could learn much.[8] My favorite words of advice for women (admittedly, to be found on the lists of one or another expert): when you reject a man's offer to have sex, he takes it as a rejection of him; men get "turned on" by a "turned on" woman; when you point out a man's mistake, you are judging him a failure, and for him nothing merits more ridicule than being a failure; a sense of humor is very sexy; and most men prefer that you sometimes be old-fashioned and feminine.

Sexually Expressing the **Total You**

By this time it should be apparent that giving physical considerations primary importance in the search for intimacy between a man and a woman, betrays a profound lack of appreciation for what human sexuality, marriage, and intimacy are all about—and ignores the primary importance of the heart and mind. This applies especially to women, but is true also for men. One clear example is the discovery in several different surveys that women do not resent impotence, sadism, or infidelity, as much as they do stinginess. Being a good provider is their first requirement in a man. In surveys that ask men those identical questions, men choose the same attribute, generosity as a good provider, as most synonymous with masculinity. Being a good lover barely makes either list.

Throughout Chapters Ten and Eleven, evidence was presented to show that so **many marriages are dull,** sexless, or unromantic, not because of sexual inadequacy or sexual ignorance, but rather *because of ignorance of the ways to express or share the* **nonsexual** *needs.*[9]

"Disorders of desire," as Bradshaw refers to them, or simply "lack of desire for genital sexual expression with another," as Barbach classifies it, are the hardest sexual problems to treat, because there are so many possible causes, virtually all having to do with nonsexual problems in the relationship. Anger or resentment, conscious or not, is just one of an endless series of possible unresolved emotional or power issues involved. In such cases, marriage counseling may be needed, not more information on sexual technique.

Perhaps this is why, as Kinsey was one of the first to discover over forty years ago, the earlier in life you start sexual activity as a woman (and therefore the less capable you are likely to be, in handling relational problems in an adult manner), the more sexual difficulties you will likely encounter, and the less satisfaction you will likely experience from sexual relationships. On the other hand, the more educated you are, the more probable it is that you will experience orgasm.[10] Kinsey, and many others since, have also provided statistics that support the statement that the more time spent separate from mother before marriage, and the more education, the lower the incidence of divorce and adultery.

Fidelity in marriage, meaning the refusal to quit trying and give up, includes continuing our efforts to maintain a reasonable state of fitness and a physical attractiveness suitable for our age! Biological deterioration is a rare cause of sexual problems compared to the much more common situation in which either the man or the woman simply decides to "let themselves go" physically, as a sign of disinterest or of rejection.

Men throughout the ages have claimed indefinite ability to perform sexually and enjoy it. Chief Justice Oliver Wendell Holmes, in addition to his fame as founder of the Constitutional law of "free speech" and writer of over 2000 opinions (still the record for the U.S. Supreme Court), was known for his fondness for the nude female figure. (In those days, the statement would likely have been the "nearly-nude" female figure.) In his eighty-first year, he was heard to lament after his regular visit to the burlesque house, that he wished he were seventy again. Victor Hugo, in the course of a speech to the French Chamber of Deputies, confessed that, at the age of eighty-four, he was no longer able to make love four times in an afternoon, but rather now only three times! This does not at all say these men, or any man, is a "great lover" because he is potent. Continued interest or performance may simply reflect that the sexual ego is intact. It does not necessarily prove anything else. In fact, the frequency of sexual intercourse is not always or necessarily an accurate measure of a couple's friendship or level of intimacy.

Getting Your Facts Straight on the Big "O"

For the last thirty years, as much has been said and written about the nature, frequency, or intensity of female orgasm as about any other aspect of this subject of sex. This was not the case thirty years ago. Then, as a newly launched obstetrician-gynecologist, I volunteered to lecture and answer questions on "Sex and Sexuality" before an audience of young, unmarried but courting, college seniors. My talk was followed by a veritable barrage of questions, from both genders in attendance, on the nature and precise characteristics of the human female sexual response! It would have been better if I had been able to give everyone a book by Masters and Johnson. But none of the books devoted entirely to the precise physical details of the female sexual response had yet been written. (Although such books do **not** guarantee improved performance or permanence in sexual relationships, perhaps no one should get married without reading at least one of them. Sex, like everything else in marriage, will present continuing challenges. It is to the benefit of everyone concerned to avoid adding total sexual ignorance to their list of problems.)

Questionnaires from various sources consistently maintain that as many as fifteen percent of women can achieve multiple orgasms in their lifetime. On the contrary, simultaneous orgasm is said to be not only an elusive goal, but also to be an undesirable one. Masters and Johnson have stated that when simultaneous orgasms do occur, they usually subtract from each person's experience of the orgasm itself, especially for the woman. This is based on theoretical analyses of female anatomy and the female sexual response. The vaginal orgasm that Freud and his follower Helene Deutsch propounded as the most mature form of female sexual response, has in recent years been generally ignored as tangential to any explanation of the female sexual response, or ridiculed as yet another "male myth." As Masters and Johnson have said, "Everyone now agrees that clitoral and vaginal orgasms are not anatomically, or physiologically, distinguishable."[11] Or are they? In 1982, *The G Spot and Other Recent Discoveries About Human Sexuality,* appeared to reassert the belief that a deep, or vaginal, orgasm is possible.[12]

Women who say they enjoy lovemaking but never experience orgasms may, in fact, be having them, since it is the essential function of an orgasm to leave you relaxed and satisfied. The spasms and contractions often described are just some of the possible characteristics of an orgasm, although admittedly the easiest ones to measure or describe. Since first taught sixty years ago, the Kegel exercises have been found to be a relatively easy way to help intensify and expand the extent of the orgasm for some women, by involving more of the pelvic muscles in the sexual response.[13]

At any rate, failure to achieve orgasm is one of the easiest sexual problems to treat, since it is not a sign of neurosis. "Inorgasmia," as it is called, is simply the result of learned sexual inhibition, lack of information on the part of the partners, or an inability to relax or to receive sexual pleasure.

The skin is the largest sexual organ, and touching all over the body before touching the genitals is the most certain route to arousal for most women. Masters and Johnson's "sensate focus" exercises have been techniques recommended for three decades for sexual dysfunction. However, a radically new, and to me a much more "human," approach to sexual problems suggests that the person who has the problem—for example, inorgasmia, premature ejaculation, or impotence—admit or "own" it as his or her own problem, not the spouse's. Once he/she has the honesty and integrity to admit and accept responsibility, the individual in question can start working on his/her OWN issues (see Schnarch, p. 217 and "Recommended Reading").

In *Sexual Intimacy*, Andrew Greeley suggests that just as Yahwah delightfully surprised Moses on the mountain, and Christ delightfully surprised his followers on Easter, so too should the wife imitate them by delightfully surprising her husband once in a while. He suggests, as an example, that she meet him at the door in the evening wearing only panties and holding a pitcher of martinis. Or, if she prefers, she can wear only the martinis.[14] Marabel Morgan, in *The Total Woman,* suggested much the same thing, though she added that the wife should make sure it is not her mother-in-law or someone else when she suddenly opens the front door.[15] Greeley adds that if the husband doesn't rush to get his clothes off, the wife could pour the martinis over him and file for divorce.

What does a man do when his wife gets nothing out of sex and perhaps regularly uses a sexual turn-off, or put down? One common example is the wife, who, at the time of union, closes her eyes and stiffens her body in apparent discomfort. The wife's actions, of course, lead the husband to believe that she hates this part of their lovemaking, or at least that he is hurting her. It is not recommended that he permanently stop trying to please her, nor is it recommended that he forsake intercourse forever. Perhaps, as a start, the husband might tell his wife that he is sorry for the apparent problem, and ask her if she has any suggestions.[16] The shoe can be on the other foot, of course. What does a woman do when her husband is a poor lover? Hopefully she will not just buy him a how-to book, or worse, just use cynicism.

Becoming the **Better Lovers** You Always Wanted to Be

Communication is often an answer to marriage problems, especially the sexual ones. Why not try the communicating techniques summarized in Chapters 10 and 11, to share your sexual needs, desires, problems, or fears? Be careful, however, to avoid cynicism, meanness, or rancor. Otherwise, those will be the messages you will communicate.

Maggie Scarf's *Intimate Partners*, or Lonnie Barbach's *For Each Other*, provide the basic physical and anatomical facts of love-making,[17] but Barbara De Angelis provides her own **"loving advice,"** which has been my inspiration for the next few paragraphs.[18]

In the "R" movies, and in the erotic or "sex-plicit" novels, the Masters and Johnson textbook models of how love is made are followed to the letter: mutual desire leads the partners quickly to arousal and excitement, which steadily and unwaveringly increases to reach a plateau, at which stage the pleasure no longer increases. This steady state of pleasure is the signal that further work must be done quickly, lest all the pleasure vanish, without either the man or the woman "achieving success," that is, ejaculation or orgasm. The whole process can be experienced by a man in two or three minutes, while for an average woman, fifteen to eighteen minutes is required. This is pleasure-, goal-, or release-oriented sex, pure and simple. For most people, this can get to be pretty boring stuff! It is easy to see how some people can reach the point of thinking that just about any "body" will do.

For persons in real life, on the other hand, the animal model should be replaced by a human model. This means one that is based on what actually happens with most of us. When normal people make love, there is a considerable variation in how aroused each feels moment-to-moment. One minute you're hot, but the next minute you're not. The key to good sex is not to worry when the sensations of arousal or bodily pleasure rise, then fall, increase, then decrease. Instead of panicking or working to maintain or increase the pleasure, rather bring in the heart and mind, and the rest of the upper half of the body, using hugs, sharing feelings, affirming, supporting, and even talking and laughing. As surely as day follows night, and within seconds, or at most a minute or two, the bodily changes signifying arousal will return, but, because all of the sexual focus is not now exclusively on the genitals, but has become more wide-spread, more of our body participates or experiences the pleasurable feelings. The process of pleasure first building, then going down, then coming back at a higher level, is repeated many times in a very satisfying way, until either one person or the other, accidentally or by a deliberate choice, experiences release, or, equally acceptable, it is agreed that both are satisfied for now, so that any further genital sexual stimulation is discontinued. Throw away the clock if you want pleasure without anxiety (which Barbara DeAngelis defines as "ecstasy"). If eventually release comes, that is fine. If not, so what? Haven't you still been making love, and having sex, possibly for more time than ever before?[19] (I have not heard women complain of pelvic pain after a prolonged "love session" in which orgasm was not deliberately sought. Pelvic pain said to be due to markedly dilated pelvic veins attributed to persistent failure to achieve orgasm, has apparently not been associated with this "ecstatic," prolonged, "love-making-without-orgasm" technique.)

An essential point to remember: communicating about sexual matters is much easier if couples have practiced and improved their general communication skills by the exercises suggested already in Chapters Ten and Eleven. The mirroring exercise and remembering to use the word "I" to begin all statements about what your needs might be, are good ways to start, unless there are deep emotional wounds being acted out sexually, in which case love letters are probably the best method to start. It is also suggested that you ask your partner directly how and when he prefers that you communicate with him. This avoids your having to guess. At these times you can remind him that the more satisfaction you get out of sex, the better it will be for him, since you will then be able to provide your own sexual energy and input to the activity.

When you are convinced that you are special and that you have a special gift to offer, namely, yourself (which of course requires that you have worked at making yourself special), and when you can also value, accept, and affirm your spouse (and make it clear that you do in some special way such as red roses for her or a back rub for him), you are setting out on the wonderful road to intimacy. If, when the inevitable conflicts arise, you show the courage to confront the problem firmly, with tact and gentleness, that road will widen and become less perilous. Whether the problem requires you to ask for something or requires you to give something, you will remember the **secret**: love and intimacy increase each time that you tell the complete truth.

Keeping Sex a Part of Your Twilight Years

A final and vital aspect of sexuality is the relationship between sexual activity or attitudes, and aging.

Myths about sexuality in the most mature segments of society have interfered with that group's enjoyment of sex for centuries. Despite all the popular articles available that insist it should be otherwise, women after seventy, for example, sometimes much earlier, often feel that it is not normal to enjoy sex so much as they do. Many feel ashamed about giving sexual pleasure such a high priority in their lives. Still, the recent "Janus Report" stated that three-quarters of the women sixty to seventy-four years of age are sexually active.[20] For most women, a fear eventually arises that intercourse may no longer be safe. However, outside of the dryness and discomfort that could result from prolonged estrogen loss, there is no reason to change anything simply because of age.[21] The vaginal discomfort is usually easily corrected with any of the following interventions: the resumption or increase in sexual activity, vaginal hormone cream, a soft vaginal ring containing estrogen that is replaced every three months, or an over-the-counter vaginal lubricant.

Getting Help For Impotence

Of course there will always be an abundance of women who answer their gynecologist's question regarding sexual difficulties with the assertion that "their husbands don't bother them anymore." Shakespeare's King Henry IV remarked, "Is it not strange that desire should so many years outlive performance?"

However, most of those women who do express anything about their husbands' cessation of sexual activity, express regret and sadness, and say they feel "abandoned." It is this area of geriatrics that is now getting more of the attention it so much deserves, both because of effective new products and because of more honest discussion of the problem. **New non-surgical treatments, pills that are taken by mouth, are now available, with at least six more coming in the next few years.** The name of the first one available is **"Viagra."** Another named **"Apomorphine"** should be available by the end of 1999. Expectations are that approximately eighty percent of men with impotence will benefit. (Note: men without impotence will derive *no* benefit from using the new meds!)

Probably at least thirty-five percent of men over sixty-five have erection problems. We will probably never know the correct percentage, because many men will deny the problem when asked. More than one woman writer has questioned with whom the men are having sex, because of the significant discrepancy that exists between the answers of the older men and the older women, when they are questioned separately about their sexual activities. Ironically, if you survey young married couples about the frequency of sexual intercourse, the women give much higher figures than the men!

Women need more, not less, physical affirmation and attention as they grow older. This fact remains true, even if their mates are now incapable of an erection. Naomi Wolf, in her most recent work (*Promiscuities,* Random House: New York. 1997) emphasizes the overwhelming consensus since the dawn of civilization that women have always been more passionate and more sexual. She asserts that "the great forgetting" of this truth is an aberration of the last 100-200 years.

Impotence does not prevent the affection and tenderness which are indispensable elements in fueling the fires of intimacy. In their writing and their teaching, women will consistently reveal that men can make love all the time simply by showing care and concern. These gifts are more important to a women than having sex, whether the woman is twenty or ninety.

A man biologically capable of sexual intercourse may have had his fragile ego damaged by his mate's attitudes or actions, which could include her seeming disinterest, lack of response, her ridicule of his past failures, her moralizing, or her personal criticism. He may be impotent because he senses that his wife regards sex as a reward or as barter for something she wants. His impotence could be a result of her refusal of sex whenever she has any grievance against him.

Unfortunately, man's belief that it is the frequency and quality of his erections that will decide his wife's respect for him is as tenacious as it is erroneous, since men are, after all, the gender with the "penis envy." This concern about the size and quality of his erections often comes into the picture as a man ages. Since sexual activity is often the only way that a man can express himself comfortably, his impotence can result in his inability to release his emotions, especially his anger, so the anger leaks out slowly and frequently as crankiness. Gradually, the marital closeness that most wives desire (but only experience when their husbands make love to them) begins to fade. This loss is felt especially by those women whose only family, or source of affirmation, is now their husband.

When Bonnie Maslin quotes the popular adage that the course of many a man's sexual history can be stated quite succinctly—"tri-weekly, try weekly, and try, weakly," she is undoubtedly correct. But the problem in the third and final stage is frequently created by the man's own response to his "failure" and rarely by his mate's reaction to it. Surely, in many cases, at least in the initial stages, the impotence is due to loss of confidence, resulting from a previous failure or failures in achieving or sustaining an erection.[22]

Despite a man's shame at losing what he considers the strongest proof of his virility, most such husbands do not simultaneously lose the desire for closeness or intimacy, though many do not consciously realize that they want and need this closeness. Both John Bradshaw and Betty Friedan claim that many men bury their feelings, because an overbearing or overinvolved mother dehumanized them or shamed them when they would try to express any "womanly" feelings.[23] This is another topic entirely. A man may act like a statue in the face of failure or pain because of a faulty relationship with his mother, but his stoicism is more likely the result of an American culture that doesn't equivocate when it defines men as "real" only if they need nobody and never cry. American society from the beginning has always admired rugged individualism above everything else. Why then should we be surprised at any man's denial of wanting to be close and intimate despite his impotence?

If a loss of confidence is the only reason for a man's impotence, a woman's patience, encouragement, or some willingness to help him achieve or sustain the erection is all that is necessary. Women in this situation should at least know that squeezing a limp penis, especially the outer half, the part farthest from his trunk, will generally prevent an erection. If an erection is present, squeezing in the same outer half, or even just the tip, may not only hurt but also make all the blood flow backward out of the penis so that the erection is lost. (This **"squeeze" technique is great if you are trying to correct premature ejaculation**.) On the other hand, gently "milking" the blood from the base of the shaft toward the middle, ideally with the penis kept down in the plane of the body, not at a right angle to it, often helps best in achieving and sustaining stiffness. Even if using these various techniques should fail, you send your husband a clear message that you care about him, that you want to be open to his needs, and that you still find him desirable. By working together, you may even discover better techniques. (Again, Maggie Scarf is recommended for detailed instructions on managing sexual difficulties, especially in older couples.)[24]

Remember the "loving advice" expressed earlier, which applies to both young and older couples: the waxing and waning of desire and arousal during sex, whether it be reflected by the loss of the erection or loss of lubrication, is in no way unusual or abnormal, or a sign that the lovemaking is faulted and going to end "unsuccessfully." This variation in desire and arousal is only predictive of how things are going to finish if one or the other sees such variation as "abnormal" or as a sign of disinterest in sex. Thus, if one partner erroneously senses "disinterest," that partner may stop making love.

As one might expect in a culture where sexual misinformation abounds, none of the scenes of allegedly "normal" lovemaking in our bestselling fiction (even the romantic, or more appropriately named "erotic," novels, written by women for women), ever seem to allow male flaccidity or declines in the heroine's apparent sexual arousal as events that can occur off and on during a love-session.[25] No wonder that so many lovers get concerned or panic when their experience is not as "good" as the couples in the books.

Unfortunately, besides the women whose husbands give up sexual intimacy because of impotence from alcohol, illness, medicines, or perceived sexual inadequacy, a large number of women are also "sexually abandoned" by their husbands through death. Forty-

one percent of all women ages sixty-five to seventy-four were widows at the time of the last census, and the death and suicide rate is at
least four-and-a half times higher for men than for women after those
ages.[26] The average age of a woman living alone is sixty-one, and of
the average male, forty-one.

Confronting the Sexual Repression

Those women of **any** age who have been sexually phobic, because they have taken a sense of their mother's disapproval of the
whole process to the marital bed, might benefit from hearing an
admonition of a great teacher and gynecologist, Dr. S. Leon Israel: "If
you think you might enjoy sex swinging from the chandeliers, you
should go for it!" For many years, I wondered why this dignified and
very proper gentleman would dare to teach such "sexual abandon."
But I have reached the same conclusions he did. Insofar as women
hold onto the sexual repressions or phobias of childhood and adolescence, they will to the same extent deprive themselves of the splen-
dors of an intimate sexual relationship. **This truth I have frequently
heard from women themselves.**[27]

William Masters and Virginia Johnson, in *The Pleasure Bond*,
wrote, "The way we express ourselves sexually—our most intimate
way of relating to another person—reflects how we value ourselves,
how we value the other person, (and) how that person values us."[28]
Thus, when "having sex" (which does not require any pre-set goals
like release or orgasm) is omitted without a physical justification,
especially for a prolonged interval, the couple is not demonstrating
that they value each other very much, and in fact, they probably
don't (whether they admit it to each other or not). This appraisal is
especially true for the man, who has virtually no other way that is
acceptable to him to express his love or reveal his positive feelings.

Loving Without Sex

On the other hand, **one cannot dogmatically state that "having
sex" is necessary for every couple. It surely is not**. When women
have expressed to me that changing their sex life is not one of their
priorities, that it is not worth it or necessary to them or their spouse
in the context of their relationship, I point out Lonnie Barbach's

findings, from a long career of providing sexual counseling to women, that "nowhere is it written that an orgasmic, sexually active relationship is necessary to be totally fulfilled and intimately involved with a partner."[29] Comments like that support the proposition that the most important fuel for the fire of human love is the sharing of the heart and mind, and never simply the sharing of our body. Perhaps this proposition sounds obvious and simple. It is, admittedly, both. But, there is one thing this book should have made quite clear by now—**sharing of our secret thoughts, needs, or desires, is definitely not easy**.

Summarizing

The main points to remember: that women are at least as capable of sexual feeling and performance as men are; that communication is the key to all intimacy including sexual intimacy and that simply having relations with someone says nothing about real "connectedness;" that a woman's sexual experience is very likely to be enhanced by correcting her ignorance of her own body and by addressing the problem of sexual repression, again through communication with her mate; and that because sexuality involves the body, mind, and spirit, the whole process should, like a fine wine or cheese, improve with age. (Or, to borrow the metaphor that Harold Kushner prefers, sexuality is like reading a good book—the more you get into it, the better it gets.) Psychotherapist David Schnarch, in *Passionate Marriage: Sex, Love, and Intimacy in Emotionally Committed Relationships* (Norton: New York, 1997), illustrates by case histories that the level of passion, eroticism, emotional intensity, and connectedness ("the level of your human sexual maturity") correlates directly with the level of connectedness reached by the couple in non-sexual matters. He insists, as I do, that the greatest sex is between committed adults, who are independent and perceived as equals.

Chapter Fourteen will provide an amplification of the theme of the previous four chapters, that is, **the work of love**. While we can sometimes ignore good health care advice without immediate consequences, we usually pay a heavy price for a failed relationship. Learning the ways to create a bond of intimacy has been and always will be our best investment against the hatred and violence that assails all of us.

14

Creating Intimacy Magic Moment-by-Moment

"There are two convictions that are the essential prerequisites for loving communication. The first is that we must think of ourselves as gifts to be given. The second is that we must regard others as gifts, sometimes tentatively and hesitantly offered to us."
—John Powell, *Happiness Is an Inside Job*

"We make our spiritual quest with the clues and the resources life gives us. One of those clues is the people who like us the way we are. . . .We need [these] people so we can unfold and open ourselves to [them]. This makes it possible to grow and develop. . . . The paradox is, we need people who like us the way we are so we can become different from what we are. And the beauty here is that as we change, the people who like us the way we were, like us just as much, or more, than before."
—Jess Lair, *"I ain't well, but I sure am better"*

John Bradshaw describes intimacy as the "struggle in which two people learn to develop their own identities, while at the same time overcoming their separateness. . . . [A]lthough seemingly very different, these processes of individuation and togetherness are inseparable."[1]

In fact, no intimacy is possible except between individuals who value themselves in their independence, who are in most ways equal, and who can freely choose at various times to be temporarily enmeshed in each other, "to lose themselves in each other," to reveal themselves to each other, while at the same time never forgetting for an instant that they are separate and distinct persons. Each trip into enmeshment becomes a deliberate search for the mystery of the other.

Paul Tournier says that to claim that you understand your spouse is equivalent to saying you have given up any real attempt to discover him or her.[2] Growing closer in friendship and more deeply intimate requires that we reveal ever more and more of "ourselves"—our talents, fears, weaknesses, desires, needs—I refer to this as "telling the complete truth."

Anger is the key that signals that we have an unfulfilled need. This unfulfilled yearning, this unsatisfied grievance, this "wound" must be discovered and revealed lest it gather strength, cause pain, hurt others, or lock our relationship in conflict. If we would only accept the insight that anger is, in effect, a **gift** because it can alert us to our unfulfilled need. Despite the fact that we are not consciously aware of the precise source of our pain, it can still become the "hidden" motivator of our negative reactions to our partner. Recognizing this insight should make us rush to discover these most important gifts/needs/wounds/grievances, so we can share these needs with the hope that we might eventually be able to let them go. The use of these techniques is essential to the love-making and connectedness process.

Forsaking All the "Secrets and Lies"

Most people in relationships would staunchly deny that they have kept thousands of secrets from their beloved and told him/her at least that many lies. We all forget the reason that the courts of law require the truth, the whole truth, and nothing but the truth— because anything less can very well be misleading or deceiving.

Obviously, all of us have had ample experience of the difficulties of sharing the complete truth with the one with whom we are sharing our life. **The effects of exchanging intimate information can quickly reveal the quality of the relationship and whether it is being built upon a loving foundation**.

Even when communicating in business, with friends, or with our children, the misunderstandings can sometimes be monumental. One of the many added problems of communicating in an intimate relationship is that virtually all of us expect our partners to be mind-readers, which of course they are not. In addition, because of the "gender difference," when we do eventually talk to each other, we do not use the same language.

If the stakes are higher in communicating with an intimate, the rewards are greater, too. Even if your partner "hears" or acts or responds to only one of your expressed "wants," good and loving feelings result. Insights that might allow us to let go of the destructive urges that are wrecking our relationships, could well result from an openness about our needs when they are shared with a caring spouse. Of course, it is essential for us to give our immediate and ongoing acceptance of the other as her/his authentic self is presented to us by his/her confession of these needs.

Creating *Magic* Moments

Without question, a profound truth about love is that it requires continual acts of **knowing—sharing** all our thoughts, and **committing—making decisions** to do things favorable to the other. Geneen Roth, in *When Food is Love*, says that **"the discovery that being intimate is a choice that we make at every moment is as close to magic as anyone ever comes."**[3]

What choices do we have presented to us throughout every day of our lives? Simply put, every decision we make that is good for us or for our mate is an act of love. **Thus you can recapture the "feel" of love by the frequent use of whatever you consider an "expression" of love**. This could be "gift-giving," that is, the exchange of kindnesses, or expressing appreciation, or acts of touching, or a million other caring actions that the human heart and imagination can devise.

*Working on Your **Appreciation** Is a Great Way To Begin*

Susan Jeffers, in *Opening Our Hearts to Men* suggests that women who are **chronically** hostile or resentful of their husbands, may have never taken the time to think about or appreciate any of the kind things he has done for them. This is not to say that when the anger is generated it should not be shared or expressed. The previous four chapters have focused on the proper and controlled expression of our anger as the key to healing our relationships. Jeffers suggests that gathering the data to justify some loving feelings toward your husband may be the way to bring back the fifth and chief element in telling the complete truth, namely, **expressing your love and appreciation.** She describes women whose entire attitudes have changed when they have taken the time to write down, on a regular basis, the spousal actions made on their behalf. Such women soon started recognizing loving gestures that they had always missed before, defusing much of their previous anger, and making their own communication more loving. It is also a fact that one cannot be appreciative and sad at the same time. Always remember, when compiling your list of things you appreciate in your mate, that **men express their love and devotion by their actions, not their words.**[4]

*Remembering **Gender Differences** May Exist*

It is a fact that men quite often use sex, and only sex, to satisfy their needs (and obligation?) for intimacy and touching. Since men are not trained to communicate intimately in a **verbal** fashion, women should not expect that they will do so very often, or resent it if, in fact, they almost never do it.

Women become "intimate" with women friends easily, sharing all kinds of deep secrets, weaknesses, desires, disappointments, failures, even "sins." Men, on the other hand, have acquaintances, sometimes many, depending on their job and lifestyle, but share few secrets with any of them. Women almost never find a husband or a lover who can approach or match their women friends, as a "soulmate."

Men do not want to be emotionally closed, especially with their mates, but in most instances they judge the risk to be too great. And probably for a lot of good reasons: women tend to judge men to be deficient in such matters and treat them accordingly. They take mens' silences personally. John Gray, whose books about the differences between men and women have gained wide popular acceptance, writes repeatedly that women give a high priority to trying to change their men, that some women (perhaps many) abhor weakness in a man, and that rarely do such women want to know the whole truth about their mate or his failings and problems. Nor do many women welcome his **frankest** thoughts about them. (The only possible **safe** place for **frank criticism** of a woman **might be** in a love letter.) In fact, women are often enraged by the same spoken criticism from their mate that they would accept, even appreciate, from a close female friend. Harville Hendrix has written that, from the reports of countless men who have sought intimacy, "When there are future arguments, what [men] have shared in their closest moments has often been used against them." Finally, mothers and wives collude with our American tradition of insisting that a **real man** _never_ shows fear, pain, or weakness.

Women, on the other hand, tend to be quite open about their "needs," often as their way of inviting intimacy. Naomi Wolf, in _The Beauty Myth_, addresses this precise problem when she speaks of the passivity and meekness that even a women who is forceful in all her other relationships will manifest in a new romance—"the certain attractiveness to dependency, something we are so used to that it's almost synonymous with being female."[5] Undoubtedly, many men are initially quite flattered when a seemingly strong and independent woman makes satisfying his needs and wishes the most important project in her life. But there are grave dangers to intimacy inherent in such an unequal relationship. (Of course, if he quickly realizes the benefits of reciprocating in kind, the woman in question can feel reassured that the relationship probably has great possibilities.)

On the other hand, virtually every woman has met at least one man who claimed he did not need anyone. A woman would be utterly foolish to spend quality time with such a person. When a man tries to convince you that you are wrong to need each other, either run away fast, or if you are already somewhat enmeshed, write up a list of all the things you need from him. This exposition might awaken the guy to realize he does, in fact, have many of his own needs satisfied by you. Strongly suggest that he write some down and then share the list with you. If he is afraid for reasons of privacy, tell him that he doesn't have to sign it. If he can't come up with anything, he'll certainly never be passionate toward you. Most likely his needs are so buried that he can't feel passion toward anyone, and he probably needs "help" badly for the wounds that hurt so much that he must hide them even from himself.

Continuing the Loving *Every Day Is the Key*

Everyone would readily admit that "lovers have to exchange gifts." I have just written of the "magic" of being able to build quickly a deeper love by continually simply touching, expressing care and appreciation, or exchanging other "gifts." Each gift that is freely given and freely received binds us together more strongly. It is really a contradiction to call something a gift when it is given out of the giver's sense of need. Rather, the gift that generally becomes most treasured is the one that satisfies the receiver's deepest need. By the same beautiful principles of love, the gift that is treasured most by the receiver comes to produce the greatest joy in the giver. All this confirms that a gift's final value in deepening our love for each other derives from both the giver's and the receiver's responses.

Why do we ever stop exchanging daily gifts? I think it is because we are inclined to withhold the offering of gifts, including even the gift of ourselves, our time, or our talent, when we do not value any of these gifts enough. For example, we lose sight of the great worth of kind words and appreciative sentiments. Often, as a consequence of our judgments that our gifts are worth little, we may seek to gain personal value by attaching ourselves to someone else who seems to possess that which we do value. But by doing this, we place ourselves in a "need," not a "love" relationship. In attaching ourselves to another as a way to hide our own deficiencies, we fail the first requisites for intimacy—being equal but separate.

The reality of love is that it is in the giving of ourselves that we best express our love. Incredible as it may seem, the most valuable gift we possess to give **is** ourselves. When we offer this gift freely and unreservedly we become more lovable, because in making ourselves vulnerable by revealing ourselves, warts and all, **we prove our love**.

Two of the classic expressions of love remain true—"I experience my greatest joy when I am giving you something that brings you joy," or "I love you so much that I must do something to prove my love." Men especially, when they are in love, have a burning desire to **do** something, ideally to give their beloved what she would most like to receive, that which would bring her the greatest happiness. Hopefully, those men who have read Section Two are now able to recognize that **what their mates want most is** *them*.[6]

Summarizing

The main points: To achieve intimacy, the myriad differences in the style of communication manifested by men in comparison with women must be overcome; suggested aids are using the techniques of love letters, mirroring or duplicating, wish lists, diaries of progress or of appreciation, compatibility lists, or planning times for "making love";[7] developing **adult** methods for revealing and sharing your **anger**, that is, your **hidden needs,** with your beloved;[8] mastering the **art of negotiation, especially** for the matters of greatest importance;[9] and by **seeking counseling** if any or all of these suggestions fail to remove the tension and conflict from your relationship.

Be wary, however, of any counselor who suggests, after you have tried some or all of our techniques for communicating, that you need to "improve your communicating skills." Once "you've been there, and done that" without benefit, more work on yourself—an examination of conscience, perhaps looking at your weaknesses and deepest feelings—might be a better starting point.

Millions of people just like you, with the same problems, have created enough joy and consolation by these works of love, to share unprecedented happiness with each other.

Section 3
Completing Your Active Choices

FACING THE FINAL CHALLENGES

15

Deciding Your Role in the Feminist Struggle

*". . . feminism, which began with the attempt by women to claim
the rights that men were proclaiming for themselves, is moving
irrationally, and at high political risk, toward the repudiation
of any notion of right beyond that of personal experience."*
—Elizabeth Fox-Genovese, *Feminism Without Illusions*

*"Yet we as observers should know that the way sexuality and
particularly rituals surrounding sex are used can tell us something
not so much about sex per se as about the society."*
—Mary Douglas, 1975

Some feminists are outspoken in their objection to what I have
given chief emphasis in Section Two, namely, giving one's first
priority to creating an intimate relationship with a man in marriage.
In fact, many vehemently and persistently deny that a woman
should seek, or, in fact, needs to be loved (at least by a man) as her
highest goal.

While **I readily agree with the part of the feminists' position
that demands that women should be free to seek other goals, even
as their first priority**, and will get to that truth momentarily, I wish
first, however, to offer some concluding thoughts on the theme of the
previous section, namely, **creating love.**

It is surely ironic that, unlike men, for whom respect is probably most desired, women in every **recorded** age and culture have found their greatest happiness in being accepted, or loved, without conditions. And for most women, this has meant a man's love!

Undoubtedly, part of the position of those feminists who call the thoughts of Section Two into question, is a reaction to those **men who callously preach that woman's highest goal is to give love,** and that providing love to husband and children constitutes her fulfillment. I believe that this statement, that women's primary role in life is to give love, is no more true for women than it is for men. When Susan Jeffers writes that "Woman's main craving in life is not to be loved, but to love. . . . [We] are the source of the experience of love, not our mate,"[1] she is **not** siding with the **narrow male view** that women should exist solely for others. Rather, she is claiming **something that applies to all of humankind, namely, that it is often more joyous or "better" to give than to receive**. As Rabbi Harold Kushner so correctly observes, "Human beings have a need to be good, to be helpful, to be generous." Nearly all would agree, I think, that we **all** have a need to **love,** and "when you have learned how to live (and to love), life itself is the reward."[2] It is probably true that some confusion arises because women recognize more often than do men the truth that the act of giving creates wonderful feelings of love. (In the words of St. Francis, "It is in giving that we receive [joy and peace]." In the words of the Talmud, "A person possesses what he gives away.")

However, even the celibate saints needed constant love and affirmation from their God! Thus, despite all the wonderful spiritual truths about "love," **every woman knows from the depth of her heart that she has no life worth living if she does not also receive love from someone in return**.

Acknowledging the Truths of the Feminist Message

However, there is another truth involved that needs to be included in our discussion of life, love, and living: **A woman's desire to love and to receive love must not remain, because of sexual stereotyping in the home, in education, at work, in government, and in religion, her only path to fulfillment.**

As Karen Horney said six decades ago,

"For centuries, love has not only been women's special domain in life, but in fact has been the only . . . gateway through which they could attain what they desired. . . . [W]omen realized that through love, and love alone, could they attain happiness, security, and prestige."[3]

An educated and wise person will readily acknowledge that the **greatest human power is the ability to love,** and that it is **in expressing that love that we are most fully human and most fully alive**. Many, too, can see that the highest truth for everyone is that **a "connection" with another must exist for that power to love, and for our expressions of that love, to be sustained.** Unfortunately, it is the fourth and final truth that is rarely acknowledged and generally forgotten: one must also **proclaim that every woman has the right to seek other goals, to accept other challenges, and to pursue other dreams**.

While all the statements of the preceding paragraphs are correct and true, the last is especially crucial for women. **Reducing a woman's whole existence to giving and seeking love is tyrannical, incorrect, unjust, and cruelly dehumanizing if the woman herself would seek something more!** And this is precisely where **the women's movement is most needed,** namely, to **empower and support, then assuage the guilt such aspirations in a woman (which may be goals of fame and glory) can still engender**.

Speaking to Those Women for Whom Marriage Is Not the Only Goal

I have made it quite explicit that a woman's responsibility for her own happiness can extend beyond the quest for personal intimacy with another person. **For many women, the need to function in society, to compete with men, and to use all of her talents (not just the "feminine" ones) is shown to be equally essential to their fulfillment.** Betty Friedan, in her manifesto, *The Feminine Mystique,* that recharged the modern feminist movement, gave her first chapter the title, "The Problem That Has No Name," in which she refers to the senselessness and emptiness of life that results when a woman comes to condemn herself for having been "only" a housewife/ mother.

The fact that this identical scenario of unfulfillment could de-scribe the lives of millions of American women in this century was the spark of reality that reignited the feminist movement in 1963. I had many such patients through the years who were brilliant human beings, but doomed by their gender to depend on the needs, grati-tude, or appreciation of their families to justify their continued existence. One such wonderful women, Ingrid (her husband was equally delightful) was the only patient I ever visited regularly in her home. I am convinced that by verbally expressing my love and appreciation of her wonderful gifts, added to the steadfast support of her husband and my wife, Ingrid was literally kept alive and functioning for fifteen years past the time (after her children were raised, married, and essentially gone from her life) that she had decided that her value, her usefulness, as a human being was lost. For, when my career was moved too far away for my wife and I to continue our visits, she deteriorated rapidly. Within a few months, her daughter called and asked me to please visit her and "see what I could do." (I had rescued her from several serious physical problems fifteen years before as part of a very detailed health maintenance program that Ingrid had been faithfully following all the years since that time.) When I saw Ingrid, I saw what her daughter had recog-nized. Ingrid, only eighty-three and now without any serious dis-ease, had "decided to die." It was as clear to me as to her daughter that Ingrid considered that her life and her considerable talents had been wasted, and that her only excuse for living—taking care of others—was now ended. She died within two months of that visit, while I was away at a medical conference.

Why is it that many such women, who have worked so hard, and given so much, get so disheartened and fail to see any accomplish-ments in their lives? Why is it that, despite a lifetime of selfless dedication, they feel, by their own accounts, that their life was "wasted"?

Doing Something About "the Problem"

The original feminists sought primarily to work for freedom and equality by changing the laws and by working within the "patriar-chal" system, even though they realized it was a system in which men have always dominated, in government, religion, work, and marriage.

The traditional form of feminism in America has had a proud history of advancing human rights for other minorities, in addition to those of women. Feminists played a major role in the movement to abolish slavery in the first half of the 19th century and a similar role in the early years of the blacks' civil rights struggle in the 1950s and '60s.

Harriet Taylor, one of the earliest and most influential feminists, undoubtedly collaborated with her husband, John Stuart Mills, on the ideas contained in his 1869 treatise, *The Subjection of Women*. Within forty years of its publication, and because of the many organized women's groups it spawned, the right to vote was accorded to women in America, Great Britain, and many of the countries of Europe. However, during the Depression, World War II, and the first two postwar decades, feminism as a civil-rights movement for women was silent.

In 1963, Betty Friedan's book clearly set out the feminist case: women have been made dependent, vulnerable, and passive and have been exploited, manipulated, and dominated by men and by the structures of society that men have created. Friedan spotlighted the unwritten "rules" required for all women. Besides the obedience, subservience, passivity, or dependence, additional prerequisites for optimal results in their assigned role included attractiveness and slenderness.

Generations of women have spoken of the boredom, emptiness, frustration, bitterness, and despair that results when women's freedoms to be authentic and "whole" are restricted. "Slavery" to one role, that of housewife/mother, has always been a central **part of the feminists' grievance.**

In addition, some women ultimately become their own greatest enemy when they punish themselves with depression for any anger, resentment, or rage they feel as a direct result of the restricted role assigned to them in life.

However, for many women, their own final, self-destructive, response to the feminine mystique is indeed "tragic." Reacting to their perception that they have done little of value, and that they are no longer needed for anything or anyone, they passively allow themselves to be overcome by the tasks of responsible living, to the extent that they become totally dependent on others for care. This occurs long before their physical health would require it, and long before their actual death.[4]

Women's massive return to home and hearth after the Second World War did not produce the result expected, that is, a generation of wonderful children. Nor did it produce an era of happy mothers. The sacrifice of the mothers' talents and abilities as human beings, apart from their total dedication to being wives and mothers, caused countless women to describe their existence as boring, oppressive, unchallenging, monotonous, unrewarding, unappreciated, unrespected, belittling, lonely, and "inhuman." Their lives were filled with feelings that they described as comparable to being "buried alive" or of "living in a concentration camp."[5] By sacrificing their capacities for intellectual growth to the demands of family, millions of housewives apparently felt dehumanized. (In 1955, tranquilizers didn't exist. Yet by 1959 the annual consumption of tranquilizers, almost all by women, was 1.15 **million pounds.**)

Recognizing the Accomplishments of the Women of the *Sandwich Generation*

The "sandwich" generation is the name applied to those women, born between 1920 and 1945, who have rendered more primary care to children, spouses, and aging parents than any other group in history. At present, ninety-five percent of the disabled Americans over sixty-five are **not** in nursing homes. For most of these, this is the result of the love and care they receive from the women in the family, which is no small contribution to the society.

However, because the demands on those born after 1945 are undoubtedly and uniquely burdensome, and as each successive decade seems to require that more time and energy be spent outside the home, it is certain that women will never again be able to supply such a high percentage of primary care in this country.

Today, no one would dare attempt to define an "ideal" woman. Nearly everyone claims the concept of femininity is passé, but women spend billions every year to conform to its dictates. Because the western cultural tradition has defined those characteristics it claims are essential to the feminine gender, for example, dependence, docility, cooperativeness, gentleness, nurturance, and attractiveness, some feminists urge abandoning the entire tradition itself, and starting over. In addition, some feminists, like Simone DeBeauvoir, Gloria Steinem, Marilyn French, Susan Faludi, Mary Koss, and Peggy McIntosh, have fought to eliminate all gender differences, and seek to make a political issue out of every supposedly-feminine quality.[6]

Examining Sexuality and the *Contradictions* in Feminist Theories

I have no intention of entering into the debate about abortion, sexual preference, or sexual freedom (the issues that come most quickly to mind in every discussion of feminism), having already made reference to the fact that there is no lack of feminists who have given up on men and on male/female sexual relationships. There are also those who would abandon our entire western cultural tradition, claiming it is built on male principles or male values. These women would substitute what they claim is the only criteria for what is valid, namely each woman's own personal experience. They see diversity and pluralism as desirable. Their key to ending male "thought-control," or the intellectual domination that justifies men's bodily domination, is to make the answer to every question indeterminate.

Fortunately, the majority view is not to repudiate our cultural heritage, including the religious ones, nor even to continue to shame and blame men for past oppression. Rather, the most recent trend is toward putting more effort into discussions of specific feminist issues, in fact initiating more civil debates, with less energy being expended and wasted on fighting.

As a suggested agenda for such discussions, Elisabeth Fox-Genovese, the noted historian, in *Feminism Without Illusions,* raises many questions that the leaders of the women's movement should not ignore. Her book concerns itself with some **"basic contradictions" of feminist theory and practice,** the most obvious being the fact that the **most frequently expressed "feminist" position on a woman's right to abortion as an unassailable individual right is 180 degrees opposed to the official feminist position on virtually all other political, legal, or social issues**.

Clearly, the feminist movement has fought to make the government **more powerful**, sometimes radically socialistic, in the movement's attempts to eliminate both public and private pornography and prostitution, as well as to establish de-facto equality in the home, politics, religion, and in the workplace.[7] Attempting to achieve equality in the workplace, feminists propose whenever possible the use of affirmative action programs that would give women more opportunities by giving equally qualified men fewer opportunities. The feminist agenda typically supports the implementation of a system of compensation for various jobs, based not on a free market system of supply and demand, but rather on an arbitrary and inevitably disruptive system of comparative worth, which means for example that "women's work," such as that of being a librarian or secretary could be compensated at the same or higher level as "men's work," such as construction or trash collection. (The level of compensation would depend on whatever the legislators would decide.) Some aims of the feminist movement would require inequitable allocation of community resources. Examples include governmental provision of daycare and health care centers as well as the increased allocation of limited police resources for the protection of women and children in the home and bedroom.

In striving for a change to stronger government, the feminists ignore the fact that their proposals would require interventions by a state so powerful that it could ignore the individual rights of others, especially of men. Admittedly, at the heart of the feminist agenda has been women's struggle to free themselves, and their children, from any form of male domination. An unfortunate consequence of the new laws that remove a man's authority over his wife in the marriage is that the male is simultaneously freed of any obligation to protect his family, when such protection is no longer in his own best interests.

Another unwanted consequence of feminist demands that the state protect women and children from men's domination everywhere, including the home and bedroom, has been the creation of state agencies that claim the right to monitor the way parents raise their children. **Thus, by removing the barrier between what is public responsibility and what is private**, they have, as Fox-Genovese writes, carried the **radical-feminists** "battle cry" to its logical conclusion: **"If the *personal* is *political*, then, by an implacable logic, the *private* must now be *public*."**[8]

The issue of abortion is a different matter entirely as the pro-choice feminists steadfastly maintain the position that the state should be **less powerful, in fact, powerless** to interfere in any woman's pregnancy. The hard-fought legal battles have already been won that finally allow women the private use of their bodies and of their sexuality without state interference, a right that men have always claimed. Now, the right demanded is for the state to allow, or in fact protect, their total control of the destiny of their unborn child.

Quite correctly, pro-choice advocates now see the legal victory on the abortion issue in "Roe vs. Wade" as a very limited one because the woman's control of the fate of her unborn child applies only to the time when the baby is "previable," defined as the time when the prevailing scientific opinion is that the unborn child cannot survive outside the mother's body. This previable portion of the pregnancy, because of seemingly inevitable scientific advances, keeps getting shorter and shorter and could someday no longer exist. Even during that "private interval" from conception to viability, the pro-choice advocates correctly see the governments on various levels raising obstacles or placing limits to a pregnant woman's choice of abortion.

Using the argument that the maternal-fetal entity is protected from government control by the mother's right to privacy has rightly been seen by many on the pro-choice side to be a very foolish one, especially after women have finally ended their status as a man's private property.[9]

In an attempt to establish a solid legal foundation for the pro-choice position, Eileen McDonagh, in *Breaking the Abortion Deadlock: From Choice to Consent*, (Oxford University Press: New York. 1996) insists that "Roe vs. Wade" placed the abortion debate on an unresolvable issue, namely, **what the fetus is,** whether a living human being that is not yet a person under the law, or a living human person. This led to the decision of the court to use "viability" as the dividing line between **legal** and **illegal abortions.** As a result of this, and subsequent decisions affirming the Supreme Court's position, all abortions, defined as "deliberately terminating a pregnancy with the intent to kill the fetus," should eventually be illegal as the technology is developed to keep a developing fetus or even the earliest embryo developing on the path to clear human personhood independent of the mother.

The only correct legal approach to the abortion issue, Ms. McDonagh insists, is for the courts and legislatures to consider **what a fetus does.** "Like it or not, abortion kills human life . . . whether or not human life is synonymous with personhood. . . . [But] once the fertilized ovum is recognized as **the agent responsible for the massive bodily transformations of pregnancy,** the primary legal issues become a **woman's right to consent to a relationship** with this intruder, **not its status as a person.** Since women cannot escape from the intrusion in any other way, they are entitled to employ deadly force, as well as state assistance, to stop it. . . . [The due process provisions of the 14th amendment] guarantee that no fetus [as a private party] has a right to intrude on a woman's body and liberty by making her pregnant without her consent . . . [and along with the equal protection provisions of the same amendment, makes] the fundamental job of the state . . . to stop [these] private parties from intruding on others, and this translates into the obligation of the state to provide abortion to women as a mandatory remedy, not a discretionary benefit."

Breaking the Abortion Deadlock ends by asserting that using another person's body (in this case, the mother's body) to preserve, protect, and defend one's own (that is, the body of the fetus) requires the consent of that other person (the mother). "This is the basic precept of the American political system."

Admitting that a cultural shock is inevitable when abortion is viewed in this way, author McDonagh insists education will dissolve our biases, and the laws will eventually be changed to conform to the new realities!

Getting Back to the Decisions That Must Be Yours

In the third millennium, the myriad choices available to the majority of women will make their personal and career decisions most difficult and conflicted. Obviously, only a fool would try to impose choices upon them. The problem that remains for women, in the short term at least, is that the joy, satisfaction, and delight that men regularly experience in their "life's work" continue to elude many women. Men, for the most part, readily find challenges they consider worthy of their time and effort. Women, on the other hand, now find it extremely difficult to find the same degree of satisfaction and joy being a housewife/mother or from a life devoted almost entirely to a career. One would have to be magnificently uninformed to say that the first is fulfilling enough to the modern woman or that a career outside the home is not many times harder for women than it is for men.

Especially in the nineties, being **"just a mother and a house-wife" seems for more and more women an admission that they are not accomplishing enough**. Surely for some women at least, the nurturing relationships could be secondary or even incidental to a life with specific goals and accomplishments.[10]

Putting the Feminist Issues in Perspective

By way of summary, a few observations seem pertinent. Perhaps most germane is the answer to the question: who is speaking for the feminist cause? Surely, there are "spokespersons" for feminism purporting to speak for the majority of women when they clearly do not, and who use a woman's stand on abortion, sexual preference, and even marriage, as a **litmus test** for deciding whether or not she is part of the **feminist** struggle. Admittedly, a basic feminist value is that each woman become independent and knowledgable enough to author her own distinctive life-vision.[11]

Since having a **choice** of being a housewife/mother and/or having a career vastly complicates, rather than simplifies, a woman's life, the future challenge for women seems awesome. It is in this vein that Susan Jeffers has written that the women's movement "is about responsibility . . . becoming the best we can. . . . Looked at this way, the women's movement has nothing to do with men."[12] Rather, whether discussing feminism or your life, **the issue is responsible choices, both great and small, lifelong and temporary, that each must make.**

16

Making Your Own Judgment Regarding Life's Meaning and Purpose

"A thought transfixed me: For the first time in my life, I saw the truth as it is set into song by so many poets, proclaimed as the final wisdom by so many thinkers, the truth that Love is the ultimate goal to which man can aspire. Then I grasped the meaning of the greatest secret that human poetry and human thought and belief have to impart: The salvation of man is through Love and in Love."
—Viktor Frankl, *Man's Search For Meaning*[1]

". . . (I)t may seem that only the big events are ultimately important. But to the soul, the most minute details and the most ordinary activities . . . have an effect far beyond their apparent insignificance."
—Thomas Moore, *Care of the Soul*

The central focus of this book has been **active choices**, meaning decisions that require you to **do** something. In prior generations, women had few, if any, choices and little time or energy to search for options outside the home. All that has changed. Now the type of life a woman experiences is very much the result of her own choices. Therefore, an early priority should be to invest as much time and effort as she can on the tasks suggested in this book.

In Section One, fifteen or twenty health suggestions for preventing bodily ailments were provided. In Section Two, the entire emphasis was on healing relationships, especially on creating one permanent and intimate "connection." In Chapter 15, information was provided to help and encourage you to choose some role in the feminist movement.

However, the final active choice, which has been saved for this chapter, could possibly be the most vital decision of your entire life: your answer to the question, **"What is life's meaning and purpose?"**

Just as women are turning increasingly to women physicians for answers to their health problems, so are they also looking to feminist spokeswomen for new answers to their questions about religion and moral issues. As a consequence, this final chapter is primarily an exhortation to women to retain what is reasonable from past traditions and to reject anything that seems to create new problems.

Accepting the *Supernatural* in Your Life

Harold Kushner writes, "'What does life mean?' is a hard question to answer, but an even harder one to avoid answering." In *Creating Love* and *The Road Less Traveled,* both John Bradshaw and Scott Peck insist on the concept that Love is life's highest goal but also life's hardest task, and that the very narrow path of Love is littered with pain and anxiety. William James, the philosopher and psychologist, wrote that when we deliberately choose suffering for ourselves, by self-denial, we are choosing the path to human happiness and fulfillment. He claimed, in fact, that this self-denial is so basic a human need that it could even replace man's need to wage war. While all these ideas seem true enough, they do not really answer the basic question, nor do they really teach us **how** to live and love. Most important, they fail to motivate us.

Rather, it is your understanding of who you are, why you are here now in this world, and what you think will happen to you, if anything, after your death, that does affect the way you handle the daily demands of living, especially the pain and suffering. Your thoughts on life's meaning also influence your response to what others do to you, and how you will treat others. Equally important, your answers to these questions determine how much you esteem yourself, and therefore, as we have seen, how much value you place on your love.

Traditionally, women have derived comfort and personal esteem from a belief that there was a totally just and forgiving God who loved them. But as Elisabeth Fox-Genovese points out, "Various feminist projects have begun to erode our confidence in the culture we have inherited . . . especially our religion."[2] **In book after book, the same isolated "chauvinistic" texts are cited to support a theory that the Bible is a human construct.** The assertion is made that it is not a divinely inspired story of the human-divine relationship, but rather part of a conspiracy at the dawn of recorded history and intended to justify and sustain a patriarchal, or male-dominated society.[3] **Despite these challenges to the Bible, as Riane Eisler admits, it is a fact that what the ancient texts foretold, the time of deliverance from hate and oppression, for Hebrew and Gentile alike, could and indeed should have been achieved, if only Jesus Christ's "central message"—the *repudiation of all notions of dominance*—had been accepted.**[4]

In fairness to the feminists' claim, it must be acknowledged that throughout all of human history, both before and since the Christian era, women have suffered more than men. The record itself is a political story, that is, a tale of relationships defined by power, of might makes right, and the domination of the weak by the strong. Every age has had its individual victors and victims. The prevailing principle for controlling human actions has been that the "ends," defined as having the power, have been used to justify any "means" for getting that power.

Precisely because the lesson of the past shows so clearly that power, on a day-to-day basis, usually defines what is right, it is futile and dangerous for the feminist movement, which seeks to protect women from domination and victimization, to adopt as its primary goal the elimination of **all** supposedly "patriarchal" or male-dominated institutions or systems, including the religious ones. Thus, when Mary Daly, Simone DeBeauvoir, Gloria Steinem, Kate Millett, Susan Faludi, and others dismiss the religious tradition as beyond repair, they are, I believe, not only demonstrating poor judgment, but they are also being dangerously shortsighted.

It seems clearly fallacious in the light of the facts to allege that women have been "subjected" by the Judeo-Christian tradition, when this tradition, in fact, has been a guarantor and protector of women's dignity, as an essential part of its dogma. **That the dogma has sometimes failed to protect women should be a judgment on the attitudes and observance of individual men, and not an accurate or faithful reflection on the rightness of the dogma.** When the religious tradition is studied as a whole, and the isolated "chauvinistic" texts already referred to are viewed in the light of the overall text, one does not see domination or oppression, but rather love and concern. That love has been expressed by those who believe and whose character reflects the gospel message, in their relationships: of truth, justice, faithfulness, forgiveness, commitment, reconciliation, reverence, and honor.[5]

While many feminist writers find problems for women in the biblical account of creation, it should be stressed, in order to be accurate, that nothing in the first two chapters of Genesis supports a hierarchical view of man and woman. In fact, one finds there that with each creative act, God made a higher form of being, so that one could logically say that Eve represented God's final triumph, not an afterthought. Eve was referred to as man's "helpmate," which throughout the Old Testament was a word used mostly to refer to God, not to a servant. God should be viewed to be as much a woman as a man, both sexes having been "made in God's image." The Bible, in fact, contains numerous references to God as Mother.[6] It is quite correct to pray to God as our Mother. (For Christians it is traditional and theologically sound to speak of God as the Father of His Son, Jesus Christ, since Jesus had a **human** *mother.* Making the concept of paternity even more confusing is the belief that the "third person of the Trinitiy," the "Holy Spirit," and not "God the Father" was the spouse of Mary. What should be manifestly apparent from these attempts to apply gender to God is the **utter incomprehensibility** of an *eternal being,* lacking nothing, who exists outside of time and space.)

Those women who reject all the present religious traditions because of their perception that they are all systems created by men, and that they all oppress women, or at least treat them as lesser humans, must now seek, as a result of this rejection, new answers to who they are, why they are in this world, and what happens afterward. Since the answer we choose to accept for each of these questions determines our ongoing response to life's demands, ultimately our answers affect both our health and our happiness. For all these reasons then, the questions cannot be ignored.

When the objection is made that religion has not always reverenced and protected women, even when society seemed to be entirely under religion's control, the answer must surely be that religion, like God, cannot take away man's free will.[7] Whether an infinite God interferes with man's freedom or men do it, it still constitutes tyranny. Despite what the basic assertion of humanism proclaims, that is, that the newborn human being is noble and good, and only later is corrupted by society, we know that history has proven that such a claim is absurd, a myth. The story of mankind shows convincingly that real sin, greed, selfishness, and aggression are ever-present choices of the human heart.

Since the lesson of history is clear, we can confidently assert that those feminists who would abolish most established religions are also being short-sighted in regard to their own welfare. We can predict that destroying or undermining religion will simply give birth to substitutes even less friendly to women.

Looking Briefly at the Message to **Men**

A large part of this book has been devoted to compiling a **wishlist** on behalf of women and children. I have dared to invite men to strive for greater reverence of women, and to develop more sensitivity to women's need to have men **verbally** communicate their love and appreciation. Hopefully this has not been a sermon delivered to the men already converted, that is, only to those who have already accepted that message in their own lives.

I have also exhorted men to cease demanding that wives, daughters, and co-workers still be made to "conform" to absurd "feminine" standards that stifle their development as persons and prevent them from pursuits they might wish to undertake. Women must not, in Stendhal's words, continue to be "lost to humanity " because of these outdated restrictions.

Summarizing . . . Where We Stand

The matter of women's "position" in society is officially being reported each ten years in the United Nations publication, *State of the World's Women*. The 1975 and 1985 evaluations were nearly identical.

Women comprise one-half of the world's population, work twice as many hours as men for one-tenth of the pay men earn, and acquire one-hundred times less property.[8] The 1995 report showed little economic progress, not to mention the failure to decrease the incidence of atrocities inflicted worldwide. These crimes, shameful enough to stir the coldest of hearts, were spotlighted at the International Conference on Women, held in Beijing, China, in 1995.[9]

While no "report" can accurately measure the fears that American women experience daily as a result of our violent culture, my focus on "women's active choices" is prompted by my firm conviction that women's happiness, and men's too, not to mention the fate of this planet, depends almost entirely on women healing their relationships with their mates. Employing patience and exercising great respect for men's sensitivity, each woman must try to guide her mate to an awareness of the pain that keeps him unfeeling and which motivates his destructiveness. As a reward for such "work," she might discover a man who has become more caring, more feeling, more gentle, and more joyous.

Even though marriage often continues to be an institution that legitimizes a man's imperious tendencies, or that allows him to maintain a sexual dominance, it is the woman who must empathize, or feel with him, the terrible emptiness or void that becoming a man produces, and which results in his inability to be intimate with anyone.

Obviously, the challenge for the 21st century is to make American society safe for everyone. History's message is quite clear, namely, that whenever the rights and dignity of any group is ignored or left unprotected, the dignity of everyone else in that society is also diminished.[10]

However, **the most important truth for each one of us to remember, accept,** *and act upon* **is that each "good" human relation-**

ship, each "bond" of intimacy, produces much more than the countless *personal* benefits of genuine love. These bonds represent the only antidote, the only defense, the only hope humanity has to survive the violence and save our world.

JAS-1997.

Appendix

WARNING! *by Jenny Joseph*

When I am an old woman I shall wear purple
With a red hat which doesn't go, and doesn't suit me.
And I shall spend my pension on brandy and summer gloves
And satin sandals, and say we've no money for butter.

I shall sit down on the pavement when I'm tired
And gobble up samples in shops and press alarm bells
And run my stick along the public railings
And make up for the sobriety of my youth.

I shall go out in my slippers in the rain
And pick the flowers in other people's gardens
And learn to spit.

You can wear terrible shirts and grow more fat
And eat three pounds of sausages at a go
Or only bread and pickle for a week
And hoard pens and pencils and beermats and things in boxes.

But now we must have clothes that keep us dry
And pay our rent and not swear in the street
And set a good example for the children.

We must have friends to dinner and read the papers.
But maybe I ought to practice a little now?
So people who know me are not too shocked and surprised
When suddenly I am old, and start to wear purple.

When I Am An Old Woman, I Shall Wear Purple
(Ed. Sandra Hartman Martz) Papier Mache Press,
135 Aviation Way, #14, Watsonville CA 95076 (1991)

245

NOMOGRAM FOR BODY MASS INDEX

Directions: Determine the weight and height and connect the two values by a straight line. The point of intersection with the central line is the value for the "body mass index." The "acceptable," "overweight," and "Obese" ranges are indicated. (See page 115 of text for explanation of use of this value.)

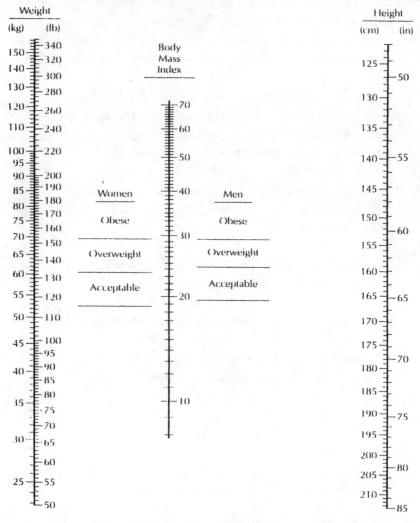

Nomogram copied from *Clinical Endocrinology and Infertility*. Fifth Edition. Speroff, Leon., Robert Glass., Nathan G. Kase. Williams and Wilkins: Baltimore. 1994. page 653.

FORMULA FOR CALCULATING PERCENT BODY FAT

For use and significance of percent body fat for women. See especially Chapter Eight, page 115.

Percent Body Fat = Constant A (hip in inches) + Constant B (waist in inches) – Contant C (height in inches)

$\dfrac{\text{Percent Body Fat - 22}}{100}$ x weight (lbs.) = number of pounds over/under ideal weight

Hips		Abdomen		Height	
In.	Constant A	In.	Constant B	In.	Constant C
30	33.48	20	14.22	55	33.52
31	34.87	21	14.93	56	34.13
32	36.26	22	15.64	57	34.74
33	37.67	23	16.35	58	35.35
34	39.06	24	17.06	59	35.96
35	40.46	25	17.78	60	36.57
36	41.86	26	18.49	61	37.18
37	43.25	27	19.20	62	37.79
38	44.65	28	19.91	63	38.40
39	46.05	29	20.62	64	39.01
40	47.44	30	21.33	65	39.62
41	48.84	31	22.04	66	40.23
42	50.24	32	22.75	67	40.84
43	51.64	33	23.46	68	41.45
44	53.03	34	24.18	69	42.06
45	54.43	35	24.89	70	42.67
46	55.83	36	25.60	71	43.28
47	57.22	37	26.31	72	43.89
48	58.62	38	27.02	73	44.50
49	60.02	39	27.73	74	45.11
50	61.42	40	28.44	75	45.72
51	62.81	41	29.15	76	46.32
52	64.21	42	29.87	77	46.93
53	65.61	43	30.58	78	47.54
54	67.00	44	31.29	79	48.15
55	68.40	45	32.00	80	48.76
56	69.80	46	32.71	81	49.37
57	71.19	47	33.42	82	49.98
58	72.59	48	34.13	83	50.59
59	73.99	49	34.84	84	51.20
60	75.39	50	35.56	85	51.81

From *The Complete Book of Physical Fitness*,
A.G. Fisher and R.K. Confee.

A MEDITATION ON MOTHERING

Mothering Myself
In a society preoccupied with how best to raise a child
I'm finding a need to mesh what's best for my children with
    what's necessary for a well-balanced mother.
I'm recognizing that ceaseless giving translates into giving
    yourself away.
And, when you're giving yourself away, you're not a healthy
    mother and you're not a healthy self.

So, now I'm learning to be a woman first and a mother second.
I'm learning to just experience my own emotions
Without robbing my children of their individual dignity by
    feeling their emotions too.
I'm learning that a healthy child will have his own set of
    emotions and characteristics that are his alone.
And, very different from mine.
I'm learning the importance of honest exchanges of feelings
    because pretenses don't fool children,
They know their mother better than she knows herself.

I'm learning that no one overcomes her past unless she
    confronts it.
Otherwise, her children will absorb exactly what she's
    attempting to overcome.
I'm learning that life is meant to be filled with as much
    sadness and pain as happiness and pleasure.
And allowing ourselves to feel everything life has to offer is
    an indicator of fulfillment.
I'm learning that fulfillment can't be obtained through giving
    myself away
But, through giving to myself and sharing with others,
I'm learning that the best way to teach my children to live a
    fulfilling life is not by sacrificing my life.

It's through living a fulfilling life myself.
I'm trying to teach my children that I have a lot to learn
Because I'm learning that letting go of them
Is the best way of holding on.

by Nancy McBrine Sheehan, quoted from
*Women's Bodies, Women's Wisdom: Creating Physical and
Emotional Health and Healing* by Christiane Northrup,
Bantam Books: New York, 1996, pg. 428-429

The Schaller Family Recipe for
POTATO PANCAKES

For each three medium-size Idaho potatoes, add one whole egg and one-half teaspoon of salt, and liquefy in the blender. When making large quantities—for example, twelve potatoes—an extra egg or two is suggested.

Put about one-half inch of cannola oil (or liquid vegetable oil) in a fry pan and bring to maximum heat while the potato mixture is draining in a colander. Most of the liquid should be drained before the potato mixture is put in the fat.

Using a metal slotted spoon that holds about three or four tablespoons (available at any supermarket), carefully drop about twenty *separate* spoonfuls of mixture into the hot fat. About ten seconds after being in the fat, each pancake should be flattened and "ridged" with a flat-edged pancake turner. (The smaller and thinner the pancakes are made, the crispier and tastier they become.)

When browned on one side, turn over. Do not put ridges (nooks and crannies) on this side, but rather, after ten seconds, use the smallest-pronged fork you have (or even a metal probe you use to tie up chickens), and punch multiple holes in the pancakes.

Remove when done, and put on paper towels to absorb all the fat. Eat as soon as possible, using hot apple sauce as your pancake "syrup."

GOOD EATING!

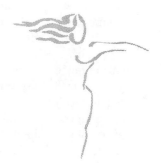

Chapter Notes

PREFACE

1. (pg. xi) The "active" ingredient in **Lydia Pinkham's Compound** was probably the hormone-like natural plant steroid supplied by a root of the Trillium, or liliaceous genus. The manufacturer harvested the herb in North Carolina, where the local inhabitants called it "Beth's root."

The phytoestrogen (plant estrogen or "weak-estrogen") equivalent available in Europe for forty-five years and now available in the United States is an extract of the rhizome (underground part) of a plant called **Cimicifuga racemosa**, popular name, "black cohosh." In a "randomized double-blind study," the use of a dose of 40mg per day of the commercially available product called **Remifemin** proved to be superior to 0.625mg of conjugated estrogen in normalizing the vagina and improving the scores on the Hamiton Anxiety Scale (HAMA), as well as being comparable in improving the Self-Assessment Depression Scale (SDS) and the Profile of Mood States (POMS). "The clinical experience confirms that **Remifemin is extremely well tolerated and does not introduce any adverse effects." (Menopause, vol. 1, No. 3, 1994, p. 173-4. Raven Press: New York.)** Now available at most health food stores as 20mg tablets to be taken twice a day, this herbal "drug" should be taken only upon the advice of a knowledgable health care provider and **never in pregnancy or while breast-feeding.** These cautions should be observed before you take any medicinal herbs.

For information on **"Vitex,"** the most popular herbal remedy in Europe for **PMS, menopause, hormonal "problems," even nausea in pregnancy,** write to **Botanica Press: Capitola, CA 95010,** Box 742.

2. (pg. xiii) Sandra Lee Bartky sees contemporary American women living in a "prison," by being subject to the disciplines of "femininity"

throughout their daily lives. "The woman who checks her make-up half a dozen times a day to see if her foundation has caked or her mascara run, who worries that the wind or rain may spoil her hairdo, who looks frequently to see if her stockings have bagged at the ankle, or, feeling fat, monitors everything she eats, has become, just as surely as the inmate [in a prison], a self-policing subject, a self committed to a relentless self-surveillance . . . a form of obedience to patriarchy." **ref. 5, p. 75.**

Nancy Friday writes, "the fashion and cosmetics industry didn't create women's dissatisfaction with their bodies. Commerce merely preys upon an already-learned insecurity, putting a dollar sign in front of the hope that someday we may find something that makes us smell, taste, and feel good about ourselves . . . we can't believe anyone would want us as we are." **ref. 36, p. 141.**

Catherine MacKinnon rejects femininity as we know it, because "accepting it would mean acceptance or even desiring male domination." **ref. 73, p. 110.**

3. (pg. xv) **Depression** affects about forty percent of Americans at least once in their lives, with slightly more than two-and-a-half times as many women being affected as men. Even when men are depressed, they can frequently mask the condition with drug and alcohol abuse or workaholism.

This book, especially Section Two, will provide little permanent help to anyone with a major depression. Rather, **professional psychiatric help is urgently needed.**

The specific criteria for depression are:

1. Depressed mood most of the day, nearly every day, as stated by patient ("sad," "empty") or observed (crying, tears),
and/or
2. Anhedonia (that is, markedly diminished interest or pleasure) in all, or almost all, activities most of the day, nearly every day.
plus any four of the following:
1. Significant weight change(+/- 10 pounds in a two-week period) when not dieting.
2. Sleeping disturbance—too much or too little.
3. Extreme restlessness or listlessness.
4. Totally fatigued day after day.
5. Feelings of worthlessness or excessive or inappropriate guilt every day.
6. Diminished ability to think, to concentrate, to make any decisions, day after day.
7. Recurrent thoughts of death, or suicidal ideas, or plans for or attempts at suicide.

For depression to be diagnosed, one or another of the first two choices and at least four of the last seven must be present for at least two weeks in the absence of any serious triggering cause such as death of a loved one or a recent diagnosis of cancer. (Quoted in **ref. 94, p. 23-24**)

Perhaps Hamlet' simple description of depression could prove useful to you: "How weary, stale, flat and unprofitable/ Seem to me all the uses of the world."

Depression and anxiety play a large part in those patients (again more frequently female than male) initially diagnosed as cases of **chronic fatigue syndrome,** but in whom no disease, viral infection, or immune system changes are found. (See Notes Ch. 3, 1.)

SECTION ONE—STAYING HEALTHY

THE FIRST CHALLENGE: Selecting the Simplest and Least Expensive, But Most Useful Health Strategies

Introducing Section One

1. (pg. 4) Besides the information provided on "Alternative Medicine" in the "Resources" segment, the reader might wish to read about some of the precautions that are included among the current articles:

Relieving Chronic Pain Without Drugs. Readers Digest. November, 1996. pp. 135-39. (Sue Browder.)

The Healing Power of Herbs. Good Housekeeping. November, 1996. pp. 104ff. (Sharon Waxman.)

Alternative Medicine. Town and Country. January, 1997. pp. 97-104. Diane Guerney.)

Remember that herbs shouldn't be taken by children, pregnant women, or nursing mothers unless specifically approved by their physician. **See also Ch. Notes, Preface, #1.**

1 Being Kind to Your Skin

1. (pg. 8) For up-to-date information on lactose intolerance, **see Ch. Notes, Ch. 5, #13.**

Bacterial Vaginosis should be treated because recent evidence indicates it can lead to pelvic pain and infection.

"Vaginal" odors, especially as women's bladders become less efficient with aging, are usually due to urinary odors that are the result of eating vegetables. The worst offender is asparagus. A herbal remedy often recommended for recurrent vaginal "problems" is a clove of garlic dipped in vegetable oil that is inserted into the vagina and changed every twelve hours for a few days!

2. (pg. 15) Jane Hirschman and Carol Hunter present their work as a "Complete Handbook for women who want to free themselves from body hatred and from the dieting it spawns." **ref. 55, Introduction.**

2 Attending to Five Other Little Things

1. (pg. 19) "Enviracaire" by Honeywell (HEPA filter); "Jenn Air Silent air purifier" (800-236-6139 or 800-777-8848); "Living Air" or "Airwise," which produce ozone, a theoretical problem to some "experts." A $500-600 machine, the size and weight of a gallon of water, can purify up to 2500 sq. ft. (610-347-6005, 800-987-9247, or 800-874-9028); "Vitar," an electrophoretic air cleaner that utilizes a washable filter and doesn't produce any ozone (609-397-3636 or fax 609-397-2626).

2. (pg. 22) A baby aspirin daily might protect against colon cancer, just like estrogen. **See also Notes, Ch. 5, 12.**

3. (pg. 27) Quoted in **ref. 31, p. 37.**

4. (pg. 27) Guidelines for **Asymptomatic Patients:** baseline breast x-rays at age 35 and repeats every year from age 40. (If mother or sister had breast cancer, test at least yearly from age of 30.)

5. (pg. 28) **ref. 55, p. 147.**

6. (pg. 29) **ref. 49, p. 38.**

7. (pg. 31) **ref. 83, p. 151.** See also **ref. 55, p. 148, 153.**

8. (pg. 32) **ref. 83, Chapter Five, and p. 165; and ref. 59**, many references to progesterone throughout the book. See also **ref. 55, p. 149.**

9. (pg. 33) **Kegel Exercises** refers to exercises for the lowermost muscles of the female pelvis. These muscles extend from the pubic bone to the coccyx, or tailbone, and "wrap around" the bladder opening, the lower vagina, and the anal canal and anal opening. Each group of "wrap-around muscles" can and should be exercised separately, at least from the first sign of weakness in stopping the flow of urine or a bowel movement, or the inability to contract the muscles that close the lower vagina. This last group of muscles can be evaluated by placing several fingers into the vagina and "squeezing" them with the vaginal muscles. Experts insist that there are two groups of muscles involved in **continence** and that it is necessary to exercise both groups by alternating contracting and relaxing these muscles repetitively very briefly with prolonged contractions lasting five to ten seconds. See also **ref. 2, p. 151-154, 157, 262.**

3 Handling the Problems Your Ovaries Hand You

1. (pg. 37) Estrogen deficiency or menopause can explain extreme fatigue, as can the **Chronic Fatigue Syndrome.** This condition, according to the Centers for Disease Control, affects 175,000±75,000 Americans. This condition is a specific disorder first recognized medically in the 1980s. People affected are truly disabled and cannot work. Commonly there is a low-grade fever, muscle aches and weakness, recurrent sore throats, painful lymph nodes, joint pains, and headache. Sleep doesn't help the fatigue, and often concentration and short-term memory are impaired. The precise cause of this disorder is unknown, but the immune system is involved.

An AMA survey showed that twenty-nine percent of women and nineteen percent of men who were randomly surveyed in the waiting room of a general medical clinic complained of chronic fatigue. If a person's chronic fatigue lasts over a few weeks and is severe, treatable causes should be sought, even though typically no cause is found. In eighty percent, however, one finds a more than normal amount of depression and anxiety. It is suggested, as with all one's emotional or relational problems, that increasing your awareness of your own feelings, and actually keeping a journal of your energy level (use a scale of 0-10) at 8 a.m., 4 p.m., and 8 p.m., will eventually lead you to better insight into your specific problems. A good idea is to focus on your energy patterns, especially the things that increase it in you.

4 Coping With Premenstrual Tension

1. (pg. 45) **Mood swings** should be easily distinguished from **PMS** by asking a few simple questions. In the former, hyperactivity alternates with the *blues* throughout the cycle, with the most symptomatic time usually *coinciding with the period.* In PMS, by contrast, the most symptomatic time is *the week before the period,* and "blessed" relief comes with the period. An overactive thyroid gland must be ruled out if mood swings occur, especially when they seem not to correlate with the phases of the menstrual cycle.

2. (pg. 46) **Migraines usually start in adolescence. "Classic" migraines are unilateral, that is, one-sided. (Contrary to what is commonly taught and believed) migraine headaches are preceded by an "aura" or warning only 20% of the time. When an aura occurs, it is usually a visual one. A migraine is often accompanied by nausea and vomiting or fear of sound and/or light.** These so-called "sick headaches" are generally disabling. When they cluster around day 10-14 of the men-

strual cycle, the days of menstruation, or the day or two before menstruation, they are almost certainly **triggered** by a fall in estrogen production. For the same reason, menopausal estrogenic hormones taken intermittently, or in generic formulations, in which the strength of each pill is allowed to vary as much as 60%, can actually be responsible for periodic migraines. True **sinus headaches** are very rare, and obviously wouldn't be intensified by light or sound. Thus, most sinus headaches are, in fact, migraine headaches. Migraines frequently produce pain in the sinus areas. It has been now fairly well-accepted that nearly **one of every five women suffer from migraine headaches.**

Headaches that become a **daily** occurrence in patients who had previously been periodic migraine sufferers have been found, in ninety percent of the cases, to be the result of **rebound** from the overuse of plain aspirin/tylenol, or these analgesics combined with caffeine, barbiturates, or other pain relievers that are frequently taken by the migraine sufferers. When such self-medications are slowly discontinued, the daily headaches stop.

In contrast, **headaches that are on the back, top, or in front of the head,** while more frequent, do not typically have any of the disabling features of a migraine, and, if due to hormones at all, are **most likely when estrogen is temporarily low or absent, not fluctuating**.

3. (pg. 47) Mary Valentis and Anne Devane write that the goal for women is to "achieve authenticity without hurting others or [themselves]. . . . Rage is the gateway to self-assertion, deeper psychological development, and emotional well-being. . . . Rage has successfully exposed and fought sexual harassment, the glass ceiling, and a medical establishment that has ignored women's issues." **ref. 113, Introduction, especially page 9.**

While **rage** has united some women, especially against men, it **has been very divisive of the feminist movement,** not to mention the damage created in each woman's closest relationships, as is detailed in Chapters Ten to Twelve.

4. (pg. 48) Most authorities, I believe, agree basically with my assertion that a **deficiency of progesterone (not the absence of progesterone) is somehow contributory to PMS**. **ref. 83, p. 108, 121, 124-25**. Some, however, say PMS involves a deficiency of estrogen in the presence of progesterone. **ref. 92, pg. 15 and 372.**

5. (pg. 49) Anorexia Nervosa occurs to some degree in 2-5% of white adolescent females and young adults. When severe, this condition represents a true psychiatric disorder that can be fatal. It is a major cause of amenorrhea or absence of periods in adolescents. (**see Notes, Ch. 8, 6.**)

6. (pg. 50) **ref. 1, p. 98.**

7. (pg. 53) Foods can influence our moods, feelings, and emotions by changing the level of **natural brain chemicals** like norepinephrine or serotonin, or other mood-elevating substances produced by the brain. Of course, the same can be said for drugs like "Prozac," "Zoloft," and "Serzone," or vitamin B6, dopamine, estrogen, melatonin, progesterone, and testosterone, as well as herbs like St. John's Wort, ginkgo biloba, kava, valerian root, soy powder isoflavones, evening primrose or flax-seed oils, and blue cahoosh or dong quai roots. Contrary to newly popular beliefs, **herbs** can be ill-advised or harmful, and **conventional medicines** can be life-saving. For your own protection, ask a professional.

8. (pg. 53) **ref. 83, p. 148.** Christiane Northrup's book provides ample bodymind or holistic recipes for everyday problems.

9. (pg. 55) Article by Lorraine Dusky, "The use of progesterone in PMS." **(McCall's Magazine), Oct. 1990, pg. 152ff.**

10. (pg. 55) The address of the *Women's Pharmacy* is: Women's Health Care Systems & Pharmaceuticals, 5900 Monona Drive, Madison, WI 53716 (800-999-6393).

Pro-Gest progesterone skin cream is manufactured by Professional and Technical Services, 333 Northeast Sandy Boulevard, Portland, OR 97232 (800-648-8211).

Madison Pharmacy Associates, 429 Gammon Place, Madison, WI 53719 (800-558-7046) has natural progesterone products and specific supplements for PMS.

11. (pg. 56) Not only do **I insist on natural progesterone in treatment of PMS**, but I also invariably double or triple the dose gradually from the first day of treatment to the last. I increase the dose for several reasons: (1) The normal ovary produces levels which go up rapidly and then down fairly quickly during the two weeks after ovulation. Since **progesterone**, among its many other anti-estrogenic effects, **is a natural diuretic** or a substance that helps the kidney excrete salt water better or faster, it reverses, at least partially, during the two weeks it is present, the salt-retaining effects of the body's estrogen. Thus, for two weeks, a woman with normally functioning ovaries has a natural diuretic, namely, progesterone, to prevent the swelling and weight gain that results from retained fluid. This natural process usually works well enough, especially if one is sensible about exercise, rest, and salt intake. But it does not work well enough if estrogen levels do not fall when progesterone levels fall. If excess estrogen is present, it will not only cause the retention of much more fluid, but it will also produce the classic mental effects seen in PMS, especially the aggression and rage. **When using progesterone to treat PMS, this "excess" estrogen during**

the final days of the cycle must be taken into account by increasing the progesterone. (2) In response to progesterone's presence in the blood, the adrenal gland produces its own powerful salt-retaining hormone—called aldosterone. Unless the level of progesterone keeps rising, the body begins, after a time, because of this adrenal aldosterone, to retain fluids. The weight often increases noticeably, temporarily.

Fluid retention is responsible for only part of the premenstrual bloating, which in many women actually means a change in dress size. Some of the change in abdominal girth is due to increased storage of gas in the small and large bowel, which itself has two explanations. Thus the bloating many women experience before their periods is explained by: (1) fluid retention in the lower abdominal fat pad; (2) a dilatation of the loops of the intestines as an effect of the female hormones' bowel-relaxing action, which is most prominent when the hormone blood levels are highest, which is premenstrually, and (3) increased swallowing of air as a result of smoking, nervousness, or anxiety.

To summarize progesterone use in PMS, it appears to be imperative that the natural fall in progesterone levels the week before the period be reversed, by doubling the dose of progesterone the second week of treatment. There are three reasons for this: (1) so that the aldosterone-estrogen fluid-retention effect can be blocked, thus markedly decreasing the swelling.; (2) because it is the last week of the cycle—the second week of progesterone treatment—that the estrogen excess is greatest; and (3) because progesterone, acting in the central nervous system, reverses the tendency of excess estrogen to make you "hyper" and instead promotes serenity.

See also Lee, John R., *Progesterone: The Multiple Roles of a Remarkable Hormone,* Sebastopol, CA: BLL Publishing (P.O. Box 02068), 1993.

5 Selecting Your Own Menopausal Approach

1. (pg. 58) ref. 83, p. 542.

2. (pg. 62) ref. 92, p. 215.

3. (pg. 62) Susan Faludi's exhaustively documented thesis that claims a media conspiracy starting at the beginning of the century, but especially in the 1980s, to make feminism, not the patriarchal system, the cause of all women's problems. ref. 28, p. 78-111, also p. xxii.

Ironically, Christina Sommers accuses Susan Faludi of biased reporting. Sommers claims Faludi ignores references that do not support her thesis. ref. 104, chapter 11.

4. (pg. 63) **Apple obesity**: when the maximum circumference of the waist exceeds 80% of the maximum circumference of the hips. There is a direct correlation of apple obesity to **high blood pressure, stroke, heart disease, diabetes, and breast cancer. Pear obesity**: when the waist is less than 75% of the hip circumference, correlates only with increased risk of arthritis of hips, knees, and ankles.

5. (pg. 64) Bergkvist, L., et al, "The risk of breast cancer after estrogen and estrogen-progestin replacement." (**N. Engl. J. Med.**, vol. 321, pg. 293-7, 1989.)

Estrogen's theoretical connection with breast cancer risk does not apply to **progesterone**. To the contrary, many studies suggest progesterone protects against breast cancer. Many patients with breast cancer, especially those who are **post-menopausal**, and therefore most likely to have **non-genetic tumors**, give a history of prolonged insufficient progesterone production. Early exposure to the large amount of progesterone in pregnancy can be protective against breast cancer for a lifetime. Studies suggest that one successful pregnancy, before age twenty, might reduce the risk of breast cancer as much as fifty percent, with two successful pregnancies, before age twenty-three, reducing the risk as much as seventy-five percent. **ref. 49, p. 90-107.** Studies equating natural with artificial progesterones are misleading because they are not at all the same hormones. (cf. "The use of estrogen and progestins and the risk of breast cancer in postmenopausal women," **The New England Journal of Medicine, June 15, 1995.**) The use of estrogen intermittently, not continuously (a method abandoned by most physicians around the world now) was totally unnatural.

Infertility, late pregnancies, no pregnancies, induced abortion, apple obesity, and the *biggest risk factor of all,* **namely advancing age, are all conditions where estrogen is present while progesterone is low or absent, and each increase the risk of acquiring breast cancer.**

How might progesterone protect against breast cancer? The essential function of progesterone is to modulate, modify, and in some cases enhance or complete the effects of estrogen on multiple organ systems. To cite just several effects at this point:

(1) In the breast and uterus, it completes and matures the tissues and prepares them for pregnancy. Its withdrawal results, in the case of the womb, in a "neat" period—that is, one that is not too heavy or too long—and, in the case of the breast, the completion in growth of potential milk-producing cells.

(2) In the kidney, it reverses estrogen's antidiuretic, or salt-retention effect, thus helping the body to get rid of retained fluid.

(3) **In the brain, progesterone tones down estrogen's tendency to stimulate the mind, and so tends to produce serenity.**

6. (pg. 65) Bergkvist, L., Adami, H.O., Persson, I., Bergston, R., Krusemo, U.B., "Prognosis after breast cancer in women exposed to estrogen and estrogen-progestin replacement therapy." (**Amer. Journal of Epidemiology, vol. 130, pg. 2, 221-228, Aug. 1989.**)

The differing conclusions about the relationship between hormones and breast cancer expressed in the **New England Journal of Medicine** article of June 15, 1995 and the **Journal of the American Medical Association** article of July 12, 1995 are but two of the thousands of studies over the past fifty years that have failed to "prove" the hormone connection. Most clinicians believe that because a definite link has not been shown in all that time, any relationship, if any, must be small indeed. Eight international experts on hormones and breast cancer reach the same conclusion. See "Demystifying the Hormone/ Breast Cancer Connection" (**Women's Health Digest, vol. 1, number 3, Summer 1995.** This is a quarterly medical journal for lay women, written by medical experts in simple language, and is available through **WOMEN to WOMEN AMERICA, 222 SW 36 Terrace, Gainesville, FL 32607.**)

7. (pg. 65) **See also Notes, Ch. 5, 5.** Another recent article reported that use of hormones for more than five years increased breast cancer risk. (**NEJM, June 15, 1995.**) Many aspects of this ongoing study render its findings suspect. Recall bias is a real concern when trying to decipher events from both the near and distant past. The skill, honesty, dedication, and motivation of the investigators in this study are not in question. Studies need to be done prospectively, with controls and randomization, and that kind of study requires many millions of dollars.

Like the report from Sweden above, the NEJM report of 1995 never clearly separates the patients into groups based on the precise or unique reasons the hormones were prescribed, nor does it detail any information whereby these differences could be taken into account. It is not possible to evaluate, by questionnaires, the reasons for hormone replacement. The patients on hormones, and for the longest time, may have been those who were most hormonally deficient. Experts who have compared the various groups have documented that they were not comparable in many important ways. (See **OB/GYN Clinical Alert 12:25-26; American Health Consultants: Atlanta, GA; 1995.**)

The authors of the NEJM study admit that in another study by other clinical investigators, in which natural and not artificial progesterone was used, the incidence of breast cancer was found to be lower in users than in non-users. The last difficulty I see with this report was the use of hormones in an unnatural way, that is, intermittently, not continuously. The preferred technique is to give the same low dose of each, every day, not just to prevent uterine bleeding but to prevent breast difficulties.

(See **Women's Health Digest, volume 1, number 3, Summer 1995, page 200.** Address of publisher provided in Note six, above.)

The reports that have kept American women wary of hormonal treatment of the menopause **never offer an explanation for the finding frequently observed that women who take female hormones of any kind, in any dose, for any length of time, and who then stop them for at least two years, had a lower risk of breast cancer than those who never used them in the first place. Even more convincing to those who reject the theory that hormone treatments increase the number of breast cancer deaths are the numerous studies which demonstrate that the risk of spread of breast cancer has been significantly less, with longer survival, when** *previous* **users of hormones are compared with** *never-***users.**

Any study on breast cancer risk and hormone use should certainly include how many people died during the time of the study, regardless of the cause. The Swedish study did that and found that there were only half as many deaths among the hormone users.

8. (pg. 70) Dr. Helfant discusses the incredibly powerful "body-mind" communication, as he sees it, in treating heart disease. **ref. 51, p. 33-41.**

9. (pg. 70) **ref. 73, p. 31.**

10. (pg. 71) Alfie Kohn's *Punished By Rewards* makes a solid case for the utter failure of using the creation of self-esteem as a substitute for using **challenging educational techniques. ref. 63.**

11. (pg. 73) **ref. 99, p. 35.**

12. (pg. 73) **ref. 13, p. 9.**

13. (pg. 74) Tests for Menopause:

I found from clinical studies in my own laboratory that one of the earliest signs of *permanent* estrogen decline is an elevation of the **ratio** between the blood level of the woman's total cholesterol to the blood level of HDL—or "good" cholesterol. For women, this ratio should be lower than 4.5, ideally lower than 3.5.

Those women who see "no need" for hormone treatment when menopausal symptoms start, or when periods cease, and whose cholesterol values are normal, should at least have a simple two-view x-ray of the hand, which has been placed beside an aluminum-alloy reference wedge. Utilizing computer analysis, this technique, called radiographic absorpsiometry (RA), provides a good assessment of bone density and fracture risk, and at a cost of less than $100. Dual-energy x-ray absorpsiometry (DEXA) is more expensive, but much more generally available at this time. There is much less radiation exposure with DEXA than with CT bone scans, which are available almost everywhere. DEXA tests take less than ten minutes to document osteoporosis of spine and/or hips. (Yates, A.J., P.D. Ross, and E. Lydick, "Radiographic Absorpsiometry in the Diagnosis of Osteoporosis," **The American Journal of Medicine, 1995, vol. 98, supp. 2A, pp. 415-475.**)

The Food and Drug Administration has approved **Miacalcin,** a nasal spray, and **Fosamax,** an oral tablet, for the treatment of osteoporosis. A half-dose (5mg.) of the tablet is also approved for the prevention of osteoporosis in women at high risk. A DEXA test of the radius, spine, and hips, after at least one year of treatment, provides an assessment of treatment success. For optimal handling of the osteoporosis problem, even women on the best treatment, which is hormone replacement, should be evaluated for osteoporosis at some time in their lives to ensure they are not part of the twenty percent of women whose bones to not benefit from estrogen.

Calcium, magnesium, and boron are also needed to prevent and manage osteoporosis. Problems with **lactose intolerance** have probably been overemphasized, scaring too many women needlessly away from dairy products. Virtually everyone can have a cup of milk per day without symptoms. A cup of yogurt is a good source of calcium, having 100mg. more calcium and half the lactose of a cup of milk. Hard cheeses contain minimal amounts of lactose, which is removed naturally in the cheese-making process.

Ethnic background has a marked relationship to lactose intolerance. Scandinavians tolerate lactose best, middle Europeans do well, but Southern Italians and those of African, Asian, Native American, or Jewish descent very likely to tolerate lactose poorly.

Measuring the blood levels of specific ovarian and pituitary hormones rarely answers any specific clinical questions, especially since the levels normally vary day-to-day (some change hour-to-hour). Testing is also expensive. The chief value of measuring the pituitary "FSH" and "LH" is that if both are elevated, **the woman can be assured that pregnancy is no longer possible.** If a peri-menopausal woman is taking oral contraceptives and wants to know if she can discontinue them without risking pregnancy, an FSH level should be done on the last three days of the pill-free week. If the level is in the menopausal range, she can discontinue pill use. (Ideally, she will have already decided which menopausal options she wants to initiate in the place of the birth control pills.)

Failure to consider and treat permanent estrogen deficiency until periods have stopped for one year or until pituitary hormones are elevated is risky. Besides all the classical menopausal symptoms described in Chapters Five and Six, there is often significant weight gain, loss of scalp hair and increase of facial hair, as well as significant bone loss, reduced circulation to the brain and unwanted changes in the cholesterol pattern. Waiting until the pap test reflects total loss of estrogen condemns the patient to very symptomatic bladder and vaginal problems.

Thyroid problems occur ten times more often in women. Hypothyroidism (underactive) often starts in the forties and mimics menopause. **Hyperthyroidism** (overactive) often starts during the thirties. **How does thyroid dysfunction often present clinically?** Unexplained weight gain, especially when accompanied by marked fatigue, difficulty in speaking and thinking, and new problems with constipation, calls for an immediate blood test (sensitive TSH) to rule out an underactive thyroid. Fine hand tremors, a pulse over 100 while sleeping, warm sweaty palms, and unexplained weight loss call for the same test to rule out an overactive thyroid.

14. (pg. 74) Ohkura, T., Y. Teshina, K. Isse, et al, "Estrogen Increases Cerebral and Cerebellar Blood Flows in Post-menopausal Women," **Menopause, 1995, vol. 2, pg. 13-18.**

15. (pg. 79) See Note 11, this Chapter, regarding DEXA test and **Fosamax** treatment.

16. (pg. 80) Three studies showing that **estrogen lowers the risk of colon cancer** can be found in the same issue of the **Journal of the American Cancer Institute 1995, vol. 87, pg. 517-523, 1039-1040, and 1067-1071.** Many articles give the possible mechanisms for this beneficial effect of estrogen. One explanation is that estrogen decreases the excretion of bile acids, which are considered "cancer-causing."

17. (pg. 81) **ref. 6** provides hundreds of examples of **postmenopausal women who "got a life."**

18. (pg. 81) **ref. 40, p. 498.**

6 Doing Something About Estrogen Loss

1. (pg. 82) Dr. Wilson is "recalled" (without praise) by Friedan in **ref. 40, p. 140, 474-475.**

2. (pg. 83) Found in **Ob/Gyn Clinical Alert, vol. 13, pages 17-19, July 1996,** edited by Leon Speroff, (published by American Health Consultants.)

3. (pg. 84) **ref. 29, p. 230-234.**

4. (pg. 84) **ref. 101, p. 35.**

5. (pg. 87) Betty Friedan opposes hormonal treatment of the menopause on principle, while Gail Sheehy sees it to be of great possible value when needed. **ref. 101 and ref. 40.**

Several books recommended for your reading about the menopause, and which are written by middle-aged women who have experienced it: *Understanding Menopause: Answers and Advice For Women in the Prime of Life* by Janine O'Leary Cobb, **(Plume, New York, 1993)**; Sadja Greenwood's *Menopause, Naturally (updated): Preparing for the Second Half of Life,* **(Volcano Press, Volcano CA, 1992)**; Lonnie Barbach's *The Pause: Positive Approaches to Menopause,* **(Signet, New York, 1993)**. Betty Kamen's *Hormone Replacement Therapy: Yes or No?* seems to stand alone, especially in its claims for the wonderful things that natural progesterone skin cream can do. **(Nutrition Encounter, Box 5847, Novato CA 94948, 1995.)**

Four other books are also recommended: 1) Judith Reichman's *I'm Too Young to Get Old: Health Care for Women Over Forty,* **Random House; New York, 1996.** Doctor Reichman is a gynecologist who is sympathetic to both sides of the hormone issue; 2) The same can be said for another gynecologist, Christiane Northrup *(Women's Bodies, Women's Wisdom: Creating Physical and Emotional Health and Healing,* **Times Books: New York, 1996)** (Both these books stress the **bodymind** relationship, as do the final two books.); 3) *Healing Mind, Healthy Body: Using the Mind-Body Connection to Manage Stress and Take Control of Your Life* by Alice D. Domar and Henry Dreher, **Henry Holt: New York, 1996**; and 4) *The Relaxation Response* by Herbert Benson, **William Morrow: New York, 1975.**

6. (pg. 90) For example, since the **number one benefit of estrogen replacement is to prevent cardiovascular disease**, shouldn't every woman be tested for her risk of such diseases and offered treatment accordingly? Yet some providers do not see the need: Recently, during a panel discussion involving gynecologists and family practice physicians—on the subject of hormones and menopause—I stated that I **never prescribe any estrogen without first testing the cholesterols**. One physician, who had earlier remarked that he prescribed whatever form of estrogen that he happened to have samples of at that moment, was so upset by my practice of checking the lipids first, that he mocked my suggestion later, behind my back, citing the "bother" and the expense. My reasoning for checking cholesterol first was this: if the number one benefit of estrogen was to prevent cardiovascular disease, shouldn't we make sure that a risk existed, and, if it did, that our treatment would correct the problem. Another gynecologist, at a different meeting on the same subject, said I should not bring cholesterol into the discussion of hormone replacement. He referred to himself as an expert on the subject and stated that absolutely nothing had yet been

proven about the clinical benefits of estrogen's cholesterol effects. Is there any wonder we have a communication problem?

These attitudes reminded me of those shown by one of the surgical professors in medical school, in the 1950s—a smoker, who was trying to convince the class that the connection between smoking and lung cancer was still unproven. He ended his lecture by stating, "You wouldn't live any longer by giving up smoking; it would only seem longer." He was wrong.

Since 1948, when Doctor William Castelli, director of the famous Framingham Heart Study, initiated investigation of blood lipids and cardiovascular diseases, there have been thousands of articles showing an almost invariable connection between the cholesterol fractions and diseases of the heart and circulation. In my own practice I found over the past ten years that **estrogen alone could restore the premenopausal cholesterol values in nineteen of every twenty postmenopausal women in whom it was discovered to be elevated.**

7. (pg. 91) See *Menopause,* **The Journal of the American Menopause Society, vol. 1, no. 4, p. 227-231, 1994.**

8. (pg. 91) Reported at the 67th meeting of **The American Heart Association in Dallas, Texas, November, 1994.**

9. (pg. 94) Non-hormonal therapies for menopausal and postmenopausal problems of all kinds, both mental and physical, are described in great detail in *Handbook For Herbal Healing: a Concise Guide to Herbal Products* by Christopher Hobbs. Everything seems to be covered for women's needs, from abdominal pain to yeast infections. **Ref. 55, p. 145-158.**

Remifemin, a herb discovered and developed in Germany as a treatment for menopause and used for forty-five years in that country and many others in Europe and in Australia, is now available in the United States. (See **Ch. Notes, Preface, #1.**)

The number of **Registered Acupuncturists** in the state of Pennsylvania rose from fifteen in 1987 to 292 in 1996. (In this state, **licenses** are not given to acupuncturists. They must work under direct supervision of a physician or see only those patients referred by a licensed physician.

In Pennsylvania, **Chiropractors** are licensed (3500 of them). One study in 1990 showed that Americans spend three times more money ($13.7 billion/yr.) on "unconventional therapy" than on physicians.

See also resources: **Alternative Medicine; Pain Treatment.**

10. (pg. 94) **ref. 73, p. 126-133.**

11. (pg. 94) **Dehydroepiandrosterone (DHEA) has been touted as the anti-aging, anti-cancer, anti-degenerative disease miracle drug.** It has much of this capability in animal (rodent) studies, but animals produce

little of this hormone naturally, while humans produce a lot. The amount humans produce keeps going down as they age. Any value in human beings of supplying this substance has yet to be proven. See **Time Magazine, Sept. 23, 1996, p. 66ff.** Now DHEA can be purchased over the counter at the pharmacy. Reports in 1997 and 1998 claim DHEA may increase pancreatic, ovarian, and prostate cancer risks.

7 Exercising: Your Secret to a Better Life

1. (pg. 98) **ref. 89, p. 83.**

2. (pg. 106) About A.D. 200, Rabbi Judah ha-Nasi completed the enormous task of compiling and editing the **Mishnah,** which is the record of centuries of interpretation of the **Torah.** In the 300 years following, rabbis in Galilee and Babylonia continued to expound on the precepts of the Mishnah. These discussions, known as the **Gemara,** also include digressions on legal and nonlegal subjects, including stories about rabbis, stories by rabbis about characters and events in the Bible, medical treatments, and science. The Gemara was eventually combined with the texts of the Mishnah to form the **Talmud.** Talmudic study remains central to Orthodox Jewish religious life. **(ref.** *The Bible Through the Ages;* **Reader's Digest Association, Inc.: Pleasantville, New York. 1996.)**

8 Throwing Away All Your Diets

1. (pg. 108) **ref. 95, p. 2.**

2. (pg. 108) **ref. 90, p. 55.**

3. (pg. 109) Quoted in **ref. 90, p. 39.**

4. (pg. 110) **ref. 95, p. 2.**

5. (pg. 112) **ref. 104, p. 132-134. See 6, next.**

6. (pg. 113) Fortunately, **the statistics that have circulated in recent years, placing the yearly deaths from anorexia at more than one-hundred thousand, seem now to have been inaccurate**. The actual figure is more likely one hundred every year, still a horrible indictment of a society that insists that, to be feminine, a girl/woman must treat her body as **the enemy**. (Incredibly inflated statistics on other "crimes against women" have also been accepted and quoted at all levels of education, in government policy discussions, and in legal proposals for "remedial" legislation. Biased reporting of feminist issues, as Christina Hoff Sommers strongly affirms in *Who Stole Feminism: How Women Have Betrayed Women,* has done great harm to the feminist struggle for equal-

ity in all things under the Law. Sommers chooses to prove her point by going to the original source of various blatantly wrong feminist assertions, concluding with an analysis of Susan Faludi's *Backlash: The Undeclared War Against American Women* and Naomi Wolf's *The Beauty Myth.* These tremendously popular works wrote of a backlash against women—by the media, by the political system, by the patriarchal construct of what constitutes beauty, and finally by a large number of women themselves—who, they claim, have been duped by men and are now the main, though unwitting, enforcers of the push to get women back to their "acceptable" roles. These two books, utilizing statistics and "facts" that Sommers calls into question, did however succeed in inciting many American women to anger, if not rage. **ref. 104, Ch. 11.**

Sommers maintains also that when feminist sources exaggerate or distort the facts concerning the plight of women "in order to help recruit adherents to the gender feminist cause . . . (and) if the figures are not true, they almost never serve the interests of the victimized women they concern." **ibid, p. 188-208.** "The actual number of anorexic deaths may be as low as **one hundred.**" (emphasis Sommers) **ibid, p. 233.**

Naomi Wolf's later work, *Fire With Fire: The New Female Power and How to Use It,* calls for the abandonment of the strident rhetoric of the "victim-feminism" of the past twenty-five years and the individual moral agendas that have divided the movement. She pleads for a feminism that does not attack men solely on the basis of gender. **ref. 118, p. 316-318.**

While these issues are basic to my prescriptions for your happiness and personal fulfillment, **in the specific matter of what is your best weight, the issues of feminism or femininity should not be applied to the calculation.** The Harvard Eating Disorders Center "estimates" that 1,000 anorexics die each year. Quoted by Marie McCullough, staff writer, in **"A new campus fad: Bulimia by the group," The Philadelphia Inquirer, pg. A1, A8, Feb. 14, 1996.**

If one's aversion to food becomes an addiction, that individual can become delusional, seeing herself as fat and refusing to eat, when in fact she looks like a recent survivor of a death camp. As the addiction increases, it eventually becomes virtually impossible to convince the anorexic to change. Even if deaths are typically the result only in severe addiction, enough permanent physical damage or failures in development occur in even the milder cases to make this problem a serious and common one indeed.)

The following **eating disorders mini-[screening] test** is taken from the same *Inquirer* article.

Do you: 1) Restrict your calories to fewer than 500 a day or skip two or more meals a day?

2) Eat a very large amount of food within a two-hour period while feeling out of control? (At least two times a week for three months)

3) Use laxatives, vomiting, excessive exercise, or other purging behaviors to lose or control weight?

4) Stay at home or avoid social situations to maintain your eating or exercise schedule?

The same article states that a "yes" to **any** of these questions may indicate an eating disorder requiring professional help.

7. (pg. 113) **ref. 90, p. 27.**

8. (pg. 115) **ref. 55, p. 64-78 and p. 111-129.**

9. (pg. 115) *Neuropsychology of Weight Control: Study Guide,* p. 28, (Sybervision Systems, Inc., Fountain Square, 6066 Civic Terrace, Newark CA 94560.)

10. (pg. 116) Despite my belief that the body mass index (B.M.I) is inferior to even simple waist measurements, a nomogram for calculating your body mass index is reproduced on page 245 of the Appendix. A straight line is traced with a ruler between the height and weight. The point of intersection with the central line gives the B.M.I. A value of 25 is average, 28 or more warrants treatment, and a value of 30 or more, corresponding to 30% or more excess weight, is the point at which excess mortality can be demonstrated.

9 Facing the Health Problems of Adolescence

1. (pg. 123) **ref. 90, preface. See also ref. 75, p. 236 for specific lyrics.**

2. (pg. 131) In Pennsylvania, a minor is anyone under 18 years of age. Issues associated with the treatment of minor patients generally fall into two categories—either consent or confidentiality.

General Consent
Under ordinary circumstances, physicians are required to get the consent of the parent or legal guardian before proceeding with non-emergency treatment of a minor. However, certain classifications of minors may consent to medical services for themselves:
- a person who has graduated from high school.
- a married person.
- a person who has been pregnant.
- a person who presents for diagnosis/treatment of pregnancy or sexually-transmitted disease, (special rules apply if an abortion is requested. See Abortion Control Act, 18 Pa. C.S.A./3201-3220)
- a minor who is a parent may give consent for her/his child.

- a minor who claims to be 18, but isn't. (The doctor has no suspicion or reason to believe the patient is lying.)

3. (pg. 131) Patricia's daughter and her husband have five children now, and they are happy. Sally's pursuit of a degree has not been abandoned, only considerably lengthened. She takes one course per semester at a local community college. Each of her subsequent pregnancies has been planned, using "natural family planning" (NFP).

Natural family planning should presently refer only to a method that uses some or all of the following: (1) the **basal body temperature chart to wait for elevations** after ovulation, (2) the **changes in the cervix itself—softer, more open, and higher up in the vagina** on fertile days, (3) the **cervical mucus changes** before and after ovulation, and (4) the one-sided **lower abdominal ache** that coincides with ovulation. Such NFP techniques are a very effective means of limiting pregnancies in a stable, permanently committed, well-motivated, and loving relationship. However, the couple should be trained in the method. Any sympto-thermal method should not be expected to work with high effectiveness for careless or unmotivated individuals. I do not recommend it if "failures" will be judged a disaster and thus aborted.

Gynecologist Christiane Northrup writes that "many couples who follow NFP as a method of regulating births become acutely attuned to each other's fertility and sexual cycles. Not only does this method afford them the means to plan or avoid conception when they desire, they often find that their intimacy and pleasure increases as well." **ref. 83, p. 228**. This finding of greater intimacy has been my experience as well. In addition to those using entirely natural methods, I cannot recall one broken marriage among the hundreds of patients over an interval of thirty years who have used my technique of "assisted rhythm" (in which I use hormones to ensure that the fertile time in each menstrual cycle remains fairly consistent).

4. (pg. 132) For more specific comments on the pill, see **Notes, Ch. 11, 11 and 19.**

5. (pg. 132) **ref. 117.** In some of the sex education classes given to our children, explicit permission to masturbate is given, as "an authentic expression of self-loving." Diagrams are provided so the little girls know how to find the clitoris. Barbara Dafoe Whitehead, in her article, "What they want to teach your child about sex," makes graphically clear that our children will be taught just about everything a person who chooses to be sexually active needs to know, by teachers with a mandate from the state legislatures or the local school boards. See Whitehead, Barbara Dafoe, "What They Want To Teach Your Child About Sex" (**The Atlantic Monthly, Oct. 1994.** Article can be found in condensed version in the **Reader's Digest, Feb. 1995.)**

6. (pg. 133) **ref. 84.** A reporter's chronicle of some schoolgirls' lives and times at two California middle schools. Not too pleasant. Compare with the situation found in many all-girls high schools as described in **ref. 75, p. 117-153.**

7. (pg. 133) Study by Marion Howard and Judith McCabe quoted in **ref. 75, p. 264.**

8. (pg. 135) **ref. 90, p 69.**

9. (pg. 136) **ibid, p. 207-8.**

10. (pg. 138) Many professionals in counseling adolescents and young adults, or who are "responsible" for their behavior away from parental control, share my views. At the Madeira all-girls high school outside Washington, where many of the people who run our government send their daughters, the director of counseling, Sophie Speidel, a famous scholar-athlete, with a master's degree in education, gives highest priority on educating her girls in sexual matters so as to help them avoid unwanted pregnancy and sexually transmitted disease. However, no condoms are provided at Madeira. When the students asked for the explanation, the answer provided was: "If you are responsible enough to have sex, you are responsible enough to go to the drugstore and buy condoms yourself." (**Quoted in ref. 75, p. 133.**)

11. (pg. 138) **ref. 90, p. 70. See also ref. 75, p. 245-260.**

There is much that parents can learn by a study of the events that occurred at Lakewood High School in California since the same thing could happen anywhere in America, where the athletes are the ones that are most highly praised, and the girls, if they are praised at all, are affirmed for their abilities to please or attract a male.

After one generation of active feminism, "girlpower" is still not a priority at home or at school!

12. (pg. 140) quoted in **ref. 25, p. 133.**

SECTION TWO—HEALING YOUR RELATIONSHIPS
THE SECOND CHALLENGE: Accepting the Work of Love

10 Looking at "Love"

1. (pg. 144) **ref. 52, 42-43.**

2. (pg. 144) In this regard, Harold Kushner, in *When All You've Ever Wanted Isn't Enough: The Search For a Life that Matters,* responds to the query regarding, "To what question is God the answer?" by saying, "The existence of God is not the issue; the difference God can make in

our lives is!" **ref. 67, p. 18.** See Ch. 16 herein for **the challenge** to decide on God's influence in your life.

3. (pg. 146) **ref. 4, p. 312.**

4. (pg. 146) **ref. 61, p. 141-2. See also ref. 4, p. 62.**

5. (pg. 149) The metaphor of the "tanks," like the identical concept of the "seesaw," is used by Barbara DeAngelis throughout the text. **ref. 21. p. 113-4, 130-1, 170. See esp. p. 123-136.**

6. (pg. 151) **ref. 61, p. 14, 37, 50-51, 151.**

7. (pg. 151) **ibid, p. 12 and Chapters 10 and 11, p. 125-199.**

8. (pg. 152) Jung's oft-repeated statements about restoring a spiritual dimension to people's lives as the only apparent successful remedy for their mental disorders, when explicitly stated in his correspondence with the co-founder of Alcoholics Anonymous, Bill W., provided the latter with insights that led him to develop his eminently successful 12-step program for alcohol addiction. Only the first step mentions alcohol. All the others have to do with higher, or spiritual realities. Nearly all the most successful addiction groups, or those groups with problems-in-common, use the same 12-step principles.

The 12-steps: We

1) admitted we were powerless over alcohol (food, drugs, sex, violence, abuse) and that our lives had become unmanageable.

2) came to believe that a Power greater than ourselves could restore us to sanity.

3) made a decision to turn our will and our lives over to the care of God **as we understood Him.**

4) made a searching and fearless moral inventory of ourselves.

5) admitted to God, to ourselves, and to another human being the exact nature of our wrongs.

6) were entirely ready to have God remove all these defects of character.

7) humbly ask Him to remove all our shortcomings.

8) made a list of all persons we had harmed and became willing to make amends to them all.

9) made direct amends to such people whenever possible, except when to do so would injure them or others.

10) continued to make personal inventory and when we were wrong promptly admitted it.

11) sought through prayer and meditation to improve our conscious contract with God **as we understood Him,** praying only for knowledge of his will for us and the power to carry that out.

12) Having had a spiritual awakening as a result of these Steps, we tried to carry this message to alcoholics, and to practice these principles in all our affairs. *(Came to Believe: The spiritual adventure of A.A. as experienced by individual members.* **Alcoholics Anonymous World Services: 468 Park Avenue South, New York, NY. 1988.**

The general psychologist principle that "an addict alone is in bad company" is stressed in AA. In the text, John Bradshaw refers to this principle as restoring the "interpersonal bridge," and Judi Hollis insists on it in treating eating disorders when she states a "sponsor" is essential for success. For this reason, many **sexually-abused women** are included in the millions of individuals who have been **freed by group therapy** from the addictive behavior that was used to separate them from their pain and sadness. Not only can groups dispel for abused women the myth of their "terminal uniqueness," they can "legitimize" for many "ordinary" women their feelings of peace, joy, and laughter—feelings to which too many women believe they are not entitled.

Many women are virtually incapacitated by cancerophobia. Christiane Northrup, a former President of the American Holistic Medical Society, quotes journalist Vivian Gornick, who says, "For a woman, coming off fear is like an addict coming off drugs." Group therapy for any problem of fear is strongly recommended.

9. (pg. 152) **ref. 4, p. 278.**

10. (pg. 152) The spiraling rates of **addiction and violent crime** in America, especially among our **youngest adolescents**, is yet additional evidence of the truth that one of society's, and education's, highest priorities should be providing support and information toward a better understanding of our motivations, human needs, and the powerful psychological forces, created in our past, that drive our personal relationships.

Besides the benefits to society at large that would result from an increase in the number of more-functional families, ample evidence exists to prove that married people themselves have been found to be happier and to live longer than those who are single, divorced, widowed, or never married. See article by Frank M. Dattilio, Professor of Psychiatry at the University of Pennsylvania, quoted in **Good Housekeeping, December 1995, pg. 72.** On the other hand, however, considerable scientific evidence has been gathered to add to the empiric observations of most health care providers, showing that marital strife has a direct, detrimental effect on health and resistance to disease. See article by Daniel O'Leary, Professor of Psychology at the State University at Stony Brook, **ibid, pg. 72. See also ref. 52, page 315.**

A recent report by the Carnegie Council on Adolescent Development, titled **"Great Transitions: Preparing Adolescents for a New**

Century," charges that as parents and society show less and less attention to the 19 million children now 10-14 years of age, very serious problems have become epidemic in that age group. The results of a 10-year study, the report says that this group is subject to the most violence, one-third have tried drugs, one-third have tried suicide, and two-thirds have used alcohol. Homicides have doubled in just seven years. Also, the rate of sexual promiscuity, smoking, and the use of marijuana has steadily increased. Quoted by staff writer, John Wostendiek in **The Philadelphia Inquirer, pg. A1, A16, November 4, 1995.**

11. (pg. 152) **ref. 21, p. 130-1.**

12. (pg. 153) **ref. 46, p. x.**

13. (pg. 153) **ref. 58, p. 161.**

14. (pg. 154) **ref. 58, p. 267.**

15. (pg. 155) **ref. 52.** This is the major theme of the book.

16. (pg. 156) **ref. 76, p. 78-103.**

17. (pg. 156) **ibid, p. 66-73. See also p. 16, 62-66, 87-93 235-256.**
One very practical example, invariably mentioned in self-help manuals for dealing with sexual problems: **withholding orgasm,** whether done consciously or not, may be the only way a woman can express her anger, or feel that she has any power at all in the relationship. The anger, or more precisely the reason for the anger, must be searched for, acknowledged, and dealt with. Once this is accomplished, the sexual problem typically vanishes.

18. (pg. 157) **ref. 21, 101-122.**

19. (pg. 157) **ref. 76, p. 78-103.**

20. (pg. 158) **ref. ibid, p. 62-66, 87-93.**

21. (pg. 159) **ref. ibid, p. 70-73.**

22. (pg. 159) **ref. 36.** Nancy Friday frequently makes the point of maternal responsibility for the daughter's reaction patterns, though the **first marriage** imagery is Bonnie Maslin's.

23. (pg. 159) **ref. 4, p. 220.**

24. (pg. 165) **ref. 21, p. 84-5.**

25. (pg. 169) **ref. 25, p. 253.**

26. (pg. 170) a) **ref. 96, p. 249-302.**

   b) **ref. 53, p. 175-210.**

   c) **ref. 80, p. 83-120.**

   d) **ref. 71.** The entire book is intended to leave little to
   the imagination.

27. (pg. 170) **ref. 46, p. 83.** Incidentally, John Gray also asserts that the
feminist contention that men are not psychologically different from
women, is "absurd." He insists that the differences are "natural" and
will never be erased by cultural or societal changes. **ibid, p. 38. See also
ref. 4, p. 312.**

28. (pg. 171) **ref. 51; ref. 52,** where it is a recurrent theme, for example **p.
23-24.**

29. (pg. 171) quoted in **ref. 116, p. 205.**

30. (pg. 172) **ref. 61, p. 239-59.** Daphne Rose Kingma has in her book a
chapter entitled "Evoking Men's Emotions," for which she provides a
"map for the journey." See also Sandra M. Schneider's chapter, "Effects
of Women's Experience on Spirituality" in **ref. 17, p. 31-48,** especially
page 40, in which **she wholeheartedly supports Carl Jung's thesis that
for a man to achieve "wholeness," he must integrate into his conscious
ego those feminine emotions he has buried in his unconscious.**

31. (pg. 172). Besides Bonnie Maslin's *The Angry Marriage* **(ref. 76),** four
concise, fundamental, yet absolutely clear texts on the **psychology of
intimacy and autonomy** are Harville Hendrix's *Getting the Love You
Want: a Guide for Couples* **(ref. 51);** his plan for **persons presently single
to improve "their act,"** *Keeping the Love You Find: a Personal Guide,* **(ref.
52);** Maggie Scarf's *Intimate Partners: Partners in Love and Marriage* **(ref.
96),** which also has **techniques of marriage therapy as well as those
specifically for correcting sexual problems;** and Scarf's *Intimate Worlds:
Life Within the Family* **(ref. 97).** All these books assert that couples usually
select each other for unconscious reasons that go back to infancy and
early childhood. Each spouse attempts to recreate, with their present
mate, their distant past, which usually means bringing back into their
emotional life the most painful parts of their relationships with their
earliest caregivers, in an effort to understand, overcome, or resolve,
those early issues or problems. For some the choice may simply be
influenced by an unconscious wish to re-experience earliest feeling and
emotions, because they are the only ones they know, or feel "safe" with.
   Hendrix states the **power struggle** stage, **which 95% of couples get
permanently stuck in,** goes through some of the same phases that
Elisabeth Kübler-Ross described in the dying patient, in her landmark
work, *On Death and Dying.* Couples will: 1) deny their shock when they
discover the real person they married; then 2) question their partners'
motives, feel betrayed, feel the pain, and get angry; if they get beyond

the anger, the era of 3) bargaining begins; the final phase 4) acceptance plays out differently in marriages, for it signifies "giving up." (The third phase is the one the marriage counselors used to keep couples fixed in, by teaching them more "civilized" ways to bargain. Couples use bargaining, or barter, all the time, sometimes consciously or overtly, often not. "If you want sex, then you have to do this. If you want me to take care of the house, then you have to do everything else." The negotiations are often the only meaningful, or authentic, communication between the spouses. When everything has failed to move the couple beyond their attempts to control, or change the other, the couple gives up. About half such marriages end entirely, with ninety percent of the rest accepting the reality that their marriage will never provide the joy and intimacy that they originally believed possible). **ref. 51, p. 81-82.**

Harville Hendrix, in *Getting the Love You Want*, prescribes sixteen suggestions or "exercises" that could change an "unconscious marriage"—in which the issues of power, conflict, and intimacy produce automatic reaction patterns, such as criticism and confrontation, and in which one's real needs and desires are hidden or unknown—into a "conscious marriage" of cooperation, empathy, and understanding, all of which can lead to a "passionate friendship."

Maggie Scarf, in her book on families, extends the insights on the intricacies of the male/female love relationship found in her earlier work to those involving parents, siblings and children, again showing how uncannily history repeats itself, most often in the ways that are least desired. Again, after showing the various ways families can function, specific therapeutic suggestions are provided for improving relationships within the family.

Connie Peck, in *How to Make Peace with Your Partner: a Couple's Guide to Conflict Management*, **ref. 88,** issues the challenge to **negotiate** your conflicting interests and concerns. She provides detailed guidance for developing the skills for successful negotiation, so that you can more often experience the "magical times when you do connect and share a brief moment of deeper understanding." **pg. 242.**

Reading John Gray's *Men, Women, and Relationships: Making Peace With the Opposite Sex*, is also a good place to begin your quest for better relationships with men. **ref. 46.**

11 Learning From Past Mistakes

1. (pg. 174) **ref. 21, p. 390-3.** Dr. Elizabeth Kübler-Ross showed that avoiding or denying death didn't help the patient's healing process. The same principle applies to any "pain." Whether one is speaking of divorce, miscarriage, abortion, or loss of a dear friend, any trauma for which one does not grieve, cannot be released.

Forgiving someone because we think it is the right thing to do becomes yet one more version of denial.

2. (pg. 174) **ref. 94, p. 123-134.**

3. (pg. 175) **ref. 52, p. 7-9, 16-17.** In an earlier book, *Getting the Love You Want: a Guide For Couples,* Hendrix offered specific techniques for saving or improving already-existing committed relationships. **ref. 51, p. 241-276.** Some of his suggestions, for example, using "mirroring" or "wish lists" to get in touch with our own and each other's feelings, along with the love letters that DeAngelis, among others, recommends, were presented in Chapter Ten.

Susan Jeffers, in *Opening Our Hearts to Men,* says that it is especially important when you are not in a relationship, to spend time learning and appreciating, then writing down, all the good things you see in yourself, including all the things you do well. She urges that you write down all the good things you do to learn or improve yourself, and also any successes you achieve, however small they seem at the time. This **appreciation of your lovability** will, inevitably, become visible to others. By these regular self-appreciation exercises, you will allow those around you to become more comfortable in your presence, and thus more likely to be friendly and affirming, whether this be your boss, co-workers, parents, children, or associates. For, **if we lack self-appreciation, we will obsessively search for it**. And there is that awful irony that the more we need love, the less lovable we are perceived. Jeffers writes that **"when we don't give ourselves credit for what is good about who we are, we set ourselves up for a feeling of inner emptiness that no man, however he may be, can fill up."** ref. 58, p. 114, 233. Obviously, people who appreciate their talents and good qualities are inclined to be more assertive, to be able to say no, and can more easily let their wishes be known.

4. (pg. 175) **ref. 4, p. 262, 266.**

5. (pg. 176) **ibid, p. 134-36, 139-41, 152, 260, 262-4.**

6. (pg. 176) **ref. 58, p. 268.**

7. (pg. 177) See *Clinical Gynecologic Endocrinology and Infertility,* Fifth edition, authored by Leon Speroff, Robert H. Glase, and Nathan G. Kase, **(Williams and Wilkins, 428 East Preston Street, Baltimore, Maryland 21202, 1994).** In 1960, 28% of women, ages 20-24, were single, and 10% of those whose ages were 25-29. In 1985, the percentages of single women in the same groups were 58.8% and 26%. pg. 692-693. However, 84% of the drop in the fertility rate during that time was due to women having fewer children, once married, and not from their simply marrying later.

8. (pg. 177) Jeanne Moorman, "a demographer in the U.S. Census Bureau's marriage and family statistics branch," quoted in **ref. 26, page 11.**

9. (pg. 177) **ref. ibid, p. 15. See also ref. 90, p. 80, and ref. 118, p. xxi.**

10. (pg. 177) **ref. 99, p. 144.**

11. (pg. 177) **ibid.** The "ten stupid things women do to mess up their life," as very loosely paraphrased from Laura Schlessinger's book of the same name, are **stupid**: 1) . . . **attachment** to a man to try to achieve your worth; 2) . . . **courtship** of a man, instead of having him court you; 3) . . . **devotion** to someone who needs or uses you; 4) . . .**passion** that guides your decisions, rather than allowing your head to guide you; 5) . . . **cohabitation** as your audition for marriage; 6) . . . **expectations** that he will have enough of what it takes for both of you; 7) . . . **conception** for your sake, not the baby's; 8) . . . **subjugation** of yourself and your children to an abusive man; 9) . . . **helplessness** in being a wimp instead of fighting for your rights; and 10) . . . **forgiving** and forgiving a jerk who'll never change.

In regard to number seven, gynecologist Christiane Northrup gave up doing abortions in the mid-1980s because she was "tired of mucking around in women's ambivalence about their fertility, and . . . was tired of performing repeated abortions on women who came back every year for the procedure." She also saw abortion as a problem resulting from a woman's sexual ignorance and a lack of self-esteem.

12. (pg. 177) Of the sixty-four billion dollars mandated by the courts for child support only fourteen billion is collected. Of the ten million women with children in fatherless homes, two-thirds get no support at all.

Now that the technology is available to prove paternity in doubtful cases, more and more support is developing inside and outside of government to hold "sperm donors" responsible financially for the rearing and education of their progeny. Since legal sanctions alone have essentially failed, people like Mary Jo Bane, Undersecretary of Health and Human Services, suggest the forces of moral condemnation be mobilized. One simple method—publishing the names in the paper and/or sending the names to their employers or neighborhoods.

13. (pg. 178) The psychology of "Romantic Love" is described in some detail in **ref. 52, p. 284-86.**

14. (pg. 178) **ref. 99, p. 148.** Laura Schlessinger calls this "using the shotgun strategy to shoot yourself in the foot." Laura, who is working on a "companion" book "about the ten ways **men** mess up their lives,"

has a syndicated radio show that is heard by more than ten million people every week, despite the fact that her message for women is to develop character, and courageously follow their conscience!

15. (pg. 179) **ref. 81.**

16. (pg. 181) **ref. 32.**

17. (pg. 181) Most of the millions of women searching for a permanent relationship in an environment where "casual sex" seems to be an essential "first step" in getting acquainted, are clearly aware of the dangers to which they expose themselves. The movie **Looking for Mr. Goodbar**, whose theme is that a good man has never been harder to find and the search has never been more dangerous, ends as the heroine in the movie, played by Diane Keaton, is being brutally murdered by her "date" for the evening.

18. (pg. 181) The **surplus of single men**: A nearly two million surplus of single men exists in those first ten years, ages 24-34, and a one-half million surplus in the later 20 years, ages 35-55. Perhaps this excess of men is yet one more reason why more and more men are seeking other men for their love relationships. **ref. 28, p. 14.** The surplus of men eligible for marriage does not apply at all to Afro-Americans. (See **The Truly Disadvantaged: The Inner City, the Underclass, and Public Policy; Univ. of Chicago Press: Chicago; 1987.**)

19. (pg. 182) A strong caution is offered: Getting "sexually" involved generally ends the process of "getting to know" the other person. At least that is the generally accepted view, as well as my own observation. **When you start having sex, you stop making love, because the courting is over.**

The oral contraceptive pill plays its own part in the "natural history" of courtship in the present era, so a short reference to the dynamics it brings to the boy meets girl story is pertinent. There is little evidence that the pill will increase a woman's success in achieving love and intimacy, though by removing the risk of pregnancy, and thus allowing her the freedom to experience a variety of partners, it should decrease her ignorance of sexual "technique." But, the initial hope, that a cheap, safe, highly reliable, and easily available contraceptive—by abolishing the contention with contraception and removing the fear of pregnancy—would lead to a greater intimacy between men and women, has not been realized. If asked this question, virtually everyone who prescribes these drugs on a regular basis would agree.

Certainly the record compiled in the thirty-five years the pill has been available, seems to show that a lack of willingness to commit to the possibility of conception, and to a permanent joint responsibility for a human life, might make a couple's sexual actions more relaxed and more recreational for a time, but the total thwarting of the possibility of any permanent consequences ultimately separates their sexual actions from their expressions of intimacy. Then, too, the path toward intimacy is blocked when either partner starts withholding anything, especially when this is done permanently or unilaterally.

Surely, any highly effective method of birth control, such as **Depo-Provera** injections, surgical sterilization, or the pill, makes *sexual independence* attainable. While to countless women around the world, "It's damn well time," the issues involved, even prescinding from any reference to God or morality, are not so simple and straightforward as **both** the "pro-life" and the "pro-choice" groups make them.

Personal fulfillment from "love affairs without strings" is a very elusive goal, and the path toward it strewn with many broken lives. Even in a "committed relationship", whether the reasons be "nature" or "nurture," women take the greater risks. Testimonials to that fact abound throughout literature. "Love, for the woman, is itself the drama; for the man, the intermission." **ref. 112. p 16.** "Too often men assume once they are married, the work of having a relationship is over. Realistically, that is when it begins." **ref. 46, p. 88.** Perhaps Geneen Roth says it best, "Nothing will change when you have met the love of your life except that you will have met the love of your life. The work begins when the infatuation ends." **ref. 95, p. 200.** Betty Friedan supplies a large part of the reason that women lose more when she writes, "If women were really **people—no more, no less—**then all the things that (keep) them from being full people in our society would have to be changed." **ref. 38, p. 9. If women are restricted to only one career, that of housewife/mother, then, when the relationship is finished, the drama is over**. History clearly shows that there has never been a shortage of men who are only too happy to take advantage of the "love" that a woman offers them and who act simply for their own sexual gratification.

True, many women enjoy recreational sex, too, as a "temporary fix," like the relief that food provides to a food addict, or as a diversion, an exciting "adventure," or as a challenge. **Some women do *use* men simply to satisfy their sexual needs. Being treated simply as a *sex-object* is every bit as dehumanizing to men as it is to women. Men don't like being used either.** Unfortunately for women's purposes, there is little doubt that the laws, customs, public attitudes or morals, and countless social and logistical differences are all stacked against them. One example of the classical **double standard**: Even among sexually active teenagers (who profess to be the most "liberated" of all) a girl who has had multiple sex partners is typically accounted "promiscuous," to put it in the gentlest terms. Perhaps even more inhibiting: the possibility of being blackmailed by being labeled a "slut" is an ever-present sword held over the heads of many adolescent girls, which prevents them in many instances from reporting harassment and abuse.

Most men eventually seek what they see as the permanence and safety of a marriage relationship. Even sexually, men want the comfort, safety, and respect of a "loving" woman, one who will be happy to have "their" children. And, apparently, this preference is beneficial to their health. Susan Faludi in *Backlash* documents the incredible health benefits and increased survival that accrue to married men. **ref. 28, p. 17.** Susan Jeffers, in *Opening Our Hearts to Men*, provides considerable evidence that **men need women much more than women need men**. Divorced men have an annual death rate that is three times that of divorced women, with suicide and alcoholism much higher in unmarried men. In fact, psychological evaluations show single women and married men doing much better than married women, with single men doing poorest. **ref. 58, p. 221.**

12 Keeping Love in the Family

1. (pg. 185) Recommended: *Spiritual Parenting: A Guide to Understanding and Nurturing the Heart of Your Child,* by Hugh and Gayle Prather. (Crown Publishers: New York.) 1996.

2. (pg. 185) **ref. 36, p. 55.**

3. (pg. 186) **ref. 116, p. 34.**

4. (pg. 187) **ref. 63.** The hypothesis of this exceedingly thought-provoking book is that rewards, including praise, are only slightly less damaging to our children and to workers and students, than are punishments. Certainly, **progress reports** that reflect both the good parts and the bad, affirmation of effort, appreciation of improvement, interest, direct teaching, and advice are better. The educators' denial that our students are marinated in "pop-behaviorism," Kohn maintains, is patently false.

Jacquelyne Eccles, a professor of psychology at the University of Michigan, has determined in her extensive research that what boys or girls achieve in their education is directly related to an extraordinary degree to their parents' expectations, as the parents reveal these hopes by their encouragement, active interest, and help. She stresses that daughters do much better academically if this aspect of their lives is given consistent and unfailing affirmation when appropriate, instead of praise being reserved for the daughters' adherence to traditional "feminine" values. Eccles believes that girls lose much from their future potential, especially at adolescence, because they "become" what the parents think they will become. This outcome is the result of the "thoughtless" signals that are constantly sent out to daughters in our culture. Even many of the staunchest feminists confess to inadvertently encouraging in their own daughters the same damaging stereotypical behaviors, for example of submission, non-aggression, conformity, and dependence, that they personally reject. Unfortunately, the young adolescent, who already feels "conspicuous" and "different" because the pubertal changes are so clearly visible to everyone, literally takes up every directive as a sponge would soak up water, so as not to be shamed or embarrassed by an unacceptable action or attitude. The "males," young and old, in her life are especially prone to notice every little change and comment on it. **(Eccles findings are discussed in Judy Mann's** *The Difference,* **ref. 75, p. 98-111. Warner Books: New York. 1996.)**

5. (pg. 187) **ref. 53, p. 62.**

6. (pg. 187) There is strong evidence that American parents will send their children long distances if the school offers them the choice promulgated by the following philosophy:

"All teachers at our school have not only pedagogical training but also detailed knowledge of the subject matter they will teach. We instill in all our children an ethic of toleration, civility, orderliness, responsibility, and hard work. Our staff has agreed on a definite core of knowledge and skill that all children will attain in each grade. We make sure that every child learns this core, and gains the specific knowledge and skill needed to prosper at the next grade level, thus enabling knowledge to build upon knowledge. Our teachers continually confer with their colleagues about effective ways of stimulating children to learn and integrate this specific knowledge and skill. The specificity of our goals enables us to monitor children, and give focused attention when necessary. To this end, we provide parents with a detailed outline of the specific knowledge and skill goals for each grade, and we stay in constant touch with them regarding the child's progress. Through this knowledge-based approach, we make sure that **all** normal children perform at grade level, while, in addition, the most talented children are challenged to excel. Attaining this specific and well-integrated knowledge and skill gives our students pleasure in learning, as well as self-respect, and it ensures that they will enter the next grade ready and eager to learn more." **ref. 53, p. 62.**

The success of the European and Asian systems have been explained as largely due to the "core curriculum," which everyone can master if he or she is willing to work hard and the parents help. Obviously, the educators in these countries believe wholeheartedly that the two keys to success are hard work on the part of the students and teacher and parental participation,. The American position, as has been demonstrated for over sixty years, seems based on the premise that the success or failure of "education" is primarily a function of "innate ability," in which case no student can be "faulted" for lack of success.

Especially noteworthy in most of the foreign educational systems, especially in Asia, is the lack of distinction made between girls and boys. Each gender is held to the same expectations. **See also ref. 64; ref. 75, p. 79-91; ref. 98, and Notes, Ch. Twelve, 1.**

7. (pg. 188) **ref. 97.**

8. (pg. 188) **ref. 86.** Camille Paglia's entire book is a chronicling in western arts and literature of maternal influence.

9. (pg. 189) **ref. 36, p. vii.**

10. (pg. 189) Judi Hollis, in *Fat and Furious,* explicitly agrees with Friday's assessment that it is the horrible state of the mother-daughter relationship, which itself results from women's inferior, subordinate, or restricted role in society and in the family, that constitutes the major problem. Hollis pioneered the hospital treatment of eating disorders and teaches that few can correct this problem on their own, but rather need a 12-step program like AA in treatment. Her suggestions include seeking a "sponsor."

Judi Hollis maintains that, as the mother hides her pain and frustration from her daughter, or secretly prays that things will be better for her, the daughter sees through the deception, and then anger and resentment foments throughout their relationship. The unresolved mother/daughter wound as the source of women's problems is the book's basic premise, even though the blame ultimately belongs to women's oppression. **ref. 56.**

11. (pg. 189) **ref. 36, p. 34.** Nancy Friday points to one immediate benefit: communicating with courage and frankness, especially about matters of sexuality, will probably get rid of some significant sexual repressions that mothers often give to their daughters and may well lead to a better overall marital adjustment. **ibid, p. 23.**

12. (pg. 189) **Mary Daly** puts her plea for mother-daughter equality, as she puts all her ideas, in an "heroic" context, using the notion of **"sisterhood" as a way of solidifying female power and rejecting all men outright.** In *Gyn/ Ecology: The Metaethics of Radical Feminism,* she provides one approach toward achieving mother-daughter equality. Summarizing the views of Jan Raymond and Nelle Morton, she addresses the "destructive binds" that patriarchy places around the "normal" mother-daughter relationship. Using Raymond's term, she labels the "feminists'" response to men's intrusions, an assertion of their "Daughter-Right." ". . . daughterhood has a universality which motherhood lacks; clearly, all women are daughters. The word daughter is less

descriptive of a role than of a given reality . . . it is the Daughter with whom we can bond. When we reach the Daughter within the mother, we break the bindings of our false inheritance; we cut our tie to the institution of patriarchal motherhood . . . we strip away the treacherous "tradition" foisted upon mothers and daughters . . . (and come) to recognize the Daughter in (our)selves, (and in) our mothers. . . ." Daly adds that by becoming "sisters in struggle," mother and daughter "become friends again." **ref. 19, p. 347.**

Between Ourselves: Letters Between Mothers and Daughters 1750-1982 (**ed. Karen Payne), Mifflin Company: Boston, 1993,** is highly recommended for those who have a difficult or impossible time giving expression to their feelings. Besides, it could provide them with a deeper insight into the world in which women live and breathe. **Women, of course, will love it because they resonate with each other in similar language.**

A "Meditation on Mothering," by Nancy McBrine Sheehan, is reproduced in the Appendix, on page 248-249. I think it summarizes that subject quite well.

13. (pg. 190) **ref. 21, p. 101-122.**

14. (pg. 191) **ref. 36, p. 35.** Nancy Friday insists that if a daughter has not been able to "cut the apron strings tying her to mother" by the time her own daughter is born, the new infant comes into the household having two "mothers"—the biologic one who is trying to make her own decisions about raising the baby, and the grandmother, for whom the biologic mother's "unconscious" mind is acting. While the mother of the baby is trying not to be influenced or controlled by her mother, she almost always is. **ibid, p. 29, 61, 147, 194.** Friday also believes that if mother and daughter had the courage to "let each other go"—by forgiving and forgetting past mistakes, stop competing and criticizing but being honest about their feelings, they could be great friends for life. **ibid, p. 199.**

John Bradshaw supports the assessments of both Judi Hollis and Nancy Friday when he says that "most of us are victims of (this) multigenerational violence." **ref. 4, p. 264.**

15. (pg. 191) **ref. 36, p. 34.**

16. (pg. 192) **ref. 67, p. 36.** Early on in her professional career, Karen Horney stood up to Sigmund Freud and his understanding of **penis envy,** basically dismissing this thesis. She insisted that such envy, if it exists at all in any particular case, was not to be seen as a sign that women wished to be men, but **simply represented their temporary and practical wish to have a better way of emptying the bladder.** She later defied, and then broke away from, the psychoanalytic "establishment"

in America, and its insistence on traditional Freudian "ego psychology," which held that the source of any psychological problem was ultimately to be found within the **ego** or psyche itself, that is, entirely within the person. Horney maintained that neuroses were rooted in social customs and norms. With another student of Freud, Melanie Klein, who also stressed the relational, or outside "object," basis for neuroses, **she helped lead the way to the present psychiatric consensus that virtually all problems are in and from relationships**, and that at no time does the mind function without using images of something outside itself. Our thoughts always include a mental "relationship" with an outside "object." Thus, in treatment, these images must be brought forth early in therapy and examined. **ibid, pg. 46.**

Horney had insisted on the distinction between basing all the psychological pathology entirely in the isolated **ego** and basing such problems on the relationships with **outside objects**. Otherwise, she said, women's apparent "psychological" inferiority to men (which, in fact, nearly everyone was then accepting) would have to be seen as a "natural" inferiority, a defect she was born with, and not the result of culture. Though not appreciated at the time, acceptance of her ideas was an important victory for women in psychological circles, and for psychiatry itself.

Soon after her break, Horney formed her own and rival organization, the Association for the Advancement of Psychoanalysis. **ibid, p. 35,** quoting *The Neurotic Personality*, pg. 139-140, (Norton, New York, 1937).

17. (pg. 192) **ref. 113, p. 38-39.** On pg. 132, these same authors quote Bly as saying in the same text, "In order to liberate the wild man in himself, the boy must steal the key from under his mother's pillow." About Bly and his work, Susan Faludi writes, "This best-seller, in hard cover by a major publisher, consisted of an assemblage of previously self-published pamphlets on 'the masculinity crisis.'" It should be stated, however, that **this oft-quoted authority on the importance of a good father verbally attacks women in his speeches and symposiums**.

In fact, Susan Faludi also states that, "as the 'prophet for New Age masculinism,' this poet of the Left . . . considers any feminine characteristics in a man . . . evidence of a disease spread by women. . . . Bly's own father was a remote and chilly alcoholic. . . . The scars of his father's neglect, and his mother's strong reaction to her husband, are visible in his works, including his 1987 manifesto of New Age masculinism, *The Pillow and the Key*." **ref. 26, p. 304-312**.

Robert Bly's most recent book **(*The Sibling Society*, Addison-Wesley, New York, 1996. 319 pp., $25)** about "the decomposition of authority," and his call "to face the children (not as equals but as adults)" has been described by David Bromvich as "an earnest warning to count the casualties, the ones who will never grow up." ("The Young Republic," in **The New Republic, Sept. 16 & 23, 1996, pp. 31-34.)**

18. (pg. 192) **ref. 116, p. 74.**

19. (pg. 193) **ref. 90, p. 118.**

20. (pg. 193) **ref. 113, p. 34, 36, 39.**

21. (pg. 193) **ref. 84.** (On a personal note, my oldest daughter, Maureen, now quite successful as a professional actuary, was assigned, in the final year of high school, a special math teacher who was hired by the school for the specific purpose of challenging her in mathematics. This one intervention literally launched her career.)

22. (pg. 194) **ref. 72.** The book provides many subtle examples of "emotional incest."

23. (pg. 194) **ref. 4, p. 116.**

24. (pg. 195) **ref. 113, p. 39.**

25. (pg. 195) **ref. 63, p. 112.** Sociologists agree that it takes years of training to turn boys into violent men. Apparently, as Paul Kivil puts it, they have to be repeatedly pushed back into their "act-like-a-man-box," which "holds" all the "manly" characteristics: aggression, being responsible and in-control, and being successful, strong, tough, courageous, active, and dominant over women. Kivil also asserts that boys-to-men are indoctrinated to use sexual means to control or intimidate women, while at the same time they are guided to deny that they are doing anything untoward at all; and they eventually learn, if confronted, to dismiss all their actions as no big deal. **ref. 63, p. 25.** Kivil's insights took form after the 1978 women's rally against violence in San Francisco, at which he heard and understood for the first time the **terror, shame, pain, anger, betrayal, and long-term scars that women carried as a direct result of the "normal" dating behavior of the typical American male.** "Of course, the link between sexuality and violence runs deep in our culture, where having sexual access to women, and having someone sexually vulnerable to us is the epitome of male power." **ibid, p. 114.**

26. (pg. 196) **ref. 113, p. 36, 39.** The authors refer to "(incest) and child molestations as among our culture's last taboos . . . (and) the worst crimes."

Rape itself, tends to be a "tragedy of youth," as one-third of all reported rapes occur between the ages of 11 and 17. **ref. 90, p. 219.** A survey of teenagers in the state of Rhode Island revealed that eighty percent didn't "know" that a man never has the right to force sex. **ibid, p. 206.**

Women are the victims of violence ninety-five percent of the time, especially when serious injury occurs. On the other hand, the majority view is that the radical-feminists are not correct in asserting that the perpetrator of abuse against women is just as likely to be your father, husband, brother, preacher, doctor, bank president, or college professor, as it is to be a "criminal type." Rather, the claim that all men, given the provocation, can be criminally violent, is clearly false. However, there may be **one exception.** Paul Kivil has worked in therapy with perpetrators of incest, and reports that he has never found any way one might distinguish them, except for the fact that virtually all experienced violence as children. **ref. 63, p. xxi.**

Unfortunately, exaggerating the rates of any of the types of violence against women and girls, as has happened repeatedly since 1970, has been very counterproductive. To cite but two among numerous examples, the assertions that one woman in every two is "battered" sometime in her lifetime and one in every four raped—some claim the figure is one in every two—is not supported by the data available. Christina Hoff Sommers, ref. 104, challenges these claims with her own documentation in her chapter entitled "Noble Lies." **ibid, pg. 188-208.** Sommers claims that the data available from independent studies already published suggest a maximum of one in twenty-five women will be forcibly raped in their lifetime. A similar decrease in the numbers for domestic violence is cited. The facts, while still showing the clearly unacceptable level of male violence that exists in America, do not provide justification for many of the key proposals of the radical-feminist agenda: labeling every male a potential rapist, who must be "socially reprogrammed" from day one, or for the institution of a whole bureaucracy of "gender-equity specialists," or "harassment monitors," to "police" every sector of society. **ibid, pg. 255-275.**

Hopefully, more precise figures on sexual violence against women will be provided by the Justice Department's Bureau of Justice Statistics. In August, 1995 they released a report for the years 1992-93 that for the first time reported results based on direct questions to women about rape, attempted rapes, and sexual assaults. Their figures show **one-half million sexual assaults per year, with one-hundred-seventy thousand rapes and one-hundred-forty thousand attempted rapes.** These figures, though much lower than had been presented by some of the feminist groups, provide extremely strong justification for the concern and anger of American women.

However, we must not overlook the fact that "It appears that **violence in lesbian relationships occurs at about the same frequency as violence in heterosexual relationships.**" Claire Renzetti's *Violent Betrayal: Partner Abuse in Lesbian Relationships,* (Newbury Park CA, Sage Press, 1994, p. 115). **Quoted in ref. 104, p. 200.** Battery between male homosexuals reflects a similar pattern.

Certainly, battery seems to always be a possibility between persons yearning for intimacy. As discussed in Chapters Ten through Fourteen of my book, intimacy requires that we divulge the secret grievances or needs that are causing us pain. As we each acknowledge these problem areas and accept them, "connectedness" increases. When differences are resisted, intimacy requires that a "satisfactory" solution be found for those differences. However, **if enough problems are buried instead of faced—thereby becoming much more powerful motivators of our reactions—anger or "violence" inevitably erupts.**

27. (pg. 197) **ref. 90, p. 230.** Maya Angelou, who stood beside President Clinton at his first inauguration and read her poem, "On the Pulse of the Morning," is the author of the best-selling autobiography, *I Know Why the Caged Bird Sings.* This Afro-American is still very active in her sixties as a playwright, producer, composer, civil-rights activist, and Reynolds Professor of African Studies at Wake Forest University. Abused as a child, she says that **"no woman ever gets over all of it. . . . I liken it to a broken wing. I cannot mend the wing, but I can still learn to fly."**

28. (pg. 197) **ref. 4, p. 48.**

29. (pg. 197) This sense of utter frustration is also evident in other areas of abuse as well. Susan Faludi asserts, in *Backlash,* that the oppression of women, the restrictions of a male culture, and the lack of equality everywhere, is more real in 1995 than it was in 1985, as men, and even many women, turn against the feminist movement. **ref. 28, p. 1-12.** For a woman's analysis of the reasons for all the defections from the feminist cause, **see also ref. 118, p. 57-134.**

30. (pg. 198) **ref. 90, p. 118, also p. 103, 117. Also p. 219, 224.**

31. (pg. 198) **ref. 36, p. 36.**

32. (pg. 198) **ibid, p. 26, 37.** A recurring theme in *My Mother/My Self* is that authentic communication between mother/daughter is almost always an essential prerequisite for learning to relate to others in an adult fashion, especially in sexual matters. "Unless we have separated from mother long before marriage, it is almost impossible to set up a healthy relationship with a man." **ibid, p. 69.** "The hardest thing to face is your mother's sexuality, and her, yours." **ibid, p. 23.** Women who are not allowed to separate from their mothers, says John Bradshaw, often become the victims of abusive men. **ref. 4, p. 220.**

Mary Ann Mayo, **ref. 80,** along with countless female writers, makes the point that ignorance of female sexuality and even genital anatomy is widespread among women. See **ref. 96, p. 208-209.** See also **ref. 80, pg. 83-119,** for help in guiding the sexual education of children and adolescents. Maggie Scarf, **ref. 96, part four,** has excellent material on sexual matters for couples in a committed relationship.

The book by Patricia Love and Jo Robinson, **ref. 71**, or that by Lonnie Barbach, **ref. 2**, might be useful for those married people who are now hopelessly bored with their "sex life," provided the couple are not engaging in one of the various forms of "angry sex." **see ref. 76, p. 38-58. (See also ref. 68, p. 473-489** for explicit sexual suggestions.)

33. (pg. 199) **ref. 104, p. 143-145.**

34. (pg. 199) **ref. 26, Introduction xxv.**

35. (pg. 200) **See Ch. Notes, Ch. 12, #12,** for the reference to the book of letters written between mothers and daughters (Ed. Karen Payne). The power of letterwriting is demonstrated with great effect.

13 Eliminating Sexual Ignorance and Repression

1. (pg. 201) Freud's "anatomy is destiny" statement that an inferior role in society is assigned to female children at birth did not mean that females were "naturally" inferior to males. Thus for Freud to state that **nurture** is the reason women are "inferior," and **not nature**, is obviously a much more optimistic statement than saying a women's nature renders her inferior. **If assignments, rules, attitudes, or styles of management are solely responsible for the "gender" differences, treating both sexes equally from birth should eliminate any female inferiority.** Unfortunately, many of Freud's closest associates ignored the vital distinction between nature and nurture, and included their bias of women's natural inferiority in their theories on female sexuality. Thus they described differences in women's response, satisfaction, and sexual performance, placing all of them at a reduced or inferior level of development, with virtually no scientific evidence for so doing. This interpretation of anatomy as destiny rightly incites the feminists to anger and retaliation, and justifies their rejection of much that has been written in this century about female sexuality.

As an example of such rejection, few feminist writers accept the assertion that women are naturally asexual, or neutral, from ages five to twelve, as boys frequently are, during their initial quest for their own identity. Nor do they accept that women revert to sexual repression with marriage, and especially after motherhood, as an effect natural to their sex.

Rather, most feminists unite in their insistence that any alleged difference in sexuality, especially an inferior one, whether in response, satisfaction, or performance is entirely the result of cultural indoctrination, and is not at all "natural." So it is society and its "feminine restraints," not biology, that gives any truth to the assertions that men have made about women's sexuality. While the consensus among the "experts" is the view proclaimed by Nancy Friday, Naomi Wolfe, or

Susan Faludi, namely that women are **not** less sexually-driven than men, there are many who claim that while women's pleasure from sex can be even more intense and wonderful than a man's, she is "naturally" less aggressive, less needful of sex, and less injured by its deprivation. One popular assertion about differences in male/female sexuality and "performance," could be divided into three basic, if somewhat facetious, statements:

(1) Men have the strongest urge toward genital sexuality at age sixteen and the urge very slowly, but inexorably, declines until their death.

(2) Women, by contrast, often have a minimal urge for genital expression of their sexual feelings when they are young, but that eventually, and it can be very variable from one woman to the next, the relentless increase in genital sexual urges begins and continues nearly to the end of her life.

(3) The result in most marriages is that there is a brief time of marital bliss when both partners have an equal desire for physical expression of their love in marital sexual intimacy. (One popular adage has it that the "time when the desire for sex is equal between the sexes, occurs at age 42 1/2, and lasts 30 minutes!) **If any of this is true, the majority now agree, its cause would be cultural, not "natural."** For another male viewpoint, **see ref. 68, p. 539-543.**

Naomi Wolf writes of the "great forgetting" in the last two centuries of the truth that women are far more sexual and passionate than men (*Promiscuities,* Random House: New York. 1997).

2 .(pg. 202) **ref. 36, p. 147.**

3. (pg. 202) **ibid, p. 23.**

4. (pg. 203) **ref. 86.** This is the thesis that Paglia's book attempts to document.

5. (pg. 204) **ref. 21, p. 13, 324.**

6. (pg. 205) **ibid, p. 340-1.**

7. (pg. 205) **ibid, p. 311.**

8. (pg. 205) **ref. 15.**

9. (pg. 206) See references given in **Notes, Ch. 10, 26.**

10. (pg. 206) Betty Friedan also points out that Kinsey's later work contradicted his earlier findings that uneducated women did "better" sexually. They do not. **ref. 38, p. 193-195.**

11. (pg. 208) **ref. 78, p. 65-6.**

12. (pg. 208) **ref. 71, p. 121,125,131,152-154, 270. Also ref. 2, p. 68-70, 75, 85, 156-157, 166, 190-191, ref. 68, pp. 466.**

13. (pg. 208) **ref. 68, p. 151-154, 157.**

14. (pg. 209) **ref. 47, p. 180.**

15. (pg. 209) **ref. 82, p. 122.**

16. (pg. 209) Closing the eyes during sex, even in the dark, but not making oneself rigid, is another thing entirely, as women writers have attested consistently. It is said to be an attempt to take the experience out of the ordinary, the limiting, the particular, and the temporary, and thus transport the entire experience to a more idyllic and more permanent level. It may also be because she is simply fantasizing about someone or something else. For the same reason, a wise man does not end the lovemaking with the question, "Was **it** all right?"—by which men generally mean, "Did you have an orgasm?"—or at least, "Did you enjoy the sex?" This is the question that infuriated Glenda Jackson in **A Touch of Class**. First of all, how particular and temporary could her lover, played by George Segal, make "it"? In addition, like many women, she concludes that setting "it" apart from all the other loving things upon which their commitment rests, makes it plain that he thinks "it" is something that he gives to her, not something she offers to him, much less something wonderful that they share with each other.

17. (pg. 210) **ref. 96 and 2.** See also **ref. 76, p. 38-58,** on "Angry Sex."

18. (pg. 210) **ref. 21, p. 23, 267-292.**

19. (pg. 211) **ibid, p. 85-92, 122.**

20. (pg, 212) quoted in **ref. 92, p. 369.** Samuel S. Janus, and Cynthia L. Janus, *The Janus Report on Sexual Behavior,* John Wiley: New York, 1993.

21. (pg. 212). Suggested vaginal lubricants, available without prescription, are **Lubrin, Gyne-moisturin, Replens, Vagicil Intimate**, and the best—**Astroglide** (which is available at only a few pharmacy chains and is expensive). Never recommended: petrolatum-based jellies.

22. (pg. 214) This unfortunate sequence for sexual performance is apparently quite common and summarizes a male attitude, reflected in a popular distinction made between depression and despair: **depression** is the first time a man can't do it twice, with **despair** being the second time he can't do it once. **See also ref 76, p. 39.**

23. (pg. 214) **ref 38, p. 282-309,** and **ref. 4,** where it is a recurrent theme.

24. (pg. 215) See **Notes, Ch. Twelve, 3 and 24.**

25. (pg. 215) "Romance" novels, read by over 20 million women in the USA, to the tune of $750 million in 1991, must be the kind of sex women prefer, or at least the kind they prefer to read about: no pornography, which is defined as violent or abusive sex that objectifies, subordinates, and dehumanizes women, but plenty of good old-fashioned values, like preserving your virginity until the right man comes along in the story and teaches you about sexual love; also, fidelity against all odds, and, in recent years, a little bit of oral sex. Unfortunately, for the ego of the "average" and "normal" woman, there is never a wavering in the sexual act itself, insofar as it concerns the march from desire to arousal to orgasm. The "dry" spells or "faltering phallus" that are part of any genuine sexual-love relationship are not allowed in erotic literature!

26. (pg. 216) **ref. 40, p. 175-76.**

27. (pg. 216) If the good doctor had read **ref. 37 or 71,** for examples of expressions of uninhibited female sexual attitudes, I think that he would have simply smiled.

28. (pg. 216) **ref. 77, p. 30.**

29. (pg. 217) **ref. 2, p. 287.**

14 Creating Intimacy Magic Moment-by-Moment

1. (pg. 218) **ref. 4, p. 316.**

2. (pg. 219) **ref. 112, p. 43.**

3. (pg. 220) **ref. 95, p. 25.**

4. (pg. 221) **ref. 58, p. 49.**

5. (pg. 222) quoted in **ref. 113, p. 96.**

6. (pg. 224) **ref. 61.** Dapne Rose Kingma's theme is that **what women want most in life is that men share themselves—what they are thinking and what they are feeling—without any bull!**

7. (pg. 224) Besides the books by Harville Hendrix, Maggie Scarf, Bonnie Maslin, and John Gray quoted in Chapter Ten, which provide information that should help anyone repeatedly manifesting destructive trends in their intimate relationships, another book is suggested **(ref. 86)** that exhorts such individuals to first **discover his or her chief "personality feature," or "weakness."** To make this discovery, a system or technique is suggested that is used in psychology and which is becoming increasingly popular in the last two decades, called the **Enneagram**—from two Greek words for "nine" and "points." The basic assertion is that indi-

viduals perform in their relationships in a characteristic, defined, and predictable way, depending on which one of only nine possible personality-types they are. Derived by the Sufi, a sect of mystics within the Muslims, the technique seeks as an early priority to have you discover which of the nine chief features—each listed and given its own number—best describes you. Once you discover your "number," you are given access to vast amounts of information, explaining the favorable or unfavorable ways persons with your personality feature, or number, typically respond to either stress, or, to the "opposite of stress," referred to as "prosperity." As an aid to memory and understanding, the system graphically portrays each individual as residing on his own particularly-numbered point on a nine-pointed star, and shows, by a few select connecting-directional lines, drawn between each point within the star, how each type of individual connects, or fails to connect, with the other personality types. Amazingly, as one consciously and honestly seeks to discover the unique way in which he relates to others, insights arrive in abundance.

Tony Schwartz, in *What Really Matters: Searching for Wisdom in America*, introduces the idea of the Enneagram in his final chapters. After first describing numerous popular psychological techniques uncovered on a five year world-wide journey to find wisdom, he concludes that "knowing your number," as it is defined in the Enneagram, could be your key to greater awareness of who you really are and thus lead you to wisdom. **ref. 100, p. 392-399.** Schwartz' wife eventually found the concepts and the details of the Enneagram, as they were taught to her, to be so helpful to her own happiness, that she resigned her previous position, and, at the time that *What Really Matters* was published, she was working full-time teaching the Enneagram approach.

(The eight couples comprising the "marriage encounter" group that my wife and I have met with for the past twenty-five years have each found the information contained in the Enneagram approach helpful for achieving deeper intimacy, not only with each other, but also with the other couples in the group. The insights that are given and received when close friends share their **numbers** can, indeed, be very striking.)

8. (pg. 224) If this book has stressed anything, it has been the **essential connection between love and anger or love/hate:**

Nancy Friday says that the best definition of love is that given by Harry Stack Sullivan: "love means that you care almost as much about the other person's safety, security, and satisfaction, as you do about your own." **ref. 36, p. 69.**

We have already seen that, as a practical matter, your attempts to get closer to your partner invariably require that he knows what you want or need, or what you do not want, and that you be selfish enough to tell him. The whole business of mirroring and the love letter of Chapters 10 and 11 was to stress that major point. Forbearance, or being silent about your gripes, can be very unloving, despite anything you may have been taught. Most of us have been trained that love means acceptance of frustration and disappointment, being tolerant and undemanding, giving up our own desires for the sake of the beloved, or in simple terms, being a martyr. Obviously this is not at all what "love" demands.

Recall that suffering selfishness constantly in silence places you on the path where your decisions to resist comment on a partner's thoughtless actions lead to resentment, then to a rejection, withdrawal, or distancing from him, and then, ultimately, to a total isolation from your mate, in your own little world of unfeeling, or of emotional numbness. Because love and hate are but two sides of the same coin—constituting, for better or worse, our relational energies and expression—any repression or suppression of these energies, which means hiding them, or being deceitful, is never good and always ultimately diminishes love. Even if silence doesn't build to a disruptive explosion, or to numbness, boredom, or depression, it will still leak out subtly in a hundred different ways equally harmful to the relationship.

Bonnie Maslin ends her book *The Angry Marriage* by affirming that "constructive anger . . . deserves its rightful place in marriage . . . as a declaration of our selfhood. . . . (T)his is me. . . . (I)t marks our separateness . . . (and allows) that the other has needs for self-determination as well . . . and seals our union." **ref. 76, p. 257.** John Gray adds, "Anger and resentment is the signal that our mate has not met our needs." **ref. 46, p. 88-89.**

However, Harriet Lerner, in *The Dance of Anger,* warns against putting our anger energy into trying to change or control a person . . . rather than putting that same energy into getting clear about our own positions and choices. . . . (W)e are able to move away from ineffective fighting only when we give up the fantasy that we can control or change anyone." **ref. 69, p. 13, 39.**

Honesty also requires that each be gracious and gentle when informing, guiding, or correcting the other, so as to enhance each others' self-esteem, not lessen it. An open dialogue on the "bad" things as well as the "good" is set forth as a primary goal in treating troubled relationships, precisely because it challenges the couple to recommit to the relationship as something more important than temporary differences. Each time this commitment is made in these contexts of stress, a spirit of safety, comfort, and acceptance is fostered, and the union is strengthened. "Fidelity" in marriage is still best defined as continued adherence to the marriage promise to keep trying.

9. (pg. 224) **ref. 88, p. 39-80.** These pages are quite detailed on the proper way to **negotiate so that both disputants win**—a skill we all definitely need to acquire.

SECTION THREE—
COMPLETING YOUR ACTIVE CHOICES
FACING THE FINAL CHALLENGES

15 Deciding Your Role in the Feminist Struggle

1. (pg. 228) **ref. 58, p. 273.**

2. (pg. 228) **ref. 67, p. 152.**

3. (pg. 229) **ref. 60, p. 35.**

4. (pg. 232) In defense of those older men and women who do little to maintain an active and social existence, and, as a result, eventually require total care and support much earlier than they might have needed such help (if only they had tried a little harder): all of us, at one time or another, act in the same foolish manner when we decide to do those various things in our lives that are intimately related to our short-term or long-term health. Obvious examples of personal neglect include smoking, excessive drinking or eating, avoiding exercise, or omitting check-ups or doctors' prescriptions. There is plenty of evidence for holistic medicine's assertion that we ultimately decide on our own death, in our own way, and in our own time.

One obvious way we play a role in deciding our own fate is by resorting to the chronic use of alcohol excessively, which is certainly a popular American form of chronic suicide. Not to mention that a recognizable suicide attempt is thirty-five times more frequent among alcoholics. **ref. 29, p. 81.**

5. (pg. 232) **ref. 38, p. 305-308.**

6. (pg. 233) Mary Ann Glendon warns of "the five dogmatic extremes that have shed more heat than light on women's issues: **sameness** feminism that insists there is no significant difference between men and women; **difference** feminism that treats men and women as virtually different species; **dominance** feminism that proclaims female superiority; **gender** feminism that regards 'male' and 'female' as mere social constructs; and the rigid **biological determinism** (associated with some critics of feminism) that would lock women into roles that were prevalent in the 1950s, the 1850s, or the time of the Babylonian captivity." Taken from a speech, "A Glimpse of the New Feminism," reproduced in *America*, **vol. 175, no.1 , pg. 14. July 1996.** Glendon is Professor of law at Harvard University Law School.

Proponents of **difference feminism** insist that the "sexuality" dif-fĉ*renc*es are so great that to attempt any reconciliation with men is futile. **"All men aĉ brutes, and all women are innocent victims,"** is the position of Catherine MacKinnon, Andrea Dworkin, and Mary Daly, among others. **ref. 34, p. 55, 56, 65, and esp. 240.**

Sameness feminists would eliminate all gender differences, making all the roles in society totally interchangeable. This view is held by, among others, Nancy Chodorow, Susan Okin, Robin West, and Cynthia Fuchs Epstein. **ref. 34, p. 52, 55.**

Elisabeth Fox-Genovese holds the **majority view, namely that equality is possible, despite the differences between the sexes.** She even stresses her conviction that if feminism is to succeed, or in fact survive, the differences in male and female sexuality must be given more prominence and attention. She emphasizes her judgment that making males and females "functionally interchangeable defies biology, history, and women's palpable needs," even if modern technology and contraception have eliminated virtually all the advantages of men's superior upper body strength and women's reproductive vulnerability. **ibid., p. 80, 250.**

However, even those who hold the majority view admit that deriving laws that take into full or fair account the differences between men and women is very difficult, and often the laws have unintended consequences. One example: changing the divorce laws, in order to make escape from domestic oppression faster and simpler, has had an unwanted consequence. Women can no longer afford to regard marriage itself as a viable "career," since their husbands can now also "leave" the marriage easily, and women generally suffer more damage financially.

Riane Eisler, in *The Chalice and the Blade*, agrees with the radical-feminists' assessment of past history—**men have been "beastly."** She, in fact, undertakes to document a **conspiracy of male-dominance.** Along with Gerna Lerner, Eisler assumes (**quoting Elizabeth Fox-Genovese' response to their teaching**), "that (Eisler's and Lerner's claim that) inequalities in all forms have somehow arisen from man's nature, (and in making that assumption, they) slight the ways in which societies construct men and women's roles and identities. . . . Patriarchy, like misogyny, exists within, not without history, and must be used with precise reference to historical relations of genders, races, and classes." **ibid, p. 143.** Going further, Fox-Genovese asserts that the "myth(ical theory) of separate values for men and women—the latter being 'by nature' nurturing, caring, (cooperative), and compassionate, and men being 'by nature' autonomous, competitive, and righteous . . . (artificially) sustains and reinforces such separate values . . . in practice."

Riane Eisler does however distance herself from the radical feminists in that she has not "given up on men," even though she **attributes virtually all manifestations of violence to the need of men to dominate not only women, but also to dominate "weaker" men.** This, she claims, necessitates "authoritarianism" in the family, in political life, between nations, and in religion.

According to Eisler's hypothesis, which she admits is still a minority view, there were groups or societies that existed for thousands of years prior to 3000 B.C.E. Only in very recent years have we begun to accurately see what those societies were all about. In these communities, located in southeastern Europe, including Greece and the Island of Crete, and in Asia Minor and the Near East, the "feminine" qualities of God were given priority, and, in fact, "informed" or controlled the lives of both men and women, within a "partnership" type of relationship. Individual activity seemed to be devoted toward promoting the good of the community, with "linking" and "sharing" the highest priority. Women's natural functions of menstruation and of childbirth were seen as god-like, or, in their mind, goddess-like, and these changes were viewed as beautifully mirroring the natural world around them, with its recurring cycles of life, death, and rebirth. Thus women, in these cultures, felt especially "connected" to the divine. In addition, no evidences were found of "ranking," or "hierarchy," or even the allocation of resources for "weapons" that would allow any group or community to "dominate" another.

The essence of Eisler's message is that if men could again accept the "partnership" model for society that existed prior to the last 5000 years, the world can still be saved. If not, then another "male" uprising will destroy the earth. ref. 27, p. 118, 171. An essential part of Eisler's message is that the mythologies of Western Civilization, in which category she places the "Bible," are all the result of a male conspiracy, and that older unwritten myths that did not include any concepts of dominance were distorted, or eliminated from the "oral" tradition, as the new written explanations of God and "creation" were used to justify and support an absolute system of male-dominance.

For an ""impassioned" overview of nearly every radical-feminist position on the Western religious traditions, as seen through the eyes of an ex-member of one of those "patriarchal" organizations, see **ref. 75, Part four, "Where It All Went Wrong," pp. 197-291.**

7. (pg. 234) The present feminist agenda reflects women's serious concern regarding the increasingly widespread dissemination of not only sexually explicit and sexually stimulating material, but also of pornography. While all these influences are very dangerous for both children and adolescents, it is pornography that carries with it a special danger to women. As presently defined, the purveyors of pornography, by material that "objectifies, subordinates, and dehumanizes" women, are undoubtedly raising the level of private and public violence toward women.

Many radical-feminists insist that private and public pornography are equally despicable, and must be prevented. **ref. 34, p. 99.**

8. (pg. 235) **ref. 34, p. 7, 99, 240.**

9. (pg. 235) In reality, the "abortion issue" is **not** about "reproductive rights" at all, since no one is interfering with a woman's right to have children. Rather, abortion deals with a **consequence** of a woman's use of her sexuality, that consequence being another human being that may or may not be a person when it is non-viable (see p. 235-6 of text).

It is undeniable that the freedom to use your personal human talents, whatever they may be, does not mean that talent can be used without regard for the consequences of such use. For example, let's compare the right to be sexually active with the constitutional right to bear arms, that is, to use a gun. The right to use either one's sexual powers or a gun is not absolute, since it does not include the right to use either in such a way as to "injure" others. In the case of the gun, you would be well-advised to consider when and where the gun is used, and at what the gun is aimed. With an unwanted pregnancy, there is the burning question of whether the living unborn that is "harmed" by an abortion is more than a "thing," specifically whether it is a human life. "Life" in Western tradition, and in the mind of our Founding Fathers, is declared the highest human value. Liberty and the pursuit of happiness mean nothing in the absence of life.

Therefore, when a mother claims that her body is absolutely hers, she is placing herself and her unborn child, and the protection of both their lives, on very dangerous ground indeed. Anything that belongs to us is our property. If **no one** can lay claim to it, then no one can be forced to protect it. Society might take precautions to protect your property, but in the absence of any absolute obligation to do so (since any "property" can be assigned a finite value), the persons arbitrarily involved in the decision to protect that property may decide that the commodity to be protected is not valuable enough. If the right to life is not **inalienable,** then it is **negotiable.**

Those feminists who desire the freedom to make free choices in everything sexual, including taking total control of their own sexuality, referring to control of the **uses of their own sexuality** and also control of the **consequences** of that use—**those women who are for** *choice*—strike a responsive chord, especially for those women whose mates never moved one muscle or expressed one thought regarding family planning, except perhaps to berate them for "becoming pregnant . . . or becoming pregnant once too often."

Unfortunately, those who insist that absolute sexual autonomy at all times is the "ideal," to be pursued relentlessly, also insist on the self-destructive notion that love relationships without commitment, solely for pleasure or release, is as much their "right" as it is a man's. In truth, while many men callously, and falsely I believe, assume that "right" and live it, it is rarely, if ever, the path to human love and intimacy. For women, the rewards are nearly always meager, at best, and quite often disastrous. That is true, at least for those who have shared their "stories" with me. **See ref. 99, especially "mistakes" #4, 5, 6, 7, 8, 10.**

Women's right to use their sexuality as they choose—to mate or not to mate, to be heterosexual, lesbian, or both, to be a prostitute, promiscuous, or even to cooperate in producing pornographic commodities for money—is all part of many feminists' agenda (though usually with the hope that their mates or daughters not be involved in the process.) **Few women, however, would agree that these "freedoms" were absolute, that is, subject to no restrictions.** The concepts of public decency and social good are still very much a priority among women, and the issue is more than a sentimental one.

The issue of reproductive right is really limited to countries like China, India, and a few others, where women are forbidden to have more children, or are sterilized or contracepted against their will. In the socialist state, children are generally considered valuable property and, as such, supported in many basic ways. However, when the state assumes responsibility to support your children, they may one day decide that a specific number of children is enough (welfare programs already have "limits"). When that happens, the issues of freedom and rights quickly become more than theory.

10. (pg. 237) Unfortunately, the hatred for men displayed by Mary Daly, Catherine MacKinnon, and Andrea Dworkin, among others, reflects their **belief that autonomy or superiority, not equality, is the answer to women's problem with men.** Such a position would obviate the institution of marriage. Camille Paglia, whom Christina Sommers describes as a "dissident feminist," writes that those feminists who profess to be anti-male, who deny "the sexual contingency of male and female, are sacrificing their natural tendencies, and desires, for the goal of female equality" (or autonomy or superiority). **ref. 86, p. 3, 10.** These women, however, are not asexual, though anti-feminists might say that they are. With a few noteworthy exceptions, some already mentioned, neither are they usually sincerely anti-male, however antagonistic they seem to be. Virtually all say they would welcome a continued relationship based on equality. It is really the slavery, dependence, or subservience that ruins male-female relationships for them. Paglia is surely correct in her assertion that sexual freedom or sexual liberation is a modern delusion, and that those feminists are dead wrong who deny the complementarity or contingency of the sexes. Yet, this denial of the need for men captured

the headlines in the feminist movement for almost a generation, starting in 1970, when the radical-feminists took center-stage. Taking their cue from Kate Millett's *Sexual Politics,* Germaine Greer's *The Female Eunuch,* and Robin Morgan's *Sisterhood Is Powerful,* and under the leadership of writers like Gloria Steinem, anti-male sentiments became the norm, and all gender differences were made cultural, not biological. They demanded that whatever personal qualities or roles were ascribed to the female sex had to be scrutinized as political issues, since **all** gender differences are ultimately and totally the result of a male-dominated or patriarchal culture. Lesbianism, or simply forsaking heterosexual relationships, were, like abortion, not moral issues at all, but rather political statements. Everything hitherto personal was now deemed to be political! Ignored in the process was the reality that the vast majority of women did find happiness in their heterosexual lifestyle, and in their lives of caring and sharing intimacy in the traditional ways, and did not choose to abort their babies, even if they respected your right to do all those things.

Moreover, the majority of women do not hold that their "stance" on any of these moral/political issues should be the basis for deciding whether they are allowed to call themselves **real feminists.**

Feminists like Gloria Steinem, Nancy Friday, Simone DeBevoir, Susan Faludi, Germaine Greer, and Susan Brownmiller, among countless others, have written, at least in some of their works, that marriage and motherhood are not essential for achieving either sexual fulfillment or for reaching the highest levels of human intimacy, going so far as to assert that, for many women, the chance for happiness is better without becoming either a housewife or a mother.

Gloria Steinem offers that "she cannot mate in captivity." Simone DeBevoir has declared that: "while love and friendship can exist in marriage, it is most often seen outside of marriage . . . [and] that marriage invites man to a capricious imperialism, [since] the temptation to dominate is . . . universal." **ref. 22, p. 465.** She states what many feminists have demonstrated by their lives—that a woman is betrayed from the day she marries. The husband "requires her to be chaste, yet passionate, to be wholly his and yet no burden . . . to establish him on a fixed place on earth and to leave him free, to assume the monotonous daily round and not to bore him, to be always on hand and never importunate, to have her all to himself and not to belong to her, and to live as one of a couple and to remain alone." **ibid, p. 478.**

Simone DeBevoir has gone so far as to suggest that women not be allowed to marry. Admittedly, we have all personally observed relationships in which Steinem's and DeBevoir's expressions of contempt for marriage might seem justifiable.

11. (pg. 237) **ref. 17, p. 318.** Joann Wolski Conn makes some strong arguments for considering Therese of Lisieux ("The Little Flower") a model feminist because she "stuck" to her own unique and original vision of spiritual development, the Church, and heaven.

12. (pg. 237) **ref. 58. p. 28.**

16 Making Your Judgment Regarding Life's Meaning and Purpose

1. (pg. 238) Frankl also writes, "The consciousness of one's inner life is anchored in higher, more spiritual things and cannot be shaken by Camp life. But how many free men, let alone prisoners, possess it." **ref. 35, p. 58.**

2. (pg. 240) **ref. 34, Introduction.**

3. (pg. 240) Feminist writers who would dismiss the Bible—and by implication, if not expressly, seek the abolition of all the "institutions" that use it, at least partly, to justify their existence—refer to brief incidents that are described identically in the Old Testament of the Christian Bible and in the books of the Hebrew Bible (though the numbers for each chapter and verse quoted are taken from a Christian Bible). **ref. 27, ch. 7.**

Number's 31:18, Deuteronomy 22:13-21 and 22:28-29, and Numbers 31:9-17 all have to do with the concept of "virgins" being some man's valuable property, even if they are "acquired" as part of the spoils of war. That only females who "had never lain with a man" were spared and taken captive after a victory was in obedience to Yahweh's command. (Everyone else was killed, so that for many generations there would not be enough enemies in that area to retaliate.) A virgin was not committed to **any** man, so could very reasonably be expected to accept the protection, present and future, of a man among the conquerors. What else virgins represented to the community, or the people as a whole, is admittedly arguable, depending upon your beliefs. Under the system prevailing in those times, the loss of virginity equated with total loss of a woman's value, at least for purposes of barter, since she was totally the property of her husband. The loss of virginity had better occur with the husband, who, thereafter and forever, had to be her protector. Death was prescribed for men or women who treated virginity lightly.

Judges 19:24-28 and Genesis 19:8 have to do with complex oriental and Near-Eastern customs of hospitality to house guests, as well as with the prevailing belief that women were of lesser value than men. The part that is always omitted in the retelling of the story from Judges, a story that tells of the "gang-rape" of one concubine, is that the violation of one woman instigated a war in which fifty to one-hundred-thousand young men were slaughtered. Apparently, the value these societies at this time placed on **any** human life was quite limited. A recent example of the belief in the expendability of our young men: the Vietnam War Memorial has 57,000 names, of which only eight are women!

Leviticus 12:6-7 typifies the Bible's judgment on women's unique natural functions as being "unclean." Like the Mosaic laws against eating pork, shellfish, and anything still containing the blood of animals, not allowing intercourse within a week of the period, and isolating a new mother from the community for a time, not to mention delaying circumcision until the boy's eighth day of life (the very day his clotting factors return to the high levels present at birth and which are again high enough to prevent hemorrhage), there were excellent health reasons for many of the "precautions" taken against women who were bleeding (or who could **potentially** bleed at any time). Nearly all the health restrictions unique to women benefited the women themselves much more than anyone else. (See also Leviticus 15: 19, 24, 28-30.)

Also a source of suspicion to those feminists who see the Bible as an entirely human work is the fact that there are two significantly-differing accounts of creation—significant at least from a feminist point of view. Which Genesis story is true? The simultaneous creation of Adam and Eve in God's image, or, like the Greek goddess Athene, who was taken from Zeus's head, the creation of Eve from Adam's rib? **(See also page 241 of text.)**

4. (pg. 240) **ref. 27, p. 120-124. See ref. 17, p. 274-286, esp. 278.** *Non-Patriarchal Salvation* by Bernard Cooke *explains* why Christ had to be killed: "he did not fit. . . . He threatened, not only the social power structure of the world, but the very notion of 'society'; for . . . he proposed and embodied a new approach to human relationships and human community, a new understanding of what it meant for a human to be a person, a new foundation for evaluating humans and their behavior. . . . A new humanity was being initiated by this 'new Adam' . . . the old patriarchal discriminations could no longer lay claim to God: 'neither Jew nor Gentile, neither master nor slave, neither male nor female.'"

5. (pg. 241) **ref. 109, Chapter 13.** For an overview of the religious tradition and feminism, **see p. 151-178.** For "students of spirituality" or anyone interested in any serious way with "women's spiritual development," see *Women's Spirituality: Resources For Christian Development*, ed. Joann Wolski Conn, Paulist Press: New York. 1986. In "Impasse and Dark Night," Constance Fitzgerald writes of the "voiceless sorrows of women long dead" quoting Alice Walker's essay, "In Search of Our Mother's Gardens"—both women referring to the throwing away of a

woman's unused and unwanted spirituality (talents) in order to survive total male oppression. **ibid. p. 307.** "The white . . . male God don't seem to listen to your prayers." Spoken by Celie in Alice Walker's *The Color Purple,* quoted **ibid. p. 303.**

Thomas C. Fox, in *Sexuality and Catholicism,* writes, ". . . the entrance for the first time of the thoughts, voices, and writings of untold numbers of educated Catholic women assures that new visions of church, already being born, will not go away, and will have greater sway in the decades ahead. . . ." **(ref. 33, p. 353)**

For "inside" information on the radical-feminists within the Roman Catholic Church, **see ref. 106.** For a concise and clear overview of the patriarchal aspects of Catholicism that some Catholic women find most "disturbing," see **ref. 33, esp. pp. 199-248, and pp. 299-333.**

6. (pg. 241) **ref. 93, p. 89.**

7. (pg. 242) The witch hunts of the 15th, 16th, and 17th centuries, especially, are cited by Mary Daly as evidence to show the utter evil and worthlessness of patriarchy. **ref. 19, p. 178-222.** Riane Eisler speaks of the witch-hunts of the 13th to 16th centuries, citing them not as evidence of mob hysteria, but more as a calculated, reasoned, legalistic form of masochism and intimidation. **ref. 27, p. 140.**

However, I agree with Naomi Wolf that "the current split, fashionable in parts of the progressive (female) community, into male-evil-sexually-exploitive-rational-linear-dominating-combative-tyranical on the one hand, and female-natural-nurturing-concensus-building-healing-intuitive-aggressionless-egoless-spirit-of-the-glades on the other hand, belies the (total) evidence of history. . . . (And it) denies the full humanity of men and women. . . . It re-creates a new version of the old female stereotype that discourages women from appropriating the power of the political and financial world to make power at last on their own." **ref. 118, p. 148-149.** "Victim feminism," besides creating male-bashing reactions, is, again in Wolf's words, "a reflex grossly unworthy of feminism, which should be the ultimate civil rights movement." **ibid, p. 151.**

8. (pg. 243) quoted in **ref. 27, p. 197.** Also, other statistics on women and children taken from the same United Nations report can be found on page 177 of Riane Eisler's book, **ref. 27.**

9. (pg. 243) Some gains were attained for women at Beijing:
India said it will increase its spending on education primarily for women and girls (six percent of its domestic product). Turkey promised to provide eight instead of five years of compulsory education for women. Our country promised a six-year, $1.6 billion program to fight violence against women.

The final Platform for Action condemned: forced sterilizations and forced abortions; perpetrators of rape by partisans in war who should be tried as war criminals; all violations of human (women's) rights— genital mutilation, sexual harassment in the workplace, domestic battering, and all violence in the home.

10. (pg. 243) Thomas Berry, who has been praised as "the Thomas Aquinas of ecological theologians," in *The Dream of the Earth*, declares that the same priority of reverence that leads to intimacy is vital to world survival, but includes a plea for **reverence of all of creation:** "The main task of the immediate future is to assist in activating the intercommunion of all living and nonliving components of the earth community. . . . (A)chieving the art of intimacy and distance, the capacity of beings to be totally present to each other while further affirming and enhancing the differences and identities of each." Quoted by Thomas Fox in **ref. 33, p. 265.**

Bibliography

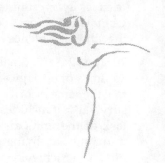

1. Adler, Mortimer J. *Aristotle For Everybody: Difficult Thought Made Easy*. Collier Books, MacMillan Publishing Company: New York. 1991. Bantam Books: New York. 1980.
2. Barbach, Lonnie. *For Each Other: Sharing Sexual Intimacy*. Penguin Books: New York. 1984.
3. ———. *Pause: Positive Approaches To Menopause*. Signet: New York. 1992.
4. Bradshaw, John. *Creating Love: The Next Great Stage of Growth*. Bantam Books: New York. 1992.
5. Bartky, Sandra Lee. *Femininity and Domination: Studies in the Phenomenology of Oppression*. Routledge: New York. 1970.
6. Bird, Caroline. *Lives of Our Own: Secrets of Salty Old Women*. Houghton Mifflin: New York. 1995.
7. Benson, Herbert., and Eileen M. Stuart. *The Wellness Book: The Comprehensive Guide to Maintaining Health and Treating Stress-Related Disease*. Simon & Schuster: New York. 1993.
8. Bepko, Claudia., and Jo-Ann Krestan. *Singing at the Top of Our Lungs: Women, Love, and Creativity*. Harper Collins: New York. 1994.
9. Berne, Eric. *What Do You Say After You Say Hello???* Bantam Books: New York. 1981.
10. ———. *Games People Play*. 34th Edition. Ballantine Books: New York. 1991.
11. Branden, Nathaniel. *The Six Pillars of Self-esteem*. Bantom Books: New York. 1994.

12. ———. *Honoring the Self: Self-Esteem and Personal Transformation*. Bantam: New York. 1985.
13. Breen, James L. (ed.). *The Gynecologist and the Older Patient*. Aspen Publishers: Rockville, Maryland. 1988.
14. Buscaglia, Leo. *Love: A Warm and Wonderful Book About the Largest Experience of Life*. Ballantine Books: New York. 1982.
15. Carter, Steven, and Julia Sokol. *Men Like Women Who Like Themselves (and Other Secrets That the Smarter Women Know)*. Delacorte: New York. 1996.
16. Chopra, Deepak. *Boundless Energy: The Complete Mind/Body Program for Overcoming Chronic Fatigue*. Harmony Books: New York, 1995.
17. Conn, Joaan Wolski, (ed.) *Women's Spirituality: Resources for Christian Development*. Paulist Press: New York. 1986.
18. Cutler, Winifred B., and Celso-Ramom Garcia. *Menopause: A Guide for Women and the Men Who Love Them*. W.W. Norton: New York. 1993.
19. Daly, Mary. *Gyn/Ecology—The Metaethics of Radical Feminism*. Beacon Press: Boston, MA. 1990.
20. Davidson, Michael W. (ed.). *Everyday Life Through the Ages*. The Readers Digest Association Limited: New York. 1992.
21. De Angelis, Barbara. *How to Make Love All the Time: Make Love Last a Lifetime*. Dell: New York. 1991.
22. De Bevoir, Simone. *The Second Sex*. Vintage Books, a Division of Random House: New York. 1989.
23. de Mello, Anthony. *Awareness: The Perils and Opportunities of Reality*. Doubleday: New York. 1992.
24. de Silva, Alvaro. (ed.) *Brave New Family: G.K. Chesterton on Men and Women, Children, Sex, Divorce, Marriage and the Family*. Ignatius Press: San Francisco. 1990.
25. Domar, Alice D., and Henry Dreher. *Healthy Mind, Healthy Woman: Using the Mind-Body Connection to Manage Stress and Take Control of Your Life*. Holt: New York. 1996
26. Edelman, Hope. *Motherless Daughters: The Legacy of Loss*. Dell: New York. 1995
27. Eisler, Riane. *The Chalice and the Blade: Our History, Our Future*. HarperCollins: New York. 1988.

28. Faludi, Susan. *Backlash: The Undeclared War Against American Women.* Dell: New York. 1992.
29. Fieve, Roland R. *Moodswing: the Third Revolution in Psychiatry.* Bantam Books: New York. 1989.
30. Folan, Lilias M. *Lilias' Yoga and You.* Bantam Books: New York. 1980.
31. Foley, Denise, Eileen Nechas, and the Editors of **Prevention** Magazine. *Women's Encyclopedia of Health & Emotional Healing.* Rodale Press: Emmaus PA. 1993.
32. Forward, Susan, and Joan Torres. *Men Who Hate Women & the Women Who Love Them.* Bantam Books: New York. 1987.
33. Fox, Thomas C. *Sexuality and Catholicism.* George Braziller: New York. 1995.
34. Fox-Genovese, Elizabeth. *Feminism Without Illusions: A Critique of Individualism.* Univ. of North Carolina Press. 1991.
35. Frankl, Viktor. *Man's Search for Meaning.* Simon & Schuster: New York. 1976.
36. Friday, Nancy. *My Mother, My Self: The Daughter's Search for Identity.* Dell: New York. 1987.
37. ———. *My Secret Garden: Women's Sexual Fantasies.* Simon and Schuster: New York. 1974.
38. Friedan, Betty. *The Feminine Mystique.* Dell: New York. 1984.
39. ———. *The Second Stage.* Dell: New York. 1981.
40. ———. *The Fountain of Age.* Simon and Shuster: New York. 1993.
41. Fromm, Erich. *The Art of Loving.* Harper: New York. 1974.
42. ———. *The Anatomy of Human Destructiveness.* Fawcett Crest Book: Greenwich, Connecticut. 1975.
43. Fuchs Epstein, Cynthia. *Deceptive Distinctions: Sex, Gender, and the Social Order.* Yale University Press and the Russell Sage Foundation: New York. 1988.
44. Fulghum, Robert. *All I Really Need to Know I Learned in Kindergarten.* Ballantine: New York. 1993. Ivy Books: New York. 1988.
45. Gil, Eliana. *Outgrowing the Pain: A Book for and About Adults Abused as Children.* Dell: New York. 1988.
46. Gray, John. *Men, Women, and Relationships: Making Peace with the Opposite Sex.* Beyond Words Publishing: Hillsboro, Oregon. 1993.

47. Greeley, Andrew M. *Sexual Intimacy.* The Seabury Press: New York. 1973.
48. Greenwood, Sadja. *Menopause, Naturally (updated): Preparing for the Second Half of Life.* Volcano Press: Volcano, CA. 1992.
49. Harris, Jay R. (ed.) *Breast Diseases.* J.B. Lippincott Company: Philadelphia, PA. 1987.
50. Helfant, Richard H. *Women, Take Heart: A Leading Cardiologist's Breakthrough Program to Help Women Combat Heart Disease.* The Putnam Publishing Group: New York. 1993.
51. Hendrix, Harville. *Getting the Love You Want: A Guide for Couples.* Harper Perennial: New York. 1988.
52. ———. *Keeping the Love You Find: A Personal Guide.* Pocket Books: New York. 1992.
53. Hirsch, E. D., Jr. *The Schools We Need: Why We Don't Have Them.* Doubleday: New York. 1996.
54. Hirschman, Jane R., and Carol H. Hunter. *When Women Stop Hating Their Bodies: Freeing Yourself from Food and Weight Obsessions.* Fawcett Columbine: New York. 1995.
55. Hobbs, Christopher. *Handbook for Herbal Healing: A Concise Guide to Herbal Products.* Botanica Press: Capitola, CA. 1994.
56. Hollis, Judi. *Fat and Furious: Women and Food Obsession.* Ballantine Books: New York. 1995.
57. Horney, Karen. *Feminine Psychology.* W.W. Norton: New York. 1967.
58. Jeffers, Susan. *Opening Our Hearts to Men: Learn to Let Go of Anger, Pain, and Loneliness and Create a Love That Works.* Fawcett Columbine: New York. 1990.
59. Kamen, Betty. *Hormone Therapy: Yes or No: How to Make an Informed Decision.* Nutrition Encounter: Novato, CA. 1995.
60. Kelley, Mary. *The Portable Margaret Fuller.* Penguin Books: New York. 1994.
61. Kingma, Daphne Rose. *The Men We Never Knew: How to Deepen Your Relationship with the Man You Love.* Conari Press: Emeryville, CA. 1993.
62. Kinsey, A.C., et al. *Sexual Behavior in the Human Female.* W. B. Saunders: Philadelphia. 1953.

63. Kivel, Paul. *Men's Work: How to Stop the Violence That Tears Our Lives Apart.* Ballantine Books: New York. 1992.

64. Kohn, Alfie. *Punished by Rewards: The Trouble with Gold Stars, Incentive Plans, A's, Praise, and Other Bribes.* Houghton Mifflin Company: New York. 1993.

65. Kübler-Ross, Elisabeth. *On Death and Dying.* MacMillan Publishing Company: New York. 1976.

66. Kurzwell, Edith. *Freudians and Feminists: New Perspectives in Sociology.* Westview Press: Boulder, Colorado. 1995.

67. Kushner, Harold. *When All You've Ever Wanted Isn't Enough: The Search For a Life That Matters.* Simon and Schuster: New York. 1987.

68. Lauersen, Niels, and Steven Whitney. *It's Your Body: A Woman's Guide to Gynecology.* (Perigee) Putnam: New York. 1987

69. Lerner, Harriet G. *The Dance of Anger: A Woman's Guide to Changing the Patterns of Intimate Relationships.* Perennial Harper: New York. 1985.

70. Lewis, Sydney. *"A Totally Alien Life-form"—Teenagers.* The New Press: New York. 1996.

71. Love, Patricia, and Jo Robinson. *Hot Monogamy: Essential Steps to More Passionate, Intimate Lovemaking.* Penguin Books: New York. 1995.

72. ———. *The Emotional Incest Syndrome: What to Do When a Parent's Love Rules Your Life.* Bantam Books: New York. 1991.

73. Lown, Bernard. *The Lost Art of Healing.* Houghton Mifflin: Boston. 1996.

74. MacKinnon, Catherine. "Desire and Power: A Feminist Perspective." In *Marxism and the Interpretation of Culture.* Edited by Cary Nelson and Lawrence Grossberg. University of Illinois Press: Chicago. 1988.

75. Mann, Judy. *The Difference. Discovering the Hidden Ways We Silence Girls: Finding Alternative That Can Give Them a Voice.* Warner Books: New York. 1996.

76. Maslin, Bonnie. *The Angry Marriage: Overcoming the Rage, Reclaiming the Love.* Hyperion: New York. 1994.

77. Masters, William H., and Virginia E. Johnson. *The Pleasure Bond.* Bantam Books: New York. 1976.

78. ———. *Human Sexual Response.* Bantam Books: New York. 1981.

79. May, Rollo. *Love and Will.* Dell Publishing: New York. 1969.

80. Mayo, Mary Ann. *Parents Guide to Sex Education.* Zondervan Publishing: Grand Rapids, MI. 1986.

81. Millett, Kate. *Sexual Politics.* Simon and Shuster: New York. 1990.

82. Morgan, Marabel. *The Total Woman.* Simon and Shuster: New York. 1975.

83. Northrup, Christiane. *Women's Bodies, Women's Wisdom: Creating Physical and Emotional Health and Healing.* Bantam Books: New York. 1995.

84. Orenstein, Peggy, in Association with the American Association of University Women. *School Girls: Young Women, Self-Esteem, and the Confidence Gap.* Doubleday: New York. 1994.

85. Pagels, Elaine. *The Gnostic Gospels.* Random House: New York. 1989.

86. Paglia, Camille. *Sexual Personae: Art and Decadence From Nefertiti to Emily Dickinson.* Random House: New York. 1991

87. Palmer, Helen. *The Enneagram: Understanding Yourself and the Others in Your Life.* Harper: San Francisco. 1991.

88. Peck, Connie. *How to Make Peace with Your Partner: A Couple's Guide to Conflict Management.* Warner: New York. 1995.

89. Peck, Scott. *The Road Less Traveled.* Simon and Schuster: New York. 1978.

90. Pipher, Mary. *Reviving Ophelia: Saving the Selves of Adolescent Girls.* Ballantine: New York. 1995.

91. Powell, John. *Why Am I Afraid to Love?* Argus Communications Co: Niles, Illinois. 1972.

92. Reichman, Judith. *I'm Too Young to Get Old: Health Care for Women After Forty.* Times Books: New York. 1996.

93. Reilly, Patricia Lynn. *A God Who Looks Like Me: Discovering a Woman-Affirming Spirituality.* Ballantine Books: New York. 1995.

94. Rosen, Laura Epstein, and Xavier Francisco Amador. *When Someone You Love Is Depressed: How to Help Your Loved One Without Losing Yourself.* The Free Press: New York. 1996.

95. Roth, Geneen. *When Food Is Love: Exploring the Relationship Between Eating and Intimacy.* Penguin: New York. 1992.

96. Scarf, Maggie. *Intimate Partners: Partners in Love and Marriage.* Ballantine: New York. 1988.

97. ———. *Intimate Worlds: Life Within the Family.* Random House: New York. 1995.

98. Schaller, James L. *In Search of Lost Fathering: Rebuilding Your Father Relationships.* Baker Book House: Grand Rapids, MI. 1995.

99. Schlessinger, Laura. *Ten Stupid Things Women Do to Mess Up Their Lives.* Harper Collins: New York. 1993.

100. Schwartz, Tony. *What Really Matters: Searching for Wisdom in America.* Bantam Books: New York. 1995.

101. Sheehy, Gail. *The Silent Passage: Menopause.* Random House: New York. 1991.

102. ———. *Passages: Predictable Crises of Adult Life.* Bantam Books: New York. 1976.

103. Smalley, Gary, and John Trent. *The Hidden Value of a Man.* Focus on the Family Publishing: Colorado Springs, Colorado. 1992.

104. Sommers, Christina Hoff. *Who Stole Feminism? How Women Have **Betrayed** Women.* Simon and Shuster: New York. 1995.

105. Stacey, Judith. *In the Name of the Family: Rethinking Family Values in the PostModern Age.* Beacon: Boston. 1996.

106. Steichen, Donna. *Ungodly Rage: The Hidden Face of Catholic Feminism.* Ignatius Press: San Francisco. 1991.

107. Steinem, Gloria. *Revolution from Within: A Book of Self-Esteem.* Little, Brown and Company: Boston. 1992.

108. ———. *Moving Beyond Words: Age, Rage, Sex, Power, Money, Muscles: Breaking Boundaries of Gender.* Simon and Shuster: New York. 1995.

109. Storkey, Elaine. *What's Right with Feminism.* SPCK: Holy Trinity Church, Marlybone Road, London NW1 4DU (Great Britain) 6th Imp. 1993.

110. Studd, John. W.W., and Roger N.J. Smith. "Gonadal Hormones and Breast Cancer Risk: The Estrogen Window Hypothesis Revisited." In *Menopause, The Journal of the North American Menopause Society.* Vol 1:49-55. 1994.

111. Swartz, Donald P.(ed.). *Hormone Replacement Therapy.* Williams and Wilkins: Baltimore, MD. 1992.

112. Tournier, Paul. *To Understand Each Other: Why Love Dies and How to Make It Live Again.* The John Knox Press: Atlanta, GA. 1977.

113. Valentis, Mary, and Anne Devane. *Female Rage: Unlocking Its Secrets, Claiming Its Power.* Crown Publishers: New York. 1994.
114. Vitz, Paul. *Psychology as Religion: The Cult of Self-worship.* Wm. B. Eerdmans Publishing Co: Grand Rapids, MI. 1994.
115. Walters, David R. *Physical and Sexual Abuse of Children: Causes and Treatment.* Indiana University Press. 1975.
116. Westheimer, Ruth, and Ben Yagoda. *The Value of Family: A Blueprint for the 21th Century.* Warner Books: New York. 1996
117. Whitehead, Barbara Dafoe. "What They Want to Teach Your Child About Sex." *The Atlantic Monthly.* (Oct. 1994). Article found in condensed version in the *Readers Digest* (Feb. 1995).
118. Wolf, Naomi. *Fire with Fire: The New Female Power and How to Use It.* Random House: New York. 1994.

ADDITIONAL READING

1. Bryan, Mark. *The Prodigal Father: Reuniting Fathers and Their Children.* Potter: New York. 1997.

     Single mothers should read this first before they send it to the father. Even the most hard-hearted "sperm donor" will cry.

2. Claude-Pierre, Peggy. *The Secret Language of Eataing Disorders.* Times Books: New York. 1997.

     Proves to me and many others that people with eating disorders are typically the finest human beings on the planet and their problem is neither their fault nor their family's. A must-read, especially if you have younger siblings or children.

3. Green, Harvey. *The Light of the Home: An Intimate View of the Lives of Women in Victorian America.* Pantheon Books: New York. 1983.

     A very detailed rendering of what daily life was like during the 100 years or so when "women knew their place" and when, from outward appearances at least, the majority of women seemed to accept it, and how nostaligia for those "good old days" is messing up relationships today.

4. Gurian, Michael. *The Wonder of Boys: What Parents, Mentors, and Educators Can Do to Shape Boys into Exceptional Men.* Putnam: New York. 1996.

   The best book yet on the reason for increasing male violence.

5. Heyn, Dalma. *Marriage Shock: The Transformation of Women into Wives.* Villard Books: New York. 1997.

   Cultural imperatives have been developed and perfected over the 300 years since the industrial revolution spawned a new class of male nobility (men with wealth) who demanded wives of which they could be proud. The complex and lofty rules and expectations for women which were often written down are still perceived as real and operative by many women when they become **wives**.

6. Nelson, Miriam E. *Strong Women Stay Young.* Bantam: New York. 1997.

   Agrees totally with my exercise program (Ch. 7) and provides clear guidelines for the anaerobic, muscle-building component.

7. Schnarch, David. *Passionate Marriage: Sex, Love, and Intimacy in Emotionally Committed Relationships.* Norton: New York. 1997.

   Schnarch's insights into "human sexuality" are recommended reading for any couple who wish to be among the "select few" whose marriages and sexual relationships live up to potential. His work has inspired my second book (for men) due for release late in 1999.

8. Shalit, Wendy. *A Return to Modesty: Discovering the Lost Virtues.* The Free Press: New York. 1999.

   Recounts how the women of her generation—the first to have sex education in the elementary schools—have been harmed greatly by the loss of innocence it foisted upon them.

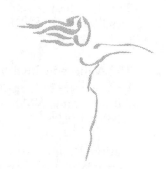

Resources

Adolescence

Girls, Inc.
National Resource Center
441 W. Michigan St.
Indianapolis, Indiana 46202

The National Coalition of
Girls' Schools
Meg Milne Moulton/
Whitney Ransome
Executive Directors
228 Main Street
Concord, Massachusetts 01742
(phone/fax) (508) 287-4485
Sponsors conferences to
familiarize girls with
technology and to assist math
and science teachers in teaching
these subjects to girls

Aging

American Geriatric Society
10 Columbus Ciccle
New York, NY 10019

Alcoholics Anonymous
P.O. Box 459
Grand Central Station
New York, NY 10163

Alternative Medicine

American Academy
of Acupuncture
5820 Wilshire Blvd., Suite 500
Los Angeles, CA 90036
(patients seeking physicians
who perform acupuncture can
call (800) 521-2262; for actual
referral, call (800) 521-2663

American Association of
Naturopathic Physicans
2366 Eastlake Ave. E., Suite 322
Seattle, WA 98102
(206) 323-7610

American Association of
Oriental Medicine
433 Front St.
Catasauqua, PA 18032
(610) 266-1433

The American Society of
Clinical Hypnosis
2200 E. Devon Ave., Suite 291
Des Plaines, IL 60018
(847) 297-3317

The Ayurvedic Institute
P.O. Box 23445
Albuquerque, NM 87192
(505) 291-9698

National Commission for the
Certification of Acupuncturists
(to see if a particular
acupuncturist is "certified"):
(202) 232-1404

American Holistic Medical
Association
4101 Lake Boone Trail, Suite 201
Raleigh NC 27607
(919) 787-5181
(For $8, they will send you a
nationwide directory of M.D.s
who practice alternative
therapies.)

The Center for Mind-Body
Medicine
5225 Connecticut Ave., N.W.
Suite 414
Washington, DC 20015
(202) 966-7338

Committee on Pain Therapy
and Accupuncture
American Socety of
Anesthesiologists
1515 Busse Highway
Park Ridge, IL 60068

Mind/Body Materials and
Herbs
Quantum Publications
P.O.Box 1088
Sudbury MA 01776
(800) 858-1808

The American Self-Help
Clearinghouse
St. Charles Riverside
Medical Center
25 Pocono Road
Denville NJ 07834
(201) 625-7101 (Information on
Support groups for various
illnesses)

(Book) Micozzi, Marc.
_Fundamentals of Complementary
and Alternative Medicine_
Churchill Livingston. 1996
Available (800) 553-5426

Office of Alternative Medicine
National Institutes of Health
9000 Rockville Pike, Bldg. 31,
Room 5B-38
Bethesda, MD 20892
(800) 531-1794

(Scientific Literature)
"Unconventional Medicine in
the United States"
New England Journal of Medicine
382: 246-53. 1993.

(Information packets)
Office of Alternative Medicine
(301) 402-2466,
fax: (301) 402-4741

Women to Women
One Pleasant Street
Yarmouth ME O4096
(207) 846-6163

Alzheimer' Disease

Alzhimer's Association
919 N. Michigan Avenue
(Suite 1000)
Chicago IL 60611
312 355-8700
800 272-3900

Cancer

American Cancer Society
1599 Clifton Road NE
Atlanta GA 30329
(404) 325-2217 OR
(800) ACS-2345 (Call last
number for help to
quit smoking)
For help with arranging
mammograms call
1 (800)-4-CANCER

(If strong family history of
breast cancer)
Strang Cancer Prevention
Center
National High Risk Registry
428 East 72nd Street
New York NY 10021
(212) 794-4900

Society of Gynecologic
Oncologists
401 N. Michigan Avenue
Chicago IL 6O611
(312) 644 6610

Cancer Information Service
(800) 4-CANCER
(Evenings) (800) 638-6694

Counseling

American Association of Sex
Educators, Counselors, and
Therapists
435 Michigan Avenue
(Suite 1717)
Chicago IL 60611
(312) 664-0828

American Psychiatric
Association
1400 K Street, NW
Washington DC 20005
(202) 682-6000

Domestic Violence

Child Abuse Hotline (24 hours)
(800) 422 4453

Child Abuse/Fmily Violence
(800) 223 6004

(Childhood Sexual Abuse)
Audiocassettes of *The Courage
To Heal: A Guide for Women
Survivors of Child Sexual Abuse.*
Harper Perennial: New York.
1989, available through
Caedmon Self-Help
Soundbooks.

Eating Disorders

Eating Disorders Hotline (24 hours)
(800) 382-2832

National Association of Anorexia Nervosa and Associated Disorders
P.O.Box 7
Highland Park IL 60036
(708) 831-3438

Overeaters Anonymous, Inc.
World Services Office
P.O.Box 44020
Rio Rancho NM 87174
(505) 891-2664

The Overcoming-Overeating Newsletter
c/o Jade Publishing
935 W. Chestnut (Suite 420)
Chicago IL 60622
(Subscription 800-299-0577)

Family

Family Resource Coalition
200 South Michigan Avenue,
Suite 1520
Chicago IL 69694
(312) 341-0900

Youth "Nineline" Hotline (24 hours)
(800) 999-9999
Referrals for youths or parents about drugs, homelessness, and runaways

General Health Information

American Lung Association
1740 Broadway
New York NY 10019

Enneagram Workshops
The Center for the Investigation and Training of Intuition
1442A Walnut Street
Berkeley CA 94704
(415) 843 7621

Hospice-National Hospice Organization
1901 North Fort Drive, Suite 307
Arlington VA 22209
703 243 5900

Information on the "Opening to Feelings" Workshops for Men
Daphne Rose Kingma
P.O.Box 5244
Santa Barbara CA 93150

Mental Health/Adult/Children Clearing House (24 hr.)
(800) 628 1696

National Health Information Center
(800) 336 4797

National Women's Health Resource Center
2440 M Street NW (Suite 325)
Washington DC 20037

Organ Donor Program
Committee on Donor Enlistment
2022 Lee Road
Cleveland Heights OH 44118

Sexual Compulsive
Anonymous
(213) 859 5585

Gynecology

CDC National AIDS Hotline
(800) 342-AIDS

CDC Nationally Sexually
Tranmitted Disease Hotline
(800) 227 8922

The Endometriosis Alliance of
Greater New York
Old Chelsea Station
P.O.Box 634
New York NY 10113-0634

HERS Foundation (Hysterec-
tomy Educational Resources
and Services)
422 Bryn Mawr PA 19004
(215) 667-7757

National PMS Society
P.O.Box 11467
Durham NC 27703
(919) 489-6577

Heart

American Heart Association
7320 Greenville Avenue
Dallas TX 75231
(800) AHA-USA1 or
(214) 373-6300

National Institutes of Health
Heart, Lung and Blood Institute
4733 Bethesda MD 20814
(301) 951-3260

Infertility/Pregnancy Loss

Abortion Survivors
Anonymous
(Support after abortion)
(619) 445-1247

American Society for
Reproductive Medicine
1209 Montgomery Highway
Birmingham AL 35216-2809
(205) 978-5000

SHARE
Pregnancy and Infant Loss
Support Group, Inc.,
St. Joseph's Health Center
300 First Capitol Drive
St. Charles MO 63301
(314) 947-6164 (Information on
support groups nationwide)

Jobs

AARP Work Force Program
601 E St. N.W.
Washington, DC 20049

(for free list of job-seeking
programs in your state, call
(800) 235-2732

Consumer Information Center
Dept. 105-B
Pueblo, CO 81009
(Enclose check for $1)

(at your library, check out the
"Occupational Outlook
Handbook," also published by
U.S. Dept. of Labor)

Success Teams
Box 20052
Park West Station
 New York, NY 10025
(see also Recommended
Reading; Sher, Barbara)

Legal

Attorney Referral Network
(24 hr.)
(800) 624 8846

Menopause

Menopause News
2074 Union Street
San Francisco CA 94123
(800) 241-MENO

North American Menopause
Society
4074 Abington Road
Cleveland OH 44106
(216) 844-3334

Natural Family Planning

Billings Ovulation Method
Association
P.O. Box 30329
Bethesda, MD 20824-0239
(301) 897-9323

Couple to Couple League
P.O. Box 111184
Cincinnati, OH 45211-1184
(513) 661-7612
(Symptothermal Method: USA
and International)

Nutritional Supplements

Nature's Wealth
800-77-NATURE
(800-776-2887)
Springfield, IL 62704

Osteoporosis

National Osteoporsis
Foundation
2100 M Street, NW
Washington DC 20037
(202) 223-3336

(Information on osteoporosis or
bone density testing)
P.O. Box 96616, Dept. M.E.
Washington, D.C. 20077-7456 or
call (202) 223-3336
(To find a bone density testing
center near you call
(800) 464-6700 between
8 a.m. to 9 p.m. (EST) Mon-Fri
and 9-5 on weekends)

Pain Treatment

Rehabilitation Accreditation
Association
(520) 325-1044

American Chronic Pain
Association
(916) 632-0922

American Pain Society
4700 W. Lake Ave.
Glenview IL 60025

UCLA Pain Medicine Center
200 Medical Plaza, Suite 660
Los Angeles, CA 90095
(310) 794-1841

Progesterone

Women's Pharmacy "Women's
Health Care Systems and
Pharmaceuticals"
5900 Monona Drive,
Madison WI 53716

Professional and Technical
Services
333 Northeast Sandy Boulevard
Portland OR 97232
(800) 648 2111

Pro-Life *and* **Pro-Choice**

The Common Ground Network
for Life and Choice
(202) 265-4300
Information is available for
starting a dialogue in your
community between those with
opposing views. An opportunity to learn that sincerity and
caring exists on both sides,
which can be used to forge an
agenda to address the problems
that lead to abortion.

Urinary Incontinence

"Femina Cones" (to teach
bladder muscle-strenthening
exercise)
Dacomed Corporation
1701 E. 79th St.
Minneapolis MN 55425
(800) 823 1108

Help For Incontinent People
(**H.I.P.**)
P.O.Box 544
Union SC 29379
(803) 579-7900 or 800-BLAD-
DER

The Simon Foundation For
Incontinence
P.O. Box 835
Wilmette IL 60091
or (800) 23-SIMON

Women's Health

American Medical Association's
*Complete Guide to Women's
Health*
1 (800) 621-8335
Order # OP840996ACD
Price $39.95

Index

abortion
  human rights issues, 235-36, 297-98n
  resources on, 319
abuse
  See also abusive relationships; child abuse
  abusive fathers, 193-97
abused children. *See also* child abuse
abusive fathers, 193-97
abusive relationships, 178-81, 284-287
  See also child abuse
  control tactics, 179-81
  father-daughter relationships, 193-97
  lesbian, 286n
  physical abuse, 178-79
  self-responsibility in, 180-81
action as emotional expression in men, 164, 221
adolescents
  alcohol use, 136
  basal body temperature charting, 124
  birth control, 131-39
  dependency issues, 190-91
  dependency needs, 190
  eating disorder patterns, 112-13
  education needs, 134-35, 280-82n, 285n
  father's importance to, 192-93, 196

  gender bias affecting, 133
  gynecological exams for, 123-24
  human values education, 134-35
  late bloomers, 126
  media images and, 122-23, 135
  menstrual cycle journals, 134
  menstruation, 124-26, 127, 134
  mother's importance to, 198-99
  parental consent to physician treatment, 268-69n
  physical exams for, 123-24
  psychological problems of, 122-35, 177-78, 190-91, 199
  puberty signs, 124-26
  pubic hair appearance, 125
  rape and date rape, 138, 197
  resources for, 313, 316
  responsibility issues, 131-32, 138-39
  self-esteem issues, 133-39
  sex education, 132-36, 202-03, 269-70n
  sexual activity concerns, 131-39, 190-91, 206
  sexual exploitation and harassment, 133-36
  sexually transmitted diseases among, 132
  smoking among, 139
  violence among, 272-73n
age
  See also aging

age *(continued)*
   as a breast cancer risk factor, 65
   cultural attitudes, 72
aging
   and brain function, 75-76
   resources on, 313
   and sexual function in men, 207
AHAs (alpha-hydroxy acids), 11-12
air conditioning, humidifiers used
   with, 18
alcholism, resources on, 313
alcohol as a hemorrhoid treatment, 25
alcohol use among adolescents, 136
alcoholism resources, 313
allergies, indoor air cleaning to
   relieve, 19-20
alpha-hydroxy acids, 11-12
Alpha-Keri oil, 12
alternative medicine resources,
   253n, 265n, 313-15
Alzheimer's disease resources, 315
anger
   in abusive relationships, 180
   anger expression techniques, 169
   connection to love, 161-63, 292-
     93n
   damaging expression of, 157,
     256n
   as a need signal, 219
   in parenting, 189-90
   as a PMS symptom, 47-48
   relationship improvement and,
     147-50
   repression in men, 149-52
   repression in women, 147-48
   role in eating disorders, 110, 111-
     12
   and sexual problems, 274
anger expression communication
   technique, 169
animal fat as a breast cancer risk,
   63-64
animal model of sexual activity, 210
anorexia, 110, 112-13, 256-57n
   effects, 112
   psychological factors, 112
antioxidants as a breast pain
   treatment, 28

appendicitis, differentiated from
   ovarian pain, 39-40
apple obesity, 63, 118, 259n
appreciation, importance of, 221,
   276n
arousal techniques (for sex), 208-12,
   214-15
assertiveness, healing qualities of,
   xvii-xix
attention to children as a parenting
   technique, 187-88
attitude
   See also emotions; moods
   as a cardiac risk, 70
   and dieting, 114-15
   fatalities created by, 70, 230
   health and, 3-4, 230, 231-32, 294n
   improving through focus on
     good influences, 58-59
   menopause affected by, 68-74
attraction of mates
   psychological dynamics, 153-55,
     158-59, 173-74
   self-knowledge and, 181-83
autonomy, importance of, 238-44

back problems, exercises for, 101
baldness at menopause, 67
basal body temperature charting,
   124
battering. *See also* abusive relationships; violence
behavioral changes resulting from
   menopause, 74-76
Beijing conference on women, 302-
   03n
Bible
   feminist theories on, 240
   God's images in, 241
   women's images in, 300-301n
bicycle riding, effects on cartilage, 98
biofeedback bladder exercise
   programs, 34
birth control
   See also birth control pills
   for adolescents, 131-39
   natural methods, 269n, 318
   resources, 318

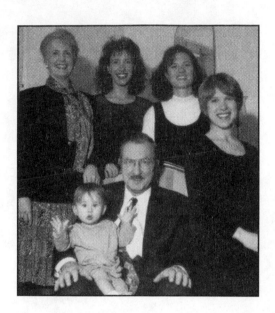

JAMES A. SCHALLER received his Doctor of Medicine from the University of Pennsylvania in 1958. While there, he was awarded membership in the Honor Medical Society, Alpha Omega Alpha. After spending four years in the Army Medical Corps, he received an "Army Commendation Medal." His residency and Post-graduate studies were completed at Misericordia Hospital and the University of Pennsylvania Graduate Medical School. He has been Certified and Recertified in his specialty by the American Board of OB-GYN, and is presently a Life Fellow of the American College of Obstetrics and Gynecology and the American Society of Reproductive Medicine. For twenty-five years he was affiliated with Nazareth Hospital where he has served as the Chairman of the Obstetrics and Gynecology department. In 1966, Dr. Schaller entered private Obstetrics and Gynecology practice.

A last note: the author invites the reader to comment, in her or his own words, where he has been accurate—or inaccurate—in his advice for getting men into the intimacy process. You may address the author c/o the publisher:

James A. Schaller, M.D.
c/o Blue Dolphin Publishing, Inc.
P.O. Box 8 • Nevada City, CA 95959